FUNCTIONAL

...OPIC

...RGERY

FUNCTIONAL ENDOSCOPIC SINUS SURGERY

The Messerklinger Technique

HEINZ STAMMBERGER, M.D.
Professor
University Ear, Nose and Throat Hospital
University of Graz
Graz, Austria

With a Contribution by
WOLFGANG KOPP, M.D.

Translated by
THOMAS J. DEKORNFELD, M.D.

Adapted and Edited by
MICHAEL HAWKE, M.D., F.R.C.S.(C)

Illustrations by
GINO HASLER

B.C. DECKER • PHILADELPHIA

Publisher

B.C. Decker
320 Walnut Street
Suite 400
Philadelphia, Pennsylvania 19106

Sales and Distribution

United States and Puerto Rico
Mosby-Year Book Inc.
11830 Westline Industrial Drive
Saint Louis, Missouri 63146

Canada
Mosby-Year Book Limited
5240 Finch Avenue East, Unit 1
Scarborough, Ontario M1S 5A2

Australia
**McGraw-Hill Book Company
Australia Pty. Ltd.**
4 Barcoo Street
Roseville East 2069
New South Wales, Australia

Brazil
Editora McGraw-Hill de Brasil, Ltda.
rua Tabapua, 1.105, Itaim-Bibl
Sao Paulo, S.P. Brasil

Colombia
**Interamericana/McGraw-Hill
de Colombia, S.A.**
Carrera 17, No. 33–71
(Apartado Postal, A.A., 6131)
Bogota, D.E., Colombia

Europe, U.K., Middle East and Africa
Wolfe Publishing Limited
Brook House
2–16 Torrington Place
London WO1E 7LT England

Hong Kong and China
McGraw-Hill Book Company
Suite 618, Ocean Centre
5 Canton Road
Tsimshatsui, Kowloon
Hong Kong

India
**Tata McGraw-Hill Publishing
Company, Ltd.**
12/4 Asaf Ali Road, 3rd Floor
New Delhi, 110002, India

Indonesia
Mr. Wong Fin Fah
P.O. Box 122/JAT
Jakarta, 1300 Indonesia

Japan
Igaku-Shoin Ltd.
Tokyo International P.O. Box 5063
1–28–36 Hongo, Bunkyo-ku,
Tokyo 113, Japan

Korea
Mr. Don-Gap Choi
C.P.O. Box 10583
Seoul, Korea

Malaysia
Mr. Lim Tao Slong
No. 8 Jalan SS 7/6B
Kelana Jaya
47301 Petaling Jaya
Selangor, Malaysia

Mexico
**Interamericana/McGraw-Hill de Mexico,
S.A. de C.V.**
Cedro 512, Colonia Atlampa
(Apartado Postal 26370)
06450 Mexico, D.F., Mexico

New Zealand
McGraw-Hill Book Co. New Zealand Ltd.
5 Joval Place, Wiri
Manukau City, New Zealand

Portugal
Editora McGraw-Hill de Portugal, Ltda.
Rua Rosa Damasceno 11A–B
1900 Lisbon, Portugal

South Africa
Libriger Book Distributors
Warchouse Number 8
"Die Ou Looiery"
Tannery Road
Hamilton, Bloemfontein 9300

Singapore and Southeast Asia
McGraw-Hill Book Co.
21 Neythal Road
Jurong, Singapore 2262

Spain
McGraw-Hill/Interamericana de Espana, S.A.
Manuel Ferrcio, 13
28020 Madrid, Spain

Taiwan
Mr. George Lim
P.O. Box 87–601
Taipei, Taiwan

Thailand
Mr. Virir Lim
632/5 Phaholyothin Road
Sapan Kwai
Bangkok 10400
Thailand

Venezuela
Editorial Interamericana de Venezuela, C.A.
2da. calle Bello Monte
Local G–2
Caracas, Venezuela

Functional Endoscopic Sinus Surgery
ISBN 0-941158-969

Library of Congress catalog card number:
90-84785

Printed in the United States

10 9 8 7 6 5 4 3 2

The authors and publisher have made every effort to ensure that the patient care recommended
herein, including choice of drugs and drug dosages, is in accord with the accepted standards
and practice at the time of publication. However, since research and regulation constantly change
clinical standards, the reader is urged to check the product information sheet included in the
package of each drug, which includes recommended doses, warnings, and contraindications.
This is particularly important with new or frequently used drugs.

Dedicated to my honored teacher

Prof. Dr. Dr. Walter Messerklinger

with gratitude and deep appreciation.

FOREWORD

This monograph has been eagerly anticipated. It is now before us in this magnificent edition. That it appears in English first is appropriate, in order that the knowledge and experience reaches the widest possible audience. In the German-speaking arena, the pioneering work in this kind of endoscopic surgery by Professor Dr. med. W. Messerklinger is already well known through his writings, which stimulated and inspired many of us.

This book could not have appeared as a compendium to the work of earlier years: it has grown and matured from the happy relationship between master and pupil. The work is before us now in this individual form and shape from the pen of the pupil, Doctor Stammberger, to whom we are grateful.

The presentation of this work in English shows Dr. Stammberger's mastery in presenting the material confidently and in a most talented fashion. It is easy to follow, understandable, and incorporates his clinical and scientific experiences. His wealth of cases and his masterful presentation of diagnosis, indications for and techniques for performance of surgery, reflect his constant self-assessment and ongoing endeavor to transmit his experiences and observations. These accomplishments are well known to us from his many clinical and scientific publications, the numerous national and international courses, and lectures and round table discussions that he has conducted or in which he participated.

The title reveals the cardinal principle of the author. The guiding thought here is the preservation of structure and the reestablishment of function by preserving the mucous membranes. To remove as little as possible and to preserve as much as possible, both of the bony structure and of the covering membranes is stated as the conditio sine qua non for a rapid and certain recovery.

The subtitle—The Messerklinger Technique—honors the master, and reflects also on the pupil who has greatly expanded the indications for this technique. Professor Messerklinger, who for many years was the chairman of the ENT department at the University in Graz, has set the standards for this technique. His impressive and constantly evolving pictorial material has been an inspiration for us, whether as moving pictures or slides. He not only familiarized us with the research aspects of endoscopy, but also with the diagnostic and surgical techniques, without which modern management of the cephalic air spaces could not even be imagined. This monograph stands to play an important role in the field of ENT education and therapy. The author of these few words has the highest regard for her own teacher, the father of modern microsurgery, Horst Ludwig Wullstein, from whom she learned from the beginning until the end of his life. His principal lesson should be treasured: ''The mucous membrane is our best friend in the microsurgery of the cranial air spaces.''

The illustrations presented here are uniquely beautiful. The brilliance and color of the photographs demonstrate not only a highly refined technique, but also the excellent cooperation and support provided by the Storz Company and its owner and developer Karl Storz. The selection of the illustrations, with their manifold pathologic processes, is very rich, as are those that depict the individual anatomic-topographic architecture of this complicated area. The captions to these beautiful illustrations are clear, terse, not too much, not too little. They contribute to the visual enjoyment of the readers and make it easy for them to follow even if they are not familiar with the subject matter. The readers should gain the impression that they are familiar with the subject from the beginning.

The monograph is divided into 14 chapters. The first three are devoted to the anatomy and physiology of this region. Two are devoted to diagnostics, to the indications, and to the functional aspects of the technique. The particular problems, mainly in relation to the coordination and interaction of the upper and lower airways, are described in detail. The last chapter is devoted to another important aspect of the technique, namely visual documentation. The still delicate and evolving issue of the handling and management of optical systems and of light sources is particularly emphasized. Endoscopy has become an irreplaceable, routine procedure. Without it, modern functional surgery is impossible.

Good postoperative results do not rest on a well-performed procedure alone. The postoperative management, tailored to the individual requirements of each and every patient is critical, and if stated, the motto of the procedure would be: ''Made to Measure.''

The goal is to arrange the surgical and functional aspects of the technique in such a fashion, and to adapt it to the individual pathomorphology of the case so that the primary focus of the disease can be discovered in its early stages. The lesson is to remove only as much as necessary, to preserve as much as possible, and to do only enough to reestablish good aeration and good mucociliary clearance.

It is hard to imagine anything more gratifying to a University Professor at the close of his or her clinical, medical activity and teaching career than to see his work maturing and advancing in the hands of his grateful pupil and to have it see the light of day, as it has done in this instance, in the form of a monograph that also incorporates the pupil's own technique.

Prof. Dr. med S. R. Wullstein

PREFACE

When I started my ENT training in 1975 with Professor Messerklinger in Graz, as the junior member of the staff, I was assigned some of the more unpleasant tasks and some which were considered burdensome by more senior colleagues. Among other things, these included assisting Professor Messerklinger during his experimental work and taking motion pictures with a 16-mm camera during endoscopic procedures in the nose. This "honorable task" was not regarded highly by the staff, since it frequently extended substantially beyond the usual working hours. It did not take long, however, until I became fascinated by this experimental and surgical technique. Until this time, the only methods that I was aware of for managing polypoid or chronic sinusitis were limited to a radical procedure, a "simple" polypectomy, fenestration of the maxillary sinus in the inferior meatus, symptomatic drug therapy, or therapeutic nihilism. The endoscope opened an entirely new world for me.

In several hundreds of cases, in which I was "forced" to operate the camera, I was able to share in the experience of seeing massive changes in the maxillary and frontal sinuses resolve within a short period of time following minor manipulation of the key sites in the lateral nasal wall. These were changes in the mucous membranes, from conditions that were described in the authoritative textbooks of the time as "irreversible." While many were still trying to modify and improve radical surgical procedures with endonasal or external approaches, a technique was developed in Graz that rendered largely obsolete major radical procedures directed towards the connecting paranasal sinuses.

By 1972 Messerklinger had almost completed a manuscript for a work on endoscopic diagnosis of the nose, although it was 1975 before it was placed with a publisher. Large and well-known publishing houses showed no interest in a manuscript that appeared to represent a purely academic activity of an ENT surgeon, rather than an innovation leading to new horizons. The work was finally published in English in 1978 under the title *Endoscopy of the Nose*. Initially, it did not receive the attention it deserved; today it is the standard and the major reference work for endoscopic diagnosis of the lateral nasal wall.

The endoscopic techniques are now well established. In combination with modern imaging techniques, particularly computerized tomography, these techniques provide diagnostic possibilities unimagined a few decades ago. The Messerklinger technique changed operations on the frontal sinus into an operation on the frontal recess and an operation on the maxillary sinus into a procedure on the ethmoidal infundibulum and/or on the clefts of the lateral nasal wall. Even in the local and medical therapy of infectious processes of the paranasal sinuses, the endoscope is of great help. Target-oriented, focused therapy of the middle meatus practically negates the use of surgical intervention, when in the past fenestration of the inferior meatus would have been almost routine.

Under endoscopic guidance, total sphenoethmoidectomy *can* be performed, when necessary. The great advantage of the Messerklinger technique, however, is that such a procedure can be largely avoided.

To put it bluntly, the endoscope is the instrument that helps us *to avoid* surgery.

The technical, surgical options offered by the endoscope go far beyond the management of inflammatory diseases. They include closure of cerebrospinal fluid fistulas, removal of certain neoplasms, decompression of the orbit, management of choanal atresia to dacryocystorhinostomy, and management of meningoencephaloceles. In the latter cases, we use the endoscope primarily as an optical instrument for the performance of generally less traumatic, but established surgical interventions.

This volume sheds "light" on the complex system of the lateral nasal wall for the interested reader. It illustrates the manifold diagnostic and therapeutic possibilities, as well as the limitations, of the Messerklinger technique.

The book had its inception through the ongoing dialogue with patients and from the questions from, and the discussions with, colleagues during lectures and postgraduate courses. I have attempted to present particularly difficult subjects, for instance the surgical anatomy of the lateral nasal wall "endoscopically." The sometimes markedly streamlined and abstract schematic drawings should help the reader to reduce the extremely complicated structures and topographic relationships to their basic components, without oversimplifying them. In various chapters, fundamental principles are repeated to emphasize their importance and give each chapter a certain degree of independence.

Standard anatomic features such as blood and nerve supply are not reiterated in this book.

For several reasons, there is no special chapter on endoscopy in children. Firstly, we are *very* reluctant to perform (this or any other) sinus surgery in children; children under 10 years of age account for less than 2 percent of our surgical cases. In contrast to adults, many other than just ethmoidal causes usually can be identified and treated (e.g., adenoids, allergies) in children's sinusitis. Secondly, *if* an ethmoidal problem is identified, it is approached the same way as in adults, by history, computed tomography, and diagnostic endoscopy (which, depending on patient cooperation, at times must be performed under general anesthesia). The indications for surgical approaches are as for in adults—the anatomic variations and stages of sinus development must be kept in mind. Thirdly, diseases more frequently encountered in children (like antrochoanal polyps or complications of acute sinusitis) are dealt with in their respective chapters. Also, special sets of instruments are available for pediatric functional endoscopic surgery. These are basically miniaturized versions of the standard adult sets and are not specifically mentioned in the Appendix. Finally, functional endoscopic surgery in children requires expert knowledge and experience and we strongly recommend that novices *not* start with pediatric cases.

First and foremost, I wish to thank my friends David W. Kennedy and S. James Zinreich for many years of intensive collaboration and for the many discussions that even today stimulate the learning process in all of us. Many of their experiences, stimuli and developments have gone into this volume and I regard them as spiritual coauthors.

In Gino Hasler I had the support of a great artist. His training was not in the medical environment, but his extraordinary ability to grasp the essentials and his ability to translate complex visual images into illustrations is outstanding.

In Graz my thanks go primarily to Dr. Wolfgang Kopp of the Radiology Clinic of the University, who wrote the major portion of Chapter 4. He and his colleagues have contributed much to this book through their unstinting helpfulness.

Among my colleagues in the Department of ENT, my particular thanks are due to Drs. Wolf, Kainz, Schröckenfuchs, and Anderhuber for their assistance during the endoscopies, their preparation of sketches and drawings to serve as bases for the finished product, and for the preparation of the anatomic dissections. Dr. Wolf also allowed me to use excellent endoscopic photographs from his collection, especially those of endonasal tumors.

Special thanks are extended to our operating room nurses and technicians who created such pleasant working conditions by their assistance, caring, and patience in technically or surgically difficult situations, and by their concern for the patients.

I wish to convey my sincere thanks to Messrs. Hans Steinmann and Joachim Lunemann, and Engineer Neumayer for their constant and efficient help with all our technical and equipment problems.

Dr. Thomas J. DeKornfeld assumed the responsibility of translating the text into English and also to do some editing on the sections written by me in English. Dr. Michael Hawke edited the text and was of the greatest help to me with advice during the planning stages of this work.

I am very much indebted to Brian C. Decker in many ways: For having encouraged and stimulated me to undertake and complete the work and for having gently coerced and motivated me to continue when I was ready to quit. He is responsible for having made this volume into such a beautiful one and he did not even give up on this endeavor when the material grew well past the original plan.

I am very grateful to Ms. Regina Thakur for her tireless work in typing and correcting the text.

Finally, and most importantly, I wish to thank my dear wife Doloris for her patience and forbearance during the four long years of work on this volume. She shielded me on many evenings and weekends from the outer world and doing this she had to give up considerable family life and personal time. Without her, this book would never have seen the light of day.

Graz, August 1990

ACKNOWLEDGMENTS

I wish to express my sincere thanks to the publishers of the following scientific publications and journals for permission to use illustrations and data from my papers originally published in these publications.

American Journal of Rhinology
Annals of Otology, Rhinology, and Laryngology
Endoscopy
European Archives of Otorhinolaryngology
HNO
HNO-Praxis Heute
Laryngologie, Rhinologie, Otologie
Otolaryngology-Head and Neck Surgery
Rhinology

CONTENTS

1   History of Nasal Endoscopy   *1*

2   Secretion Transportation   *17*
Principles of Secretion Transportation   *17*
   Secretion Transport Pathology   *25*
Pathways of Secretion Transport   *27*
   Secretion Transport in the Maxillary Sinus   *28*
   Secretion Transport in the Frontal Sinus   *30*
   Mucociliary Transport from Anterior and Posterior Ethmoidal
   and Sphenoidal Sinuses and from the Lateral Nasal Wall   *31*
   Secretory Disturbances and Tubal Function   *33*
Role of Ethmoidal Prechambers   *35*
   How can Infection Reach the Maxillary and Frontal Sinuses?   *42*
Conclusions   *45*
Summary   *46*

**3   Special Endoscopic Anatomy of the Lateral Nasal Wall
and Ethmoidal Sinuses**   *49*
Preface: A Historical Confusion   *49*
Ethmoid Bone   *52*
Bony Structures of the Lateral Nasal Wall   *54*
   Embryology   *54*
   Uncinate Process   *60*
   Ethmoidal Bulla and Lateral Sinus   *62*
   Ground Lamella of the Middle Turbinate   *62*
   Posterior Ethmoid   *65*
   Sphenoid Sinus   *67*
Roof of the Ethmoid and the Anterior Ethmoidal Artery   *70*
   Clinical and Surgical Significance   *74*

Clefts and Spaces of the Lateral Nasal Wall   76

    Hiatus Semilunaris (the Inferior Hiatus Semilunaris of Grünwald)   76

    Ethmoidal Infundibulum   78

    Frontal Recess   82

    Sinus Lateralis (Lateral Sinus)   87

4   **Radiology**   *89*

Conventional Sinus X-ray Techniques   89

Conventional Tomography   92

    Technique of Conventional Tomography   94

Computed Tomography   96

    Technique of Computed Tomographic Examination
    of the Paranasal Sinuses   98

Radiation Exposure   102

Magnetic Resonance Imaging   104

Conventional Versus Computed Tomography   108

    Three-Dimensional Reconstructions   114

Radiologic Anatomy   116

    Important Anatomic Variants   133

    Preoperative Considerations   142

5   **Endoscopic and Radiologic Diagnosis**   *145*

Preparation for Diagnostic Endoscopy   147

    Technique of Diagnostic Endoscopy   148

    Nasal Septal Deviation   156

    Concha Bullosa   160

    Variations of the Middle Turbinate   170

    Uncinate Process   173

    Ethmoidal Bulla   180

    Lateral Sinus   184

    Disease of the Ethmoidal Infundibulum   185

    Disease of the Frontal Recess   194

    Agger Nasi   200

    Haller's Cells   202

    Disease of the Posterior Ethmoid   204

    Disease of the Sphenoidal Sinus   208

    Combined Paranasal Sinus Disease on Computed Tomograms   212

Nasal Polyposis   216

    Choanal Polyps   227

    Etiology of Nasal Polyps   230

Endoscopy of the Maxillary Sinus   232

    Indications   232

    Instrumentation   233

    Technique   235

    Manipulation in the Maxillary Sinus   240

Complications   *242*

Endoscopic Findings   *245*

Histologic Findings   *253*

Differential Diagnosis   *262*

Summary and Conclusions   *268*

6   Indications for Endoscopic Surgery   273

Contraindications   *275*

Conservative Endoscopic Management   *278*

7   Surgical Technique   283

Surgical Principles   *283*

Instrument Manipulation   *284*

Surgical Technique and Options   *290*

Difficulties, Tips, and Tricks   *311*

  Local Anesthesia   *311*

  Identification of the Site of Insertion of the Uncinate Process   *312*

  Identification of the Correct Point for Perforation of the Ground Lamella   *312*

  Identification of the Sphenoid Sinus   *313*

  Identification of the Frontal Recess   *314*

  Identification of the Maxillary Sinus Ostium   *315*

  Injury to the Orbits   *316*

  Pain   *318*

8   Preoperative Preparations   321

Premedication for Local Anesthesia   *322*

Positioning the Patient   *324*

Topical and Infiltration Anesthesia   *328*

Advantages of Local Anesthesia   *332*

Endoscopic Procedures Under General Anesthesia   *333*

9   Sinus Problems and Endoscopic Solutions   335

Polypoid Rhinosinusitis   *336*

Ethmoid Disease in Sinubronchial Syndrome   *344*

Antrochoanal Polyps   *346*

Concha Bullosa   *350*

Isolated Disease of the Frontal Sinus   *356*

Frontal Sinus Cyst   *358*

Meningoencephalocele   *359*

Hyperplastic Lower Turbinate   *360*

Complications of Acute Sinusitis   *362*

Mucoceles   *365*

10   Postoperative Care   369

Postoperative Drug Therapy   *370*

Local Postoperative Care   *372*

Postoperative Problems and Complications   *377*

   Serious Complications During Aftercare   *378*

Discharge Instructions to the Patient   *379*

11   **Special Problems**   *381*

When Fenestration and Caldwell-Luc Fail   *381*

   Symptoms   *381*

   Endoscopic Findings   *382*

   Radiologic Findings   *390*

   Secretion Transport   *392*

   Conclusions   *394*

   Surgical Therapy   *396*

Mycoses   *398*

   Aspergillosis of the Paranasal Sinuses   *400*

   Aspergillus fumigatus: Ecology and Physiology   *400*

   Clinical Picture   *404*

   Radiographic Diagnosis   *405*

   Endoscopic Diagnosis   *409*

   Histologic Diagnosis   *411*

   Fungal Cultures   *411*

   Clinical Course and Complications   *411*

   Therapy   *412*

   Surgical Procedure   *412*

   Postoperative Care   *418*

   How do Aspergillus Infections Arise?   *419*

   Candidiasis   *424*

   Therapy   *426*

   Mucormycoses   *426*

   Clinical Findings   *426*

   Therapy   *427*

Allergy: Role of the Messerklinger Technique in Inhalational Allergies   *428*

Septal Deviation   *430*

Removal of Foreign Bodies   *434*

   Detection and Treatment of Cerebrospinal Fluid Leaks   *436*

Endoscopic Approach to Headaches and Sinus Disease   *442*

   Unusual Lesions   *446*

   Causes of Pain in Areas of Mucosal Irritation   *447*

   Pain Mediation   *448*

   Conclusions   *450*

12   **Asthma and Sinus Disease**   *453*

13   **Results, Problems, and Complications**   *459*

Results   *459*

Problems and Complications   *466*

  Intraoperative Bleeding   *469*

Severe Complications   *473*

14   **Documentation**   *479*

Still Photography   *479*

  Cameras   *479*

  Light Sources   *482*

  Light Cables   *482*

  Endoscopes   *484*

  Photographic Technique   *486*

  Film Selection   *488*

Video Documentation   *488*

  Videotaping Technique   *491*

Teaching Modalities   *492*

Appendix   Endoscopes and Instruments   *495*

Bibliography   *511*

Index   *519*

Chapter 1

HISTORY OF NASAL ENDOSCOPY

Throughout the history of medicine, numerous attempts have been made to illuminate and examine the inside of the various hollow cavities located within the body. The interior of the nose and the paranasal sinuses, with their narrow passages, fissures, and bony walls, places particularly heavy demands on the design of instrumentation to be used for this purpose. It is not surprising, therefore, that after some initial attempts and disappointments, this area of endoscopy developed very slowly. Nasal endoscopic examination has only recently become an important component of our diagnostic and therapeutic armamentarium.

In 1915, Killian published a review of the "History of endoscopy, from the earliest times to Bozzini" in which he recorded all the attempts to inspect the upper airways prior to the beginning of the nineteenth Century.

Philip Bozzini, in 1806 published an article describing the first "Light conductor, or description of a simple device and its use for the illumination of the internal cavities and spaces of the live animal body." With this device, it was possible to "see around the corners, inside the cavities of the human body." In this article, he comments that the area behind the soft palate can also be illuminated with this device.

Prior to the development of the cystoscope by Nitze-Leiter in 1879, a wide variety of devices were developed and used for the inspection

Material for this chapter was taken in part from a speech by Professor Dr. W. Messerklinger on the occasion of Mr. Professor G. Terrier becoming Emeritus at "Journées de Rhinologie," March 3 and 4, 1988 in Lausanne.

not only of the urethra, the urinary bladder, the vagina, the uterus, the stomach, and the rectum, but also of the larynx and the nasopharynx.

There were three basic types of equipment:

1. Devices in which the light source and the mirror were attached to or incorporated into the diagnostic instrument (Bozzini, Figs. 1.1 and 1.2; Fisher, Fig. 1.3; and Désormeaux, Fig. 1.4). Modifications were made by Cruise in 1863 and Fürstenheim and Andrews in 1867/68.

2. Instruments in which the endoscope and the mirror were combined, but the light source was separate (Langlebert's urethroscope, 1868; Segala's speculum urethro-cystique; Warwick's endoscope; Stein's photo-endoscope; Wales' endoscope, 1868, Fig. 1.5; Brunton's otoscope, Fig. 1.6); or alternatively, a speculum with mirror and a loupe (Bonnafont, 1870). This latter instrument was simplified by Hassenstein during the same year.

3. Instruments in which the endoscope, the mirror, and the light source were entirely separate. This arrangement was used almost exclusively in the early days to examine the nose and the nasopharynx.

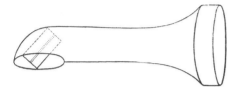

FIGURE 1.1   The endoscopic part of the Bozzini system with a mirror at the distal aperture.

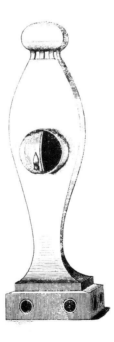

FIGURE 1.2   The light component of the Bozzini system.

2

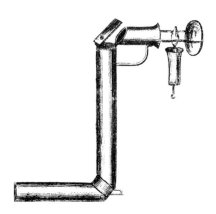

FIGURE 1.3   Fisher's endoscope.

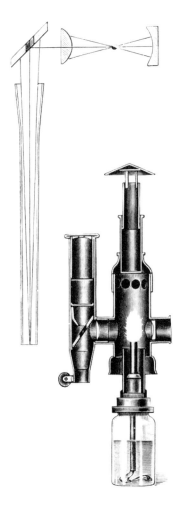

FIGURE 1.4   The Désormeaux endoscopic lamp. The optical pathway is indicated by lines in the diagram on the left.

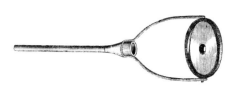

FIGURE 1.5   Wales's endoscope.

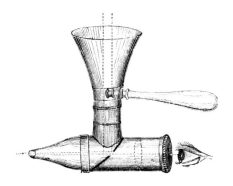

FIGURE 1.6   Brunton's otoscope.

In designing these instruments several significant technical difficulties had to be overcome:

The initial source of light was the sun and this greatly limited the opportunities for successful examinations both spatially and temporally. The success of sunlight was also dependent upon the weather. Candles and kerosene and oil lamps subsequently served as sources of artificial light. Attempts were made to concentrate or focus the light of petroleum lamps by using round wicks, 3.5 cm in diameter. Gas was also used as a source of light as was gasogene, a mixture of 95 percent alcohol and turpentine, which smoked fiercely and died rather promptly. "Limelight" was produced in a cylinder of lime that was heated to incandescence by an oxyhydrogen flame or by a mixture of oxygen and coal gas (Fig. 1.7). The fact that this crude instrument exploded every so often contributed little to its wider acceptance.

The first electric light was provided by a glowing platinum wire. Unfortunately, platinum wire only produced satisfactory and steady illumination when its generator was driven by a steam engine. This presented problems in private homes or even in the physician's residence. Furthermore, there was still considerable uncertainty about the safety of this "new" light, and there was great concern for the eyesight of both the practitioner and the patient (Voltolini).

The patient was positioned so that the light fell either directly into the organ to be examined, or was deflected by a free-standing reflector (usually a flat or concave mirror). To concentrate and focus the light, Stoerk in 1880 used a "water lens," a water-filled glass sphere that was also known as a "cobbler's sphere" (Fig. 1.8). Later, convex lenses were used to concentrate the light, which was then reflected off a mirror worn on the head of the examiner, attached to either a pair of glasses or to a headband. To keep the mirror from fogging, it was moistened with lysoform or lysol.

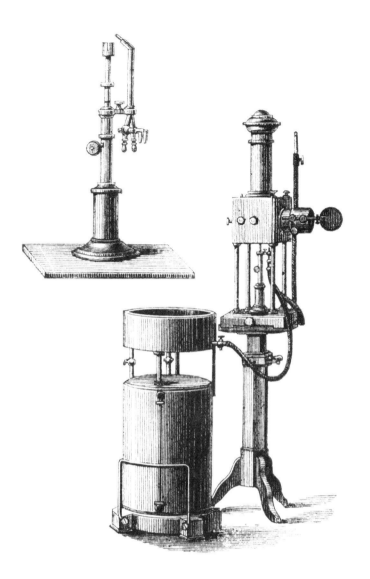

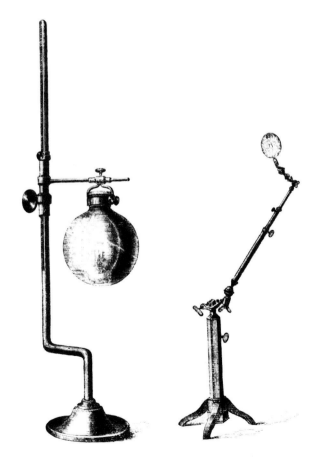

FIGURE 1.7   Ziemssen's limelight system.

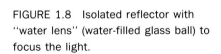

FIGURE 1.8   Isolated reflector with
''water lens'' (water-filled glass ball) to
focus the light.

Bozzini mentioned in 1806 that he was able with the aid of his light conductor to see some areas behind the soft palate. In 1838, Baumes presented to the Medical Society in Lyons a mirror the size of a two franc piece that could be used for the examination of the choanae and the larynx. In 1859 in Vienna, Czermak developed a technique similar to the laryngoscopy of Türck, which allowed him to view the nasopharynx, the choanae, and the posterior aspect of the nose with the aid of a small mirror. He called this procedure "rhinoscopy," a term still used today.

In 1860 Czermak wrote:

> As far as the examination of the nasal cavity through the nares is concerned...
> I should mention an instrument that was made for my friend Markusowsky, in
> Budapest, a few years ago, according to his own design. It should become very
> well known and should be used everywhere, since as far as I know, nothing
> like it has ever been as well received.

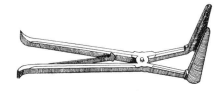

FIGURE 1.9   Markusowsky's nasal speculum.

He was talking about the nasal speculum (Fig. 1.9). Czermak was apparently not aware of the fact that speculum-shaped dilators had already been used in Pompei during the first century and that Van Hilden (1560–1643) had developed an ear speculum that was the precursor of the nasal speculum.

Our present day technique of anterior rhinoscopy was used routinely since 1868, primarily by otologists who wanted to examine the nose before introducing a catheter into the eustachian tube.

Using a Markusowsky speculum and a small mirror, Czermak was able to identify a bristle passed through the nasolacrimal duct into the lower nasal passage of a cadaver in 1860.

Wertheim made a conchoscope in 1869 to examine the anterior and middle thirds of the nasal cavity. This was a small tube, closed at one end and fitted with a mirror at a 45 degree angle, with an aperture over the mirror. The "conchoscope" also had a channel for the introduction of a sound or other instrument (Fig. 1.10).

The second stage in the development of endoscopy began with the development of the cystoscope by Nitze-Leiter in 1879. The first model still used a platinum wire light, which generated so much heat that continuous cooling with water was required (Fig. 1.11). A year later Zaufal used a similar instrument modified by Leiter for examining the orifice of the eustachian tube (Fig. 1.12). Since this instrument still required cooling with water, it was relatively large and thus found little use in practice.

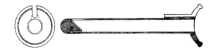

FIGURE 1.10   Wertheim's conchoscope.

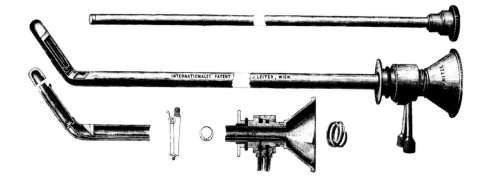

FIGURE 1.11 The first Nitze-Leiter cystoscope (1879).

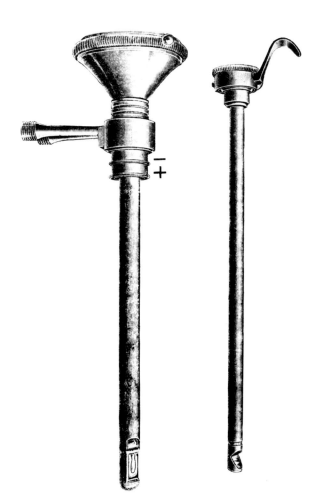

FIGURE 1.12 Leiter's modification of the Nitze cystoscope with which Zaufal examined the eustachian tube.

The strong and widespread misgivings present at this time regarding the use and safety of electricity combined with the technical difficulties in producing electricity in the required voltage and uniformity made Voltolini voice a plea in 1885 against the use of electric light. For this reason, the cystoscope was rarely used for rhinoscopy and pharyngoscopy during the last two decades of the nineteenth century.

Nevertheless, during this period significant advances and discoveries markedly increased both diagnostic and surgical interest in the nasal cavity and the paranasal sinuses.

In 1882 Zuckerkandl published his ''Anatomy of the nose and of its pneumatic attachments.'' This text was universally accepted and became the standard reference work for this field. In 1883, Koller introduced cocaine as a surface anesthetic for the eye. Jellinek extended this technique of topical anesthesia to the ear, nose, and throat area. In 1895, Röntgen discovered the rays that carry his name and in 1896 Killian described his ''rhinoscopia media.''

The ''miniature'' light bulb, introduced at the end of the last century provided a light source that generated so little heat that a cooling system was no longer required. The small size of these light bulbs permitted the construction of much smaller endoscopes. Valentin, in Bern, had an instrument with a diameter of only 4.5 mm, which enabled him to introduce it through almost any nose. He thus became the father of ''salpingoscopy'' (eustachian tube inspection) in 1903. Voss adapted the salpingoscope to allow the introduction of a sound into the eustachian tube. In 1909, Mayr reported two cases in which he was able to operate on the ostium of the eustachian tube with a sharp sound and electrocautery.

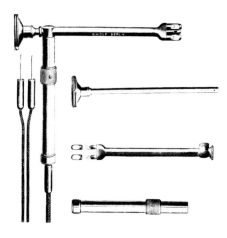

FIGURE 1.13 Flatau's endoscope with electrical light source (1909).

Flatau (Fig. 1.13) and Hays independently described an endoscope in 1909 and 1910 for ''salpingoscopy'' by the direct approach through the lower or common nasal passage. This instrument made it possible to see the nasopharynx and also allowed posterior rhinoscopy through the oropharynx. The patient could close his mouth after the insertion of the instrument. Fidenberg reported on his experiences with Hays's instrument in *Laryngoscope* in 1909 and Garel, in the same year wrote: ''Une révolution dans la rhinoscopie postérieure par le pharyngoscope de Harold Hays.''

Gyergyai (1910) and Yankauer (1912) developed a speculum that allowed them to perform a direct examination of the nasopharynx through the mouth after retracting the soft palate anteriorly.

In 1902, Hirschmann and Valentin followed shortly by Reichert, (Fig. 1.14) in 1903, were able to introduce a modified cystoscope directly into the maxillary sinus through an enlarged dental alveolus. In 1908, Sargnon published his experiences with "Endoscopie directe du sinus maxillaire par les fistules." In his investigations in 1903, Hirschmann studied 5 ethmoids from which the middle turbinate had been partially or completely resected. In a case with a chronic ethmoid empyema he was able to identify the etiologic focus and was also able to achieve a cure following several sessions of endoscopic surgery. Binder removed a foreign body from the maxillary sinus using an endoscope in 1904. Imhofer also reported the use of the endoscope for this purpose in another case in 1910.

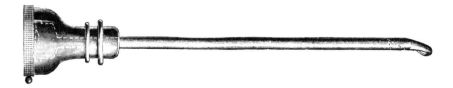

FIGURE 1.14   Hirschmann's modified cystoscope for maxillary sinus endoscopy through the dental alveolus (1903).

Although Tovölgyi described a trocar for the endoscopic examination of the maxillary sinus through the inferior nasal meatus in 1911, the only other publications dealing with endoscopy of the paranasal sinuses up until the end of the Second World War came from Dennis and Mullen (1922), Slobodnik (1930 and 1932) (Fig. 1.15), and Lüdecke (1932). All other "endoscopic" publications were limited to the description of new or modified instruments. These included Marschik (1913), Spielberg (1922), Portman (1925), Maltz (1925), Watson-Williams (1929), Slobodnik (1930), and Botey (1936).

The value of paranasal sinus endoscopy was still debated at this time. Kretschmann discussed in 1910 whether the "salpingoscope" made any contribution to the available diagnostic techniques. He concluded that "For inspection of the anterior parts of the nasal cavity, I would say no. Anterior rhinoscopy and Killian's median rhinoscopy give us a clearer picture of these areas. The natural colors of the tissues can be seen and the instrument permits far superior therapeutic measures. In some other areas, it may serve as a useful supplement." His collaborator Franke stated in 1916 that the endoscope "can also be used advantageously for the inspection of the maxillary sinus."

In an article on the diagnosis of nasal diseases Zarniko in 1925 wrote about nasal endoscopy that "It impresses me more as an interesting toy, than as a necessary diagnostic tool. I know of no results achieved by its use, that could not have been achieved by other, simpler methods." Zöllner stated in 1942 that: "Although endoscopy was invented in Germany..., the nasal endoscope has not been accepted by a wide circle of our specialty in Germany."

After the Second World War, maxillary sinus endoscopy gained the support of individuals in a number of countries (Christensen, Agazzi, Bethmann, Jimenez-Quesda, Bollobas, Aleksasin, Hahn, Nehls, v. Riccabona, Timm, Bauer and Wodak, Kawakubo, Hally, Rosemann, Pihrt, and Papurov), although it still did not achieve widespread acceptance. As late as 1956, Lüscher wrote: "A cystoscope-like antroscope can be introduced through the inferior nasal meatus that permits direct visualization of the maxillary sinus. In some cases this may make a contribution."

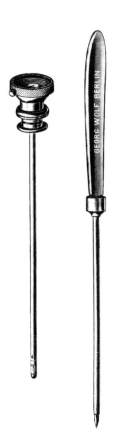

FIGURE 1.15 Slobodnik maxillary sinus trocar and endoscope.

During this time period (1951–1956), Hopkins (Fig. 1.16) made fundamental improvements in the optics of endoscopy. These included a light source that was separate from the instrument, excellent resolution with high contrast, a large field of vision in spite of the small diameter of the endoscope, and perfect fidelity of color.

Thanks to these new endoscopes, which met the highest technical requirements, endoscopy of the upper airways has enjoyed a worldwide popularity since the early 1970s. Although initially the maxillary sinus (as the largest and the most frequently affected sinus) was the focus of diagnostic interest, endoscopy was soon extended to the other paranasal sinuses. The Hopkins rod rigid nasal endoscopes made it possible to examine in detail the clefts and recesses of the nose. The ability to enter the middle meatus of the nose enabled inspection of the anterior ethmoid sinuses, the key area of infectious paranasal sinus disease. Today, nasal endoscopic examination in combination with tomography allows the identification of small, circumscribed changes in the paranasal sinuses. These small changes are frequently of considerable pathophysiologic significance.

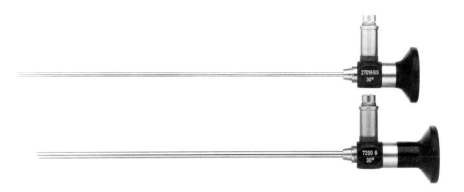

FIGURE 1.16   Modern, high-powered endoscope—a Karl Storz Hopkins' rod lens model.

Our endoscopic armamentarium has been augmented during the last decade with the nasopharyngeal scope (v. Stuckrad and Lakatos) and by the flexible fiberoptic scope (Yamashita). While these latter instruments have a firm place in the diagnostic area, they have not been able to assume a major role in therapeutic and surgical procedures.

Since a surgeon can usually operate wherever he is able to look at, these new opportunities for surgical intervention were quickly explored. Heermann began using the surgical microscope for endonasal procedures in 1954. This was soon followed by endoscopic sinus procedures that were, however, still performed according to the principles of radical paranasal sinus surgery.

Since the introduction of these new and improved nasal endoscopes, numerous publications have appeared describing their use. A complete listing of all these publications is beyond the scope of this introductory chapter. These studies have already been reported in books and other publications of which the most important ones include: Messerklinger (1969, 1973, 1978, 1987), Hellmich and Herberholdt (1971), Draf (1973, 1978), Berci and Buiter (1976), Terrier (1978), Wigand (1977, 1978, 1981), Daele and Melon (1979), Ashikawa (1982), Friedrich (1985), Brandt (1985), Yamashita (1984), and Onishi (1986). In their papers, many of these authors dealt with endonasal surgery, primarily on the large sinuses, using either the operating microscope, the rigid endoscope, or a combination of these two instruments. Although then still using a radical surgical technique, Wigand developed a technique in 1978 that spared as much of the mucous membranes as possible.

Messerklinger is credited with being the first to develop and establish a systematic endoscopic diagnostic approach to the lateral wall of the nose. His studies beginning in the 1950s demonstrated that in most cases the frontal and maxillary sinuses are involved indirectly by primary disease that originates in the narrow spaces of the lateral wall of the nose and in the anterior ethmoid. This discovery led to the development of an endoscopic diagnostic technique that focused on changes in the lateral wall of the nose and identified and isolated these changes with the aid of the rigid endoscope and tomography of the sinuses. This in turn resulted in an endoscopic surgical technique that was directed specifically at the primary disease in the ethmoid region. Messerklinger observed that the eradication of this primary anterior ethmoid disease by means of a circumscribed, limited endoscopic surgical procedure resulted in the recovery of even massive mucosal pathology in the adjacent, large paranasal sinuses within a few weeks and without operating directly on these areas.

The endoscopic diagnostic and surgical techniques described in this book are directed less towards the larger paranasal sinuses (even though recovery from disease in these areas results), but instead to the diagnosis and therapy of the primary disease that originates in the nasal cavity and the lateral wall of the nose.

David Kennedy has taken on and has popularized this technique in the United States. His colleague Jim Zinreich has made significant contributions to the further development of this technique by developing and refining some of the modern imaging techniques.

REFERENCES

AGAZZI C. Il valore dell'antroscopia per la diagnosi della affezioni del seno mascellare. Arch Ital Otol 1952; 63:182.

ALEKSASIN JV. Endoskopie der Oberkieferhöhle. Vestn Otol I T D 1954; 16:66.

ANDREWS E. The urethra viewed by a magnesium light. Med Record 1867; 8:107.

BAUER E, WODAK E. Neuerungen in der Diagnostik und Therapie der Nasennebenhöhlen. Arch Ohr Nas u Kehlk Heilk 1958; 171:325.

BERCI G. Endoscopy. New York: Appleton-Century-Crofts, 1976.

BETHMANN W. Endoscopische Bilder aus gesunden und erkrankten Kieferhöhlen. Zahnärztliche Welt 1953; 8:606.

BINDER G. Über die Extraktion eines Fremdkörpers aus der Oberkieferhöhle unter Leitung des Salpingoskopes. Arch Laryngol Rhinol (Berl) 1904; 16:173.

BOLLOBAS B. Gesichtshöhlen-Punktionstrokar und Endoskop. Zentralbl Chir 1954; 79:973.

BONNAFONT HR. Catalog chirurgischer Instrumente. Wien: Josef Leiter, 1870.

BOTEY R. Die Endorhinoskopie. Zbl HNO 1927; 9:215.

BOZZINI P. Lichtleiter, eine Erfindung zur Anschauung innerer Theile and Krankeiten. Journal der practischen Arzneykunde and Wundarzneykunst. (Berlin) 1806:24.Bd.

BRANDT RH. Endoskopie der Luft- und Speisewege. Leipzig: JA Barth, 1985.

BUITER CT. Endoscopy of the upper airways. Excerpta Medica (Amst) 1976.

CHRISTENSEN H. Endoscopy of the maxillary sinus. Acta Otolaryngol (Stockh) 1946; 34:404.

CRUISE H. Notizen über das Endoskop. Deutsche Klinik 1863.

CZERMAK JN. Der Kehlkopfspiegel. Leipzig: W Engelmann, 1863.

CZERMAK JN. Zur Verwerthung des Liston-Garcia'schen Prinzips. Wien Med Wochenschr 1861; 11:81.

DAELE J, MELON J. Les explorations functionnelles et endoscopiques en rhinologie. Acta Otorhinolaryngol Belg 1979; 33:805.

DENNIS FL, MULLEN WV. Value of direct inspection in the diagnosis of chronic maxillary sinus disease. Laryngoscope 1922; 32:300.

DRAF W. Endoskopie der Nasennebenhöhlen. Berlin: Springer, 1978.

FIDENBERG P. Pharyngoscopic studies. Laryngoscope 1909; 19:535.

FLATAU TS. Laryngoskopie und hintere Rhinoskopie bei geschlossenem Mund. Passow Beitr 1910; 3:461.

FRANKE K. Über Endoskopie des Nasen-Rachenraumes. Passow Beitr 1916; 8:284.

FRIEDRICH JP, TERRIER G. Indications et résultats de l'evidement ethmoidale sous guidage endoscopique. Schweizerische Ges für HNO. 73. Frühjahrsversammlung St. Moritz, Juni, 1986.

GAREL J. Une révolution dans la rhinoscopie postérieure par le pharyngoscope de Harold Hays. Ann Mal Oreille 1909; 35:529.

GRÜNFELD J. Zur Geschichte der Endoskopie und der endoskopischen Apparate. Wien: Med Jahrbücher, 1879.

GYERGYAI AV. Über mein Verfahren zur direkten Untersuchung des Nasenrachens und der Ohrtrompete. Z Laryngol (Leipz) 1913; 5:57.

HAHN W. Die Anwendung des Antroskops in der Kieferheilkunde. Zahnärztl Rdsch 1955; 64:175.

HALLY A. Die Antroskopie als Hilfsmittel der Diagnostik von Kieferhöhlenerkrankungen. Österr Stomat 1960; 57:326.

HASSENSTEIN P. Catalog chirurgischer Instrumente. Wien: Josef Leiter, 1870.

HAYS H. Eine neue Untersuchungsmethode für die hintere Nase, die Tuben und den Larynx mit einem elektrischen Pharyngoskop. Z Laryngol (Leipz) 1910; 2:496.

HEERMANN H. Über endonasale Chirurgie unter Verwendung des binocularen Mikroskopes. Arch Ohr Nas Kehlkopfheilk 1958; 171:295.

HELLMICH S, HERBERHOLDT C. Technische Verbesserungen der Kieferhöhlenendoskopie. Arch Klin Exp Ohr Nas Kehlkopfheilk 1971; 199(2):678.

HIRSCHMANN A. Über Endoskopie der Nase und deren Nebenhöhlen. Arch Laryngol Rhinol (Berl) 1903; 14:194.

IMHOFER R. Entfernung eines Fremdkörpers aus der Kieferhöhle mit Hilfe der Endoskopie. Z Laryngol 1910; 2:427.

JELINEK. Über locale Anaesthesie des Larynx und Pharynx durch Cocain. Wien Med Bl 1884:39.

JIMENEZ-QUESDA M. Exploratien optic de los senos maxillares y tratamiento de algunas formas de sinusitis cronicas. Cons Col Méd España 1953; 14:25.

KAWAKUBO J. Antroscopic study of pathology, physiology in chronic maxillary sinusitis. J Otorhinolaryngol Soc Jpn 1958; 61:708.

KILLIAN G. Zur Geschichte der Endoskopie von den ältesten Zeiten bis Bozzini. Arch Laryngol Rhinol (Berl) 1915; 29:347.

KILLIAN G. Über Rhinoskopia media. Münch Med Wochenschr 1896; 768.

KOLLER K. Vorläufige Mitteilung über lokale Anaesthesierung am Auge. Klin Mbl Augenheilk 1884; 22:60.

KRETSCHMANN H. Ist das Salpingoskop eine Bereicherung des diagnostischen Instrumentariums? Ms Ohrenheilk 1910; 44;757.

LANGLEBERT E. An uncomplicated urethrosocope. Lancet 1868; 768.

LÜDECKE E. Die verbesserte Antroskopie. Zbl HNO 1932; 31:507.

LÜSCHER E. Lehrbuch der Nasen- und Halsheilkunde. Wien: Springer, 1956.

MALTZ M. New instrument: the sinuscope. Laryngoscope 1925; 35:805.

MAYR K. Zur Endoskopie des Ostium pharyngeum tubae. Arch Ohr Nas Kehlkopfheilk 1909; 80:192.

MESSERKLINGER W. Die normalen Sekretwege in der Nase des Menschen. Arch Klin Exp Ohr Nas Kehlkopfheilk 1969; 195:138.

MESSERKLINGER W. Endoscopy of the nose. Baltimore: Urban & Schwarzenberg, 1978.

MESSERKLINGER W. Die Rolle der lateralen Nasenwand in der Pathogenese, Diagnose und Therapie der rezidivierenden chronischen Rhinosinusitis. Laryngol Rhinol Otol 1987; 66:293.

NEHLS G. Antroskopieerfahrung. Ein Beitrag zur Nasennebenhöhlendiagnostik. HNO (Berl) 1955; 5:158.

NITZE M. Eine neue Beobachtungs- und Untersuchungsmethode für Harnröhre, Harnblase und Rectum. Wien Med Wochenschr 1879; 649.

PAPUROV G. Sinuscopy of the maxillary sinus. (Bulgarien) Otorhino-laryngologie 1967; 4:30.

PIDOUX JM, TERRIER G. Endoskopie der Nase und der Nasennebenhöhlen bei der Frühdiagnostik der Tumoren der Nasenhaupthöhle und der Nasennebenhöhlen. J Fr Otorhinolaryngol 1977; 26:311.

PIHRT J. Bilan des examens de la cavité maxillare par la sinuscopie. Rev Laryngol Otol Rhinol (Bord) 1964; 85:781.

PORTMANN G. Le sinus-pharyngoscope. Rev Laryngol Otol Rhinol (Bord) 1925; 46:387.

REICHERT M. Über eine neue Untersuchungsmethode der Oberkieferhöhle mittels des Antroskops. Berl Klin Wochenschr Nr 1902.

RICCABONA A. Erfahrungen mit der Kieferhöhlenendoskopie. Arch Ohr Nas Kehlkopfheilk 1955; 167:359.

ROSEMANN G. Zur endoskopischen Kieferhöhlendiagnostik. Z Laryngol Rhinol 1961; 40:935.

SARGNON F. Endoscopie directe du sinus maxillaire par les fistules. Arch Int Laryngol 1908.

SLOBODNIK M. Die direkte Untersuchung der Kieferhöhle durch Endoskopie. Z Laryngol 1930; 19:437.

SLOBODNIK M. Der negative Befund bei der Probespülung der Kieferhöhle und die Highmoroskopie. Zbl HNO 1932; 30:320.

SOBEL J, FRIEDRICH JP, TERRIER G. La sinusomanométrie à débit constant. HNO (Berl) 1984; 32:482.

SPIELBERG W. New instruments for puncturing and visualizing the maxillary antrum of Highmore. Laryngoscope 1924; 33:844.

SPIELBERG W. Antroscopy of the maxillary sinus. Laryngoscope 1922; 32:441.

STOERK C. Klinik der Krankheiten des Kehlkopfs, der Nase und des Rachens. Stuttgart: F Enke, 1880.

v. STUCKRAD H, LAKATOS I. Über ein neues Lupenlaryngoskop (Epipharyngoskop). Laryngol Rhinol Otol 1975; 54:336.

TERRIER G. L'endoscopie rhinosinusale moderne. Inpharzam S.A. 1978.

TERRIER G. Die Endoskopie des Sinus maxillaris in der traumatischen und infektiösen Pathologie. Ther Umsch 1975; 32:628.

TERRIER G, FRIEDRICH J. Der Beitrag der modernen Endoskopie bei allergischen Nasen-Nebenhöhlenerkrankungen. Acta Otorhinolaryngol Belg 1979; 33:490.

TERRIER G, GUIGNARD C. La technique de l'endoscopie sphénoidale. Schweizerische Ges für ORL. 65. Frühjahrsversammlung Bad Ragaz, Juni, 1978.

TIMM C. Die Endoskopie der Kieferhöhlen. Fortschr Med 1956; 74:421.

v. TOVÖLGYI E. Der Antroskopietrokar. Arch Laryngol Rhinol (Berl) 1911; 25:144.

TÜRCK L. Klinik der Krankheiten des Kehlkopfes. Wien: W Braumüller, 1866.

VALENTIN A. Die cystoskopische Untersuchung des Nasenrachens oder Salpingoskopie. Arch Laryngol Rhinol (Berl) 1903; 13:410.

VOLTOLINI R. Die Rhinoskopie und Pharyngoskopie. Breslau: E Morgenstern, 1879.

VOLTOLINI R. Das elektrische Licht, verwendet in unserer Spezialität und die Anwendung des Cocain. Ms Ohren heilk 1885; 19:142.

VOSS. Verh Dtsch Otol Ges 1908.

WALES P. A new endoscope. Philadelphia Med Assoc Surg Rep 1868; June 13.

WATSON-WILLIAMS P. A new endo-rhinoscope or salpingoscope. Zbl HNO 1930; 14:855.

WERTHEIM G. Über ein Verfahren zum Zwecke der Besichtigung des vorderen und mittleren Drittels der Nasenhöhle. Wien Med Wochenschr 1869; 19:293.

WIGAND ME. Transnasal ethmoidectomy under endoscopical control. Rhinology 1981; 19:7.

WIGAND ME, STEINER W. Endonasale Kieferhöhlenoperation mit endoskopischer Kontrolle. Z Laryngol Rhinol 1977; 56:421.

WIGAND ME, STEINER W, JAUMANN MP. Endonasal sinus surgery with endoscopial control: from radical operation to rehabilitation of the mucosa. Endoscopy 1978; 10:2255.

WILLEMOT J. The birth of rhinological endoscopy. F méd (BR) 1987; 94(4):237.

YAMASHITA K. Endonasal flexible fiberoptic endoscopy. Rhinology 1983; 21:233.

YANKAUER S. Die pharyngeale Tubenmündung mit Beschreibung eines Spekulums und anderer Instumente zur direkten Untersuchung und Behandlung derselben. Z Laryngol (Leipz) 1912; 4:361.

ZARNIKO C. Diagnostik der Nasenkrankheiten. Handbuch der Hals-Nasen-Ohren-Heilkunde. Herausgegeben von Denker-Kahler. Berlin-München: Springer-Bergmann, 1925; 1:722.

ZAUFAL E. Zur endoskopischen Untersuchung der Rachenmündung der Tube en face und des Tubenkanals. Arch Ohr Nas Kehlkopfheilk 1909; 79:109.

ZÖLLNER F. Anatomie, Physiologie, Pathologie und Klinik der Ohrtrompete und ihre diagnostisch therapeutischen Beziehungen zu allen Nachbarschaftserkrankungen. Berlin: Springer, 1942.

ZUCKERKANDL E. Normale und pathologische Anatomie der Nasenhöhle und ihrer pneumatischen Anhänge. Wien: W Braumüller, 1882.

Chapter 2

SECRETION TRANSPORTATION

PRINCIPLES OF SECRETION TRANSPORTATION

Drainage and ventilation are the two most important factors in the maintenance of normal physiology of the paranasal sinuses and their mucous membranes. Normal drainage of the paranasal sinuses is a complex function of both the secretion and transport mechanisms, and is to a large extent dependent upon the amount of mucus produced, its composition, the effectiveness of the ciliary beat, mucosal resorption, and the condition of the ostia and the ethmoidal clefts into which the respective sinus ostia open.

In health, the mucus blanket that covers the nasal mucosa is continuously produced by the mucoserous nasal glands and the intraepithelial goblet cells. This mucus film has two layers: an inner serous layer, called *the sol phase*, in which the cilia beat and an outer more viscous layer, *the gel phase*, which is transported by the ciliary beat. Normal nasal mucus exists in equilibrium between the sol and gel phases at a pH range of 7.5 to 7.6. A proper balance between the inner sol and the outer gel phase is of critical importance for normal mucociliary clearance. Dust and other fine particles are incorporated into the gel phase under normal conditions and, together with the gel phase, are transported out of the sinuses. Under abnormal conditions, pathogens (especially viruses) may be incorporated into the cells of the mucosa itself.

Movements of the mucosa, especially pulsations in cases of inflammation or movements of the nasal fontanelles, may assist the transportation of secretions out of the maxillary sinus. An unimpeded flow of air during inspiration through the nose is a further factor, since forced inspiration creates suction or negative pressure that promotes the transportation of mucus out of the sinuses.

The cilia beat in a synchronized (transversally) and metachronized (longitudinally) manner, although the precise mechanism of this synchronization is still not fully understood. The cilia move almost exclusively in the sol phase of the secretion. The gel phase is actively transported over the sol phase like a carpet by the cilia when their tips touch this overlying "carpet" during their short active beat; there is no contact between the cilia and the gel phase during their slower recovery stroke (Figs. 2.1 and 2.2).

Nasal mucus is constantly produced. The quantity and composition of the mucus depends among other factors upon environmental conditions such as humidity, pollution, or other airborne external irritants.

The mucosal glands are regulated predominantly by parasympathetic nerve fibers, which reach the glands from the nucleus salivatorius superior via the nervus petrosus major and the ganglion pterygopalatinum as postganglionic fibers. A sympathetic afferent nerve supply may also reach the glands through their blood vessels, which are innervated by both sympathetic and parasympathetic fibers. The sympathetic fibers come from the lateral horn of the spinal cord. The postsynaptic fibers reach the skull base via the plexus caroticus. They form the nervus petrosus profundus and join the nervus petrosus major to form the nervus canalis pterygoidei (the vidian nerve) in the bony canal of the same name. Without further synapses, these fibers reach the nasal and sinus mucosa. There is some evidence that sympathetic fibers may reach the mucosa from the plexus caroticus internus via the ethmoidal arteries and the first branch of the trigeminal nerve.

FIGURE 2.1 The "bridging phenomenon" is shown on the right. When mucosal surfaces come close to each other or even into contact, the cohesive forces within the mucus blanket of the gel phase can bridge the gap, leaving the recess between the opposing mucosal surfaces filled with the more serous sol phase. This "bridging phenomenon" allows normal mucus transport to continue. Mucus transport over a bony crest with the gel phase of mucus becoming somewhat thicker due to gravity when transported upward is shown on the left.

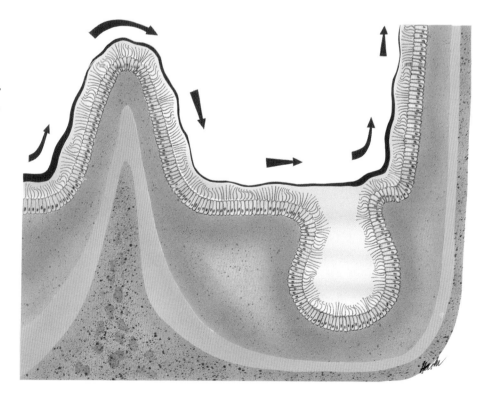

Gel phase

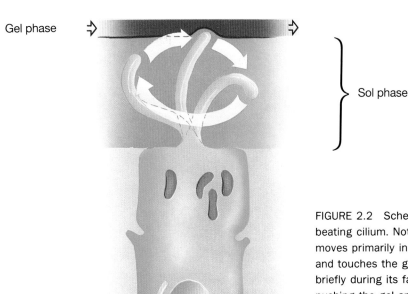

Sol phase

FIGURE 2.2 Schematic drawing of a beating cilium. Note how the cilium moves primarily in the sol phase (*blue*) and touches the gel phase (*purple*) only briefly during its fast "active beat," thus pushing the gel and the "blanket" in the direction of the active beat (to the right in this case). The slower "recovery beat" takes the cilium to the extreme left without touching the gel layer during this movement.

Recent research indicates that another group of neuromediators, the neuropeptides, are present and active in the nasal mucous membranes. Substance P appears to have a great effect on the mucosal glands, and its liberation from C fibers via local reflexes may cause massive hypersecretion, vasodilatation, and extravasation of plasma. (For details see Chapter 11.)

Under normal conditions, the mucus layer is steadily transported away. Our own endoscopic studies indicate that a healthy maxillary sinus renews its mucus layer every 20 to 30 minutes on average. The ciliary beat can be studied easily during maxillary sinuscopy. During sinuscopy, the effect of the ciliary beat on the transport of mucus, pus, blood, or other particles can be seen directly. In addition, the beating cilia can be seen in the light-reflecting areas of the mucosa. All of these mechanisms, and the variations and abnormalities of mucociliary transport in the maxillary sinus are demonstrated in our film "The Maxillary Sinus: A Clinical Entity?"

Normally, the secretion covers the mucosa in all corners of the sinuses with a homogeneous layer of more or less constant thickness. Near the ostia of the larger sinuses, the viscous layer appears to be somewhat thicker, probably because the secretion from the entire sinus converges there.

Bony crests, found protruding into the lumen of the frontal sinuses are usually traversed by the secretion without any problem (see Fig. 2.1). If the secretion becomes more viscous and consequently thicker and heavier, however, these crests may become an obstacle to mucus transport and secretion may be retained at the crest and finally drain away through the effect of gravity (Fig. 2.3).

Small mucosal defects such as a cut usually have no influence on the transportation of secretions no matter what their direction. The cohesive nature of the mucus allows the mucus "carpet" to be transported over such lesions (Fig. 2.4).

Small mucosal lesions (Figs. 2.5 and 2.6) are usually also passed by the secretion. In cases of higher viscosity of the secretion, such a defect may become an obstacle so that secretion is retained at the site of the defect. In some cases, the mucus can be pushed or pulled over the surface of this type of mucosal lesion and rest there for a while, as described by Hilding in cases of squamous cell metaplasia.

This mucociliary clearance phenomenon can also be studied in the nasopharynx at the border of the ciliated and squamous cell epithelium. At this junction, the active cilia-based transport of the mucus comes to an end, and the mucus is retained for a short while before gravity and the swallowing mechanism move it on.

FIGURE 2.3 *A*, The highly viscous secretion that is blocking the natural ostium of a right maxillary sinus. After a certain amount of mucus had gathered, it was pulled by gravity to the floor of the sinus and then slowly transported again toward the natural ostium, *B*. (30 degree wide angle lens.) t = trocar sleeve and oi = ostium internum (maxillary ostium).

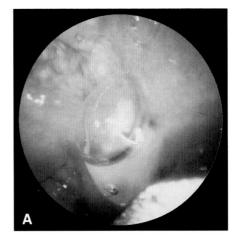
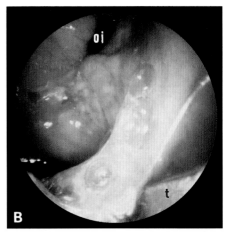

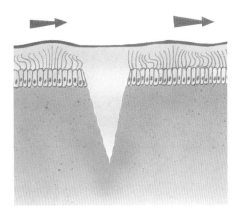

FIGURE 2.4 Unimpeded mucus transport over a small mucosal defect. Modified after W. Messerklinger.

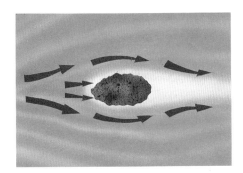

FIGURE 2.5 Mucus transport as seen from above bypassing a small mucosal lesion. Modified after W. Messerklinger.

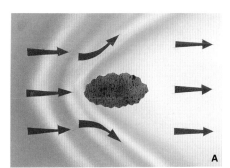

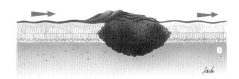

FIGURE 2.6 Mucus of a higher viscosity at a mucosal lesion as seen from above, A, and in cross section, B. The mucus may be pushed onto and sometimes pulled over the surface of the mucosal lesion. Modified after W. Messerklinger.

21

Frequently, accessory ostia are present in the fontanelles of the maxillary sinus. These accessory ostia are usually bypassed by normal secretion inside the sinus (Fig. 2.7). In cases of higher viscosity, the entire mucus layer may move over such an accessory ostium without any mucus leaving the sinus (Fig. 2.8). We have seen this happen in accessory ostia with a diameter of up to 4 mm. With larger accessory ostia, we were sometimes able to observe an active outwardly directed transport of the mucus. Usually only that portion of the secretion moving toward the middle of the ostium was transported out actively.

FIGURE 2.7 Blood-stained mucus in a left maxillary sinus bypassing a large accessory ostium to leave via the natural ostium (A, B, C, and D). In this patient, blood-stained mucus from the floor of the maxillary sinus can been seen in these "time lapse" photographs bypassing the accessory ostium in the posterior fontanelle to leave via the posterior aspect of the natural maxillary ostium. Through the large accessory ostium, the free inferior margin of the middle turbinate can be identified together with the inferior aspect of the bulla above the laterally bent middle turbinate. Note how the mucus starts to cover the accessory ostium like a veil from both directions, anteriorly and posteriorly (E). The cohesive, viscous mucus has formed a blanket that moves over the accessory ostium toward the natural ostium with little mucus leaving the accessory ostium. When the patient was asked to perform the Valsalva maneuver, the mucus blanket burst like a bubble, only to close again a few moments (F) later. (30 degree wide angle lens.) om = maxillary ostium; ao = accessory ostium; and t = trocar sleeve.

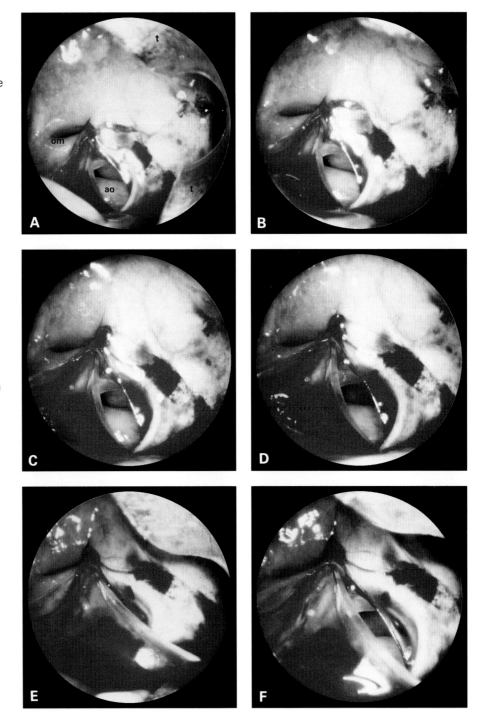

Secretion Transport Pathology

In cases of hypersecretion, mucus *flows* toward the deepest point of the respective sinus under the influence of gravity. If the composition of the mucus remains balanced, a gel layer persists on the surface. Because of cohesion, this mucus carpet on the surface may be pulled away by the still active cilia of the ''non-drowned'' mucosa (Fig. 2.13) provided that the direction of transport of the corresponding mucosal areas are not opposing each other and the cilia still beat normally. If as shown in Figure 2.13 a maxillary sinus is half filled with such secretion, the transport of the mucus layer in different directions is hindered by the cohesive forces of the gel layer at the surface level because the cilia of the still intact mucosal areas are not powerful enough to ''tear off'' the surface gel layer. Thus despite a normally functioning ciliary action, secretion transport ceases completely. If the hypersecretion is aspirated in such a case, normal transport will recommence almost immediately.

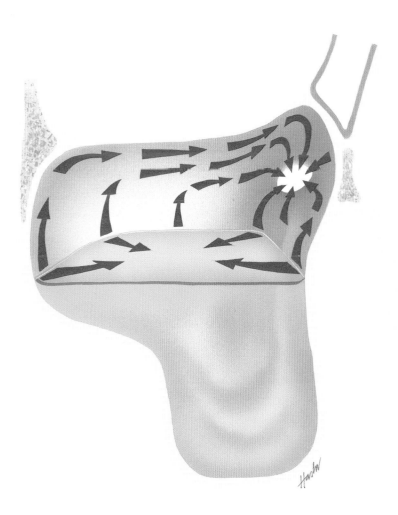

FIGURE 2.13 In this schematic drawing of a maxillary sinus half filled with secretions, the transportation of the mucus layer is held back by the cohesional forces of the gel layer on the surface. The cilia of the still intact mucosal areas are not powerful enough to ''tear off'' the gel layer from the surface. Modified after W. Messerklinger.

If the composition of the secretion is changed so that the mucus produced becomes more viscous, transport towards the ostium slows considerably and the gel layer becomes demonstrably thicker. In such cases the viscous secretion reaches the ostium although it is apparently too thick to pass through. This results in a collection of thick mucus, at the ostium, which finally flows back down to the floor of the sinus as it succumbs to the effect of gravity. Depending upon prevailing conditions, this thick mucus may be dissolved and then transported away or the trek toward the ostium may be repeated and the secretion retained in the sinus for a varying period of time (see Fig. 2.3). (See also Chapter 11.)

If there is a lack of secretion or if a loss of humidity at the surface can not be compensated for by the glands and the goblet cells, the mucus becomes viscous and the sol phase may become extremely thin allowing the gel phase to come into intense contact with the cilia, thus impeding their action. This can be studied clearly during maxillary sinuscopy in fresh cadaver heads. With continuing dehydration one can see a worm-like movement in the mucus layer with only a minimal movement of the cilia. Sometimes after the application of a few drops of saline solution this almost dry mucus is dissolved and the cilia beat again with their normal speed and pattern. In patients who have been given atropine as premedication, similar findings can be observed.

When inflamed, the mucosa of the sinuses can swell very rapidly. When performing maxillary sinuscopy in such cases, one frequently can see the entire sinus mucosa pulsate. If the patient is asked to perform the Valsalva maneuver, thus increasing the venous pressure, the mucosa often swells considerably. In addition, pronounced movements of the membranous portions of the maxillary wall in the region of the fontanelles may occur.

In cases of bacterial or viral superinfection, not only may the mucosal glands be affected, but the entire mucosal surface may be partially destroyed or paralyzed and thus unable to provide its mucociliary clearance function. A variety of ciliary or mucosal dysfunctions or malfunctions such as the immotile cilia syndrome, cystic fibrosis, and allergic rhinitis can also severely impair mucociliary clearance.

For optimal function of the mucociliary clearance system, normal ventilation, humidification, metabolism, osmotic pressure, and pH are as important as protection from external noxious stimuli. The frequency of the ciliary beat ranges from 8 to 20 beats per second with a considerable variation between individuals. The frequency of the ciliary beat is significantly influenced by the temperature of the inspired air. The optimum temperature for efficient ciliary beat is around 33° Celsius. Below 18° C the frequency slows down, stopping completely between 12 and 7° C. At 40° C, ciliary activity slows down as well, and at 43° C it stops completely. If these temperature extremes last for a short period of time, this temperature dependent cessation of ciliary activity is reversible.

General factors that also affect ciliary function include: longstanding dehydration, which leads to complete ciliary failure; medications such as atropine and antihistamines, which slow the action of the cilia completely as may contact with allergens; chemical substances or cigarette smoke; and foreign bodies.

A reduced oxygen supply also slows ciliary movement, even where the blood supply is normal. Enriched oxygenation can raise the frequency of ciliary beat by 30 to 50 percent. The best pH for ciliary activity is between 7 and 8. Below pH 6.5, ciliary activity decreases rapidly.

During maxillary sinuscopy another phenomenon can sometimes be observed: immediately after penetration into the sinus by the trocar, the ciliary beat of the entire sinus mucosa may come to a complete halt for several minutes and then gradually return to normal. This appears to be a reflex phenomenon triggered by sudden trauma to the sinus mucosa with a possible interruption of the synchronization of the cilia, although the exact underlying mechanism is not yet clearly understood.

Not all areas of the maxillary sinus mucosa transport their secretion uniformly, and from time to time the endoscopist can see one area of mucosa transporting mucus faster than its neighboring areas with that mucus overtaking the other secretions on their way to the ostium. After a few minutes, the slower areas may speed up as the faster area slows down. This phenomenon of "secretion expressways" (see Figs. 2.10 and 2.15) can be found both in cases of abnormal secretion and also in apparently normal sinuses. It is not known whether this phenomenon is an accidental finding, or an artifact caused by the light and warmth of the endoscope or the trauma of its insertion, or whether this phenomenon serves a special purpose, i.e., to avoid accumulation of the secretion at the narrow ostial passage.

PATHWAYS OF SECRETION TRANSPORT

Human nasal and paranasal sinus mucosa and their ciliary activity may survive the death of the individual for 24 to 48 hours. The cilia beat somewhat slower but in exactly the same pattern as they do in a living person. With progressing dehydration and increasing viscosity of the mucus or with the final death of the mucosal cells, the ciliary beat ceases completely, normally around the second or third day post mortem.

In his original studies, Messerklinger used fresh cadaver heads, staining the mucus with various techniques or by adding dust particles or various kinds of powders. By taking time lapse movies, he was able to follow the pathways of the secretion transport in all the paranasal sinuses. Simultaneously during sinus operations, he tried to confirm his observations using sterile dermatol powder to learn more about the pathologic conditions of the mucociliary transport mechanism.

These studies were done primarily with the operating microscope in the 1950s and the early 1960s. It was the need to study the normal and abnormal pathophysiology of the mucociliary transport pattern in patients without traumatic or invasive techniques that made Messerklinger search for a better tool for this purpose. He ultimately selected the nasal endoscope as his primary investigative instrument. Today, with powerful cold light endoscopes, the ciliary transport mechanism can be easily studied, since almost all of the mucosal surfaces can be directly visualized. Not only can the effect of ciliary action and secretion transport be observed, but the ciliary beat itself becomes easily visible in the light-reflecting areas of the mucosa.

After experimentation with a variety of stains and particles, we found that the patient's own blood provides the best substance to color the secretion. Either the few drops of blood that flow into the maxillary sinus when the trocar is inserted can be used, or in some cases we take a few drops of blood from a vein and instill them into the floor of the sinus through the trocar sleeve. Usually after 2 or 3 minutes, depending upon the prevailing mucosal pathology, the blood-tinged mucus can be followed on its way toward the ostium as illustrated in Figures 2.7, 2.12, and 2.14. Sometimes heparin or citrate is added to the blood to prevent coagulation.

One of the most important of Messerklinger's discoveries, following earlier animal studies by Hilding Sr., was the observation that the secretions of the various sinuses do not reach their respective ostia by random routes, but instead follow very definite pathways, which seem to be genetically determined. While these pathways may be impeded or even blocked by various pathologic conditions, their direction is not significantly altered.

Secretion Transport in the Maxillary Sinus

In the maxillary sinus, secretion transport starts from the floor of the sinus in a stellate pattern. The mucus is transported along the anterior, medial, posterior, and lateral walls of the sinuses as well as along the roof. All these secretion routes converge at the natural ostium of the maxillary sinus (Figs. 2.14 and 2.15). When the secretion has passed through the maxillary sinus ostium it is not yet in the free middle meatus, but must pass through a very narrow and complicated system of clefts in the lateral nasal wall.

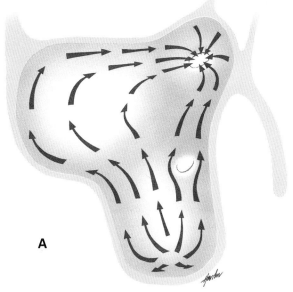

A

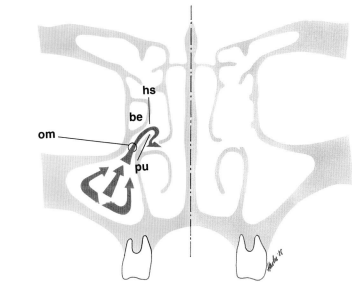

FIGURE 2.14 Schematic drawings of the normal transportation pathways of mucus inside (*A*) and moving out (*B*) of a maxillary sinus. be = bulla ethmoidalis; pu = uncinate process; hs = hiatus semilunaris; and om = maxillary ostium. Modified after W. Messerklinger.

B

FIGURE 2.15 *A*, Note the stellate transport routes all moving toward the natural ostium in a right maxillary sinus, as encountered during sinuscopy. Note (*B*) the "expressway" phenomenon.

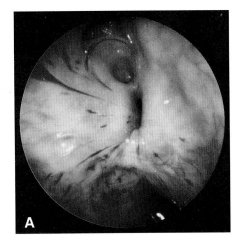

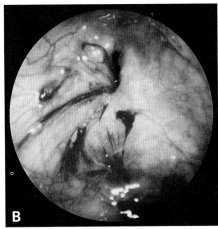

The maxillary sinus ostium normally opens into the floor of the posterior third of the ethmoidal infundibulum, which is bordered by the uncinate process medially and the papyraceous lamina of the orbit laterally (see Chapter 3). The ethmoidal infundibulum opens into the middle meatus through the hiatus semilunaris (a two-dimensional cleft bordered by the anteroinferior face of the ethmoidal bulla posteriorly and the posterior free margin of the uncinate process anteriorly). Via the hiatus semilunaris, the secretion from the maxillary sinus is transported over the medial face of the inferior turbinate posteriorly into the nasopharynx.

Secretion from the sinus is always transported via the natural ostium, even when there is one or more accessory ostium in the area of the fontanelles and even in those patients in whom a patent window in the inferior meatus has been surgically created (see Chapter 11). This is one of the reasons we no longer perform inferior meatal antrostomies. While an inferior meatal nasoantral window may well provide ventilation to a diseased maxillary sinus and consequently may help to normalize conditions in the sinus and even in the ethmoidal prechambers of that sinus, these inferior meatal windows do not achieve considerable active outwardly directed transportation of secretion (see Chapter 6).

Secretion Transport in the Frontal Sinus

The frontal sinus is the only sinus in which there is an active *inwardly* directed transportation of mucus. Along the interfrontal septum, mucus is transported into the frontal sinus, then laterally along its roof and back medially via the floor and inferior portions of the posterior and anterior wall of the sinus. The secretion then exits the frontal sinus via the lateral aspect of its ostium. Not all of this mucus leaves the sinus after one "round trip." This is the result of a whorl-like formation in the ciliary pattern, which may be present in a shallow sulcus immediately above the frontal ostium as well as inferior to it in the frontal recess. An unspecified amount of mucus comes into contact with the inwardly directed transport route again and thus may recycle through the sinus several times (Fig. 2.16).

Once it has passed out of the ostium, the secretion is then transported through a narrow cleft of variable dimensions, the frontal recess. This recess drains either directly into the ethmoidal infundibulum from above, or medial to the ethmoidal infundibulum if the infundibulum ends with a superior blind pouch. The frontal recess, depending upon the prevailing anatomic variations, may collect the secretions from the other ethmoidal compartments including secretions from the lateral sinus, from the agger nasi, from

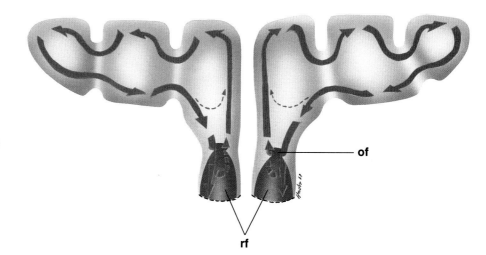

FIGURE 2.16 A schematic drawing of secretion transport inside and out of the frontal sinus. of = frontal sinus ostium and rf = frontal recess.

pneumatized middle turbinates, and from the most anterior ethmoidal cells. In addition, the mucus transport routes from the superior aspect of the head of the middle turbinate and the beginning of the middle meatus may also have a connection to the transport routes out of, and what is even more important, *into* the frontal sinus. Eventually, the secretions from the frontal sinus merge with the secretions from the maxillary sinus and together they are transported back into the nasopharynx.

Mucociliary Transport from Anterior and Posterior Ethmoidal and Sphenoidal Sinuses and from the Lateral Nasal Wall

If the ostium of an ethmoidal cell is located at its floor, then the secretion is usually transported directly toward the ostium. If the ostium is located higher up in one of the walls, e.g., in the posterior wall of the bulla ethmoidalis, then there is usually a spiral transport pattern toward the ostium. The borderline between the anterior and posterior ethmoid is the ground lamella (see Chapter 3). All cells opening anteroinferiorly to the ground lamella are anterior ethmoid cells and drain into the middle meatus. All cells that open posteriorly and superiorly to the ground lamella are posterior ethmoid cells and drain via the superior meatus into the sphenoethmoidal recess. Should there be a supreme or fourth turbinate with cells in the supreme meatus, then these cells also drain into the sphenoethmoidal recess. In the sphenoid sinus, depending upon the location of the ostium, there usually is a spiral transportation of secretion toward the ostium. The secretion subsequently passes into the sphenoethmoidal recess.

In the lateral nasal wall, two major routes of mucociliary transport can usually be identified (Fig. 2.17). The first route combines secretion from the frontal and maxillary sinuses and the anterior ethmoidal complex. These secretions usually join in or near the ethmoidal infundibulum, and from there the transport passes over the free rear margin of the uncinate process and along the medial face of the inferior turbinate toward the nasopharynx. At this point the secretions pass anteriorly and inferiorly to the eustachian tube orifice. Active transport continues up to the borderline of the ciliated and the squamous epithelium in the nasopharynx. From this point, the secretions are moved by gravity and assisted ultimately by the swallowing mechanism.

The second route combines the secretions from the posterior ethmoid cells and the sphenoid sinus. The secretions from these two sinuses meet in the sphenoethmoidal recess and are then transported toward the nasopharynx posteriorly and superiorly to the eustachian tube orifice. Occasionally minor amounts of secretion from the superior meatus near the posterior end of the middle turbinate may join the first or inferior secretion pathway. The eustachian tube is thus like a breakwater between these two secretion pathways. The secretions from the nasal septum are transported more or less vertically downward to the floor of the nose and then backwards, where in most cases they join the first secretion pathway inferior to the eustachian tube.

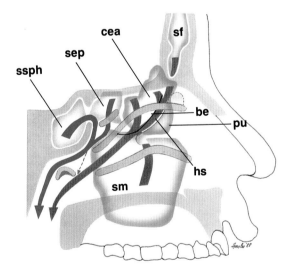

FIGURE 2.17 A schematic drawing of the normal secretion transport pathways in the lateral nasal wall. sf = frontal sinus; sm = maxillary sinus; cea = anterior ethmoidal complex; be = ethmoidal bulla; pu = uncinate process; hs = hiatus semilunaris; sep = posterior ethmoidal sinus; and ssph = sphenoid sinus.

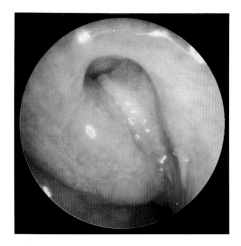

FIGURE 2.18 A left eustachian tube orifice open during swallowing.

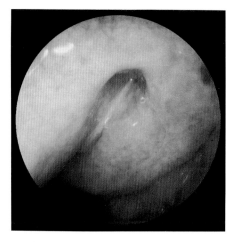

FIGURE 2.19 Right eustachian tube orifice closed. (30 degree endoscope.)

Secretory Disturbances and Tubal Function

A wide variety of diseases of the nose and paranasal sinuses may affect the function of the eustachian tube and consequently that of the middle ear. The common cold, allergic rhinitis, and acute or chronic recurrent sinusitis may lead to obstruction of the eustachian tube orifice with all the attendant consequences for the middle ear. These include ascending infections leading to acute otitis media, tubal malventilation leading to serous otitis, glue ear, or even retraction pockets. The rigid endoscope is the ideal instrument to investigate the eustachian tube orifice. With the 4-mm 30 degree lens, the opening and closing mechanism during swallowing can readily be studied. The 30 degree lens also allows observation of the eustachian tube orifice on both sides from the same inferior or common nasal meatus simply by rotating the lens to the desired position (Figs. 2.18 and 2.19). (See Chapter 5. Technique of Diagnostic Endoscopy.)

If pathologic changes occur in the nasal or paranasal sinus mucosa and the nature of the secretions alters, e.g., the purulent or highly viscous thickened secretions found in acute or chronic sinusitis, or if the composition of the mucus becomes more viscous, the normal secretion routes may undergo significant changes (Fig. 2.20). Mechanical obstructions, e.g., massive septal deviations or spurs may also alter the normal drainage routes. When such pathologic changes exist, the two major secretion routes may join before they reach the

FIGURE 2.20 A schematic drawing showing a pathologic alteration in the normal secretory transport routes out of the lateral nasal wall, resulting in large amounts of mucus moving directly over the eustachian tube orifice.

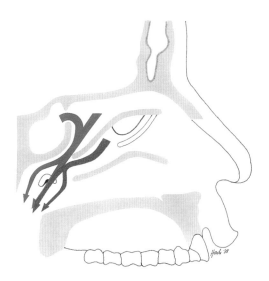

eustachian tube ostium, and one or both routes may form whorls around or even in the orifice itself. Abnormal infected secretions may then move directly over the orifice (instead of bypassing it) as demonstrated in Figures 2.20, 2.21, and 2.22. The consequences of this on the normal function of the eustachian tube may be severe (Fig. 2.23). Due to its own mucociliary clearance, a previously normal eustachian tube can remain resistant to abnormal secretions for a time. Depending on the duration and virulence of such a condition, however, tubal dysfunction will occur. Congestion and obstruction of the orifice due to inflammation of its lymphoreticular tissue with slowing down of the mucociliary clearance may result in impeded ventilation or ascending infection of the middle ear. In our experience it has proven worthwhile to look for underlying causes like these in cases of middle ear problems and tubal malfunction. It is important, however, not to rely on just one endoscopic investigation, as the pathologic condition is not necessarily present at the time of the first examination.

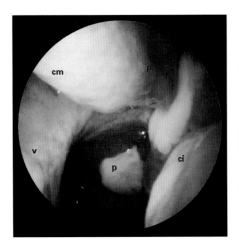

FIGURE 2.21   Note the streak of pus flowing out of the middle meatus and back into the nasopharynx in this case of acute sinusitis. p = pus; cm = concha media; ci = concha inferior; and v = vomer.

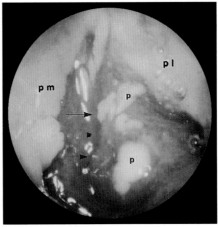

FIGURE 2.22   A close-up view of the eustachian tube on the left side of the same patient seen in Figure 2.21. Pus can be seen passing the eustachian tube medially and laterally, and also moving directly over the mouth of the eustachian tube together with thick glary secretion. The orifice is extremely narrowed by swollen, inflamed mucosa. p = pus (m = medial, l = lateral).

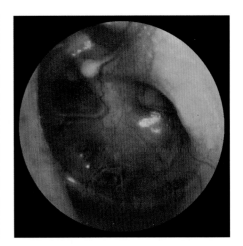

FIGURE 2.23   The tympanic membrane of the same patient as in Figures 2.21 and 2.22 showing increased vascularity and a serous otitis media.

ROLE OF ETHMOIDAL PRECHAMBERS

The two largest and clinically most important sinuses, the frontal and maxillary sinuses, communicate with the middle meatus via very narrow and delicate "prechambers." The maxillary sinus ostium opens into a cleft in the lateral nasal wall called the ethmoidal infundibulum. The frontal sinus ostium opens into an hourglass-shaped cleft, the frontal recess, which in textbooks is usually referred to as the "nasofrontal duct." This is, we believe, a misnomer, as usually no bony tubular structure corresponding to an actual "duct" can be identified (see Chapter 3).

Both of these clefts or prechambers are part of the anterior ethmoid and fulfill important tasks as long as they are healthy. In these pre-chambers the mucosal surfaces are very closely approximated, and as indicated previously, in clefts such as these the mucus, especially when more viscous or otherwise pathologically altered, can be more easily transported away and thus the sinus more efficiently drained because the ciliary beat can work in these narrow areas on the mucus layer from two or more sides (Fig. 2.24). In an ostium, the cilia can act upon the mucus in a circular fashion (Figs. 2.25 and 2.26).

If, however, the opposing mucosal surfaces in these clefts come into intense contact or are firmly pressed against each other as the result of mucosal swelling, the drainage and ventilation of the larger dependent sinuses may be seriously interfered with because the ciliary beat is immobilized and consequently the mucus is no longer transported away (Fig. 2.27). Active transportation of mucus can only continue peripheral to these areas of intense contact. If the area of contact is extensive, the ciliary beat may stop completely.

Despite the fact that these areas of contact are almost invisible clinically, small areas like these may be the underlying cause of severe problems. They can irritate the nasal function, disturb the nasal cycle and cause reactive hypersecretion of the surrounding mucosa as well as being the cause of sinus headaches or recurring infections of the larger dependent sinuses. If mucosal swelling and mucus retention occurs in one of the key areas such as the infundibulum or the frontal sinus, then ventilation and drainage of the dependent larger sinus may become impaired and the secretions of that sinus retained. When the area of blockage becomes larger or infection occurs, the retained mucus provides an ideal nutrient for both viral and bacterial growth, thus creating a vicious circle.

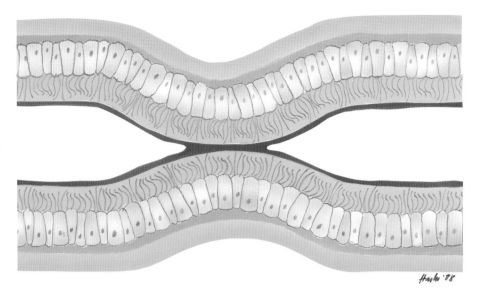

FIGURE 2.24 A schematic drawing of an ethmoidal "bottle neck" in a healthy individual. In this instance the ciliary beat can work on secretion from two sides and thus promote mucus transportation.

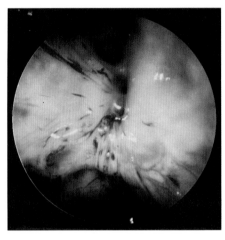

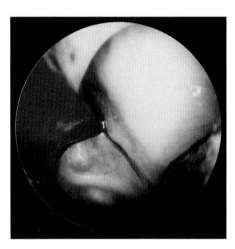

FIGURE 2.25 Thick secretions are transported through the "corner" of the ostium with ciliary activity from at least three sides in this right maxillary sinus.

FIGURE 2.26 Blood-stained, thick mucus is transported through the "inferior corner" of the natural ostium in this left maxillary sinus.

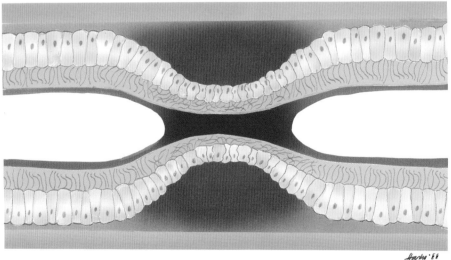

FIGURE 2.27 A schematic drawing of a diseased ethmoidal "bottle neck." The opposing mucosal surfaces are in intimate contact, with the pressure stopping the coordinated ciliary beat. The mucus between the opposed surfaces is thus no longer transported away.

In cases of poor ventilation, the pH of the involved sinus falls, which in turn slows ciliary movement and causes mucus of a higher viscosity to be produced. Because of blockage of the prechamber and ciliary insufficiency, these secretions may not leave the sinus for a considerable period of time. If, in addition, superinfection occurs, hypoxia and mucus accumulation provide ideal conditions for the growth of pathogens. Infection and toxins may additionally impair mucosal function.

The clinical symptoms in such a case are those of "typical" maxillary or frontal sinusitis. The underlying cause for the disease, however, is found in one of the ethmoidal prechambers, not in the diseased sinuses themselves (Fig. 2.28). If these ethmoidal prechambers are considerably diseased, the subordinate larger sinus simply cannot help but become involved, as its ventilation and drainage are compromised.

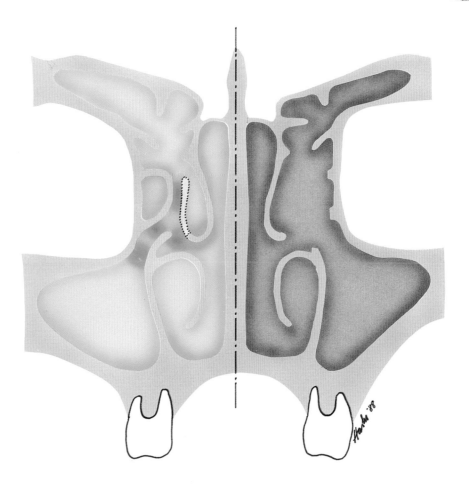

FIGURE 2.28 This schematic drawing demonstrates the key diseased ethmoidal positions (*left*). The situation after functional endoscopic sinus surgery is shown on the *right*.

Figures 2.24 to 2.32 illustrate the hidden position and the dependence upon the surrounding structures of the maxillary and frontal sinus ostia. A window cut into the middle turbinate of a cadaveric head allows visualization of the lateral nasal wall (Fig. 2.29). The free posterior margin of the uncinate process, the anterior face of the bulla and the hiatus semilunaris between these two can be identified. The maxillary sinus ostium is not visible. In Figure 2.30 the middle turbinate has been fenestrated even more and the frontal recess thus exposed. The probe now placed through the hiatus semilunaris into the ethmoidal infundibulum demonstrates the cleft between the uncinate process medially and the papyraceous lamina, respectively and the superior aspect of the medial wall of the maxillary sinus laterally. The endoscope is in position and a sickle scalpel incises the uncinate process at its anterior insertion. Only after the uncinate process has been substantially resected (Fig. 2.31) does the maxillary ostium become visible. In this specimen the maxillary sinus ostium was hidden more than one centimeter in the depth of the posterior

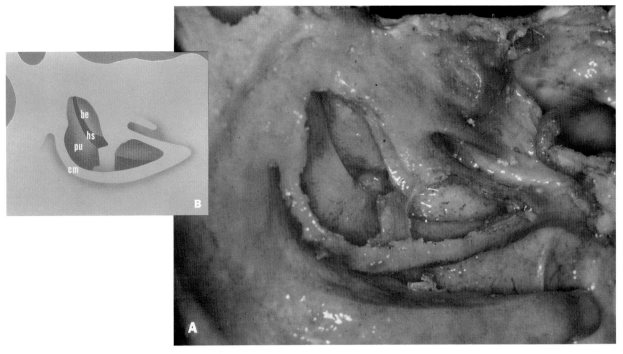

FIGURE 2.29 In this cadaver head (A), a window has been cut into the middle turbinate to allow visualization of the lateral nasal wall. The free posterior margin of the uncinate process, the anterior face of the bulla, and the hiatus semilunaris can be identified. This is also shown in the schematic diagram (B). be = ethmoidal bulla; hs = hiatus semilunaris; pu = uncinate process.

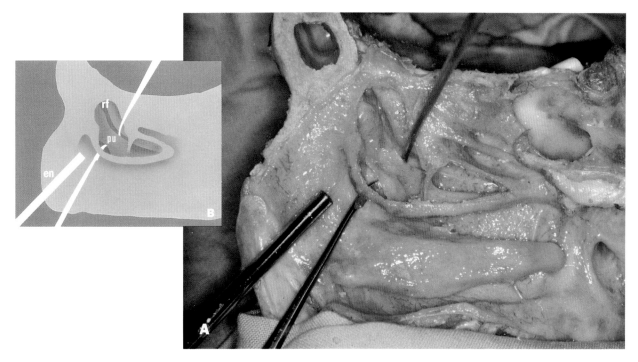

FIGURE 2.30 *A*, In this photograph of the specimen seen also in Figure 2.29, the window in the middle turbinate has been enlarged so that the frontal recess is exposed. A probe has been placed through the hiatus semilunaris into the infundibulum to demonstrate the cleft between the uncinate process and the anterior wall of the bulla. The endoscope is shown in its normal position as the sickle knife incises the uncinate process at its anterior insertion. *B*, A schematic diagram of these structures. en = endoscope; rf = frontal recess; and pu = uncinate process.

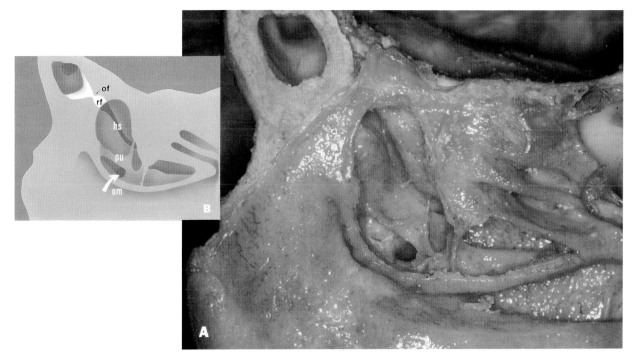

FIGURE 2.31 *A*, The maxillary ostium can only be seen after a substantial portion of the uncinate process has been resected. In this specimen, the maxillary sinus ostium was hidden more than one centimeter in the depth of the posterior third of the infundibulum at its floor. The accompanying schematic diagram, *B*, illustrates the hidden position of the frontal recess and the frontal sinus ostium. pu = uncinate process; rf = frontal recess; om = maxillary ostium; of = frontal sinus ostium; and hs = hiatus semilunaris.

third of the infundibulum at its floor. In this case, superiorly the uncinate process bends laterally and attaches to the lateral nasal wall, thus forming a blind superior end, the so-called ''recessus terminalis'' (Figs. 2.31 and 2.32). Thus, the frontal recess drains medially to the ethmoidal infundibulum (Fig. 2.32).

These pictures demonstrate that any abnormality, be it infection, allergy, trauma, tumor, or anatomic variation that blocks the entrance into the middle meatus, the hiatus semilunaris, or the infundibulum itself or narrows these already very narrow systems of clefts, may predispose to or promote a partial or complete blockage of the maxillary or frontal sinus ostia (Fig. 2.31). Depending upon the individual circumstances, e.g., if superinfection occurs, this may not only give rise to continuing problems like nasal obstruction and headaches or a postnasal discharge, but may also cause recurring acute or chronic frontal or maxillary sinusitis.

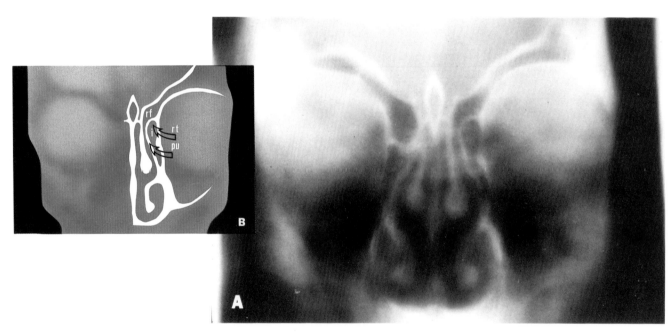

FIGURE 2.32 *A*, A tomographic cut in the coronal plane through the infundibulum anterior to the maxillary sinus ostium; shown also in, *B*, schematic diagram.

rf = frontal recess; i = ethmoidal infundibulum; pu = uncinate process; and rt = recessus terminalis.

The computed tomogram (CT) shown in Figure 2.33 clearly demonstrates this concept. Pronounced disease of the anterior ethmoid is present on the patient's right side completely blocking the ethmoidal infundibulum and there is clearly a thickening of the mucosa of the maxillary sinus. The ethmoidal disease need not necessarily be as severe as can be seen on the other side of Figure 2.33. On this side a relatively small but critically located lesion situated exactly in the infundibulum blocks the infundibulum causing an air-fluid level in the left maxillary sinus. These changes are only visible by tomography or CT scan. The plain sinus radiographs of this patient who had suffered from bilaterally recurring acute maxillary sinusitis only demonstrated a massive opacification suggesting an air-fluid level in the maxillary sinuses in the acute phases of the disease, but did not reveal the underlying causes in the ethmoidal complex. This case reinforces the fact that for the identification of the underlying causes of chronic recurring sinusitis, plain sinus X-ray films are inadequate.

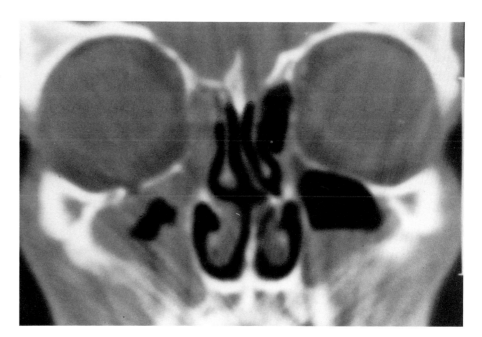

FIGURE 2.33 A CT of bilateral infundibular disease with secondary maxillary sinusitis.

How Can Infection Reach the Maxillary and Frontal Sinuses?

We have already seen that in the frontal sinus, mucus is actively transported into the sinus along the interfrontal septum on both sides. Apart from being inhaled into the sinuses, pathogens deposited by the airflow at the entrance to the middle meatus adhere to the mucus. Owing to the confluence of the secretion pathways from the entrance to the middle meatus with the pathways of the infundibulum and the frontal recess, these pathogens may be transported into the sinus where they may find ideal conditions for growth. If the self-healing capacity of the sinus mucosa or medical treatment is insufficient to clear the sinus, an acute or chronic recurring sinusitis develops.

The mechanism by which pathogens reach the maxillary sinus can be studied during maxillary sinuscopy. Thick viscous mucus can frequently be seen entering the maxillary sinus through accessory ostia in one or both of the nasal fontanelles (Fig. 2.34). Once this mucus has entered the maxillary sinus it is then transported upward along the natural pathways inside the sinus toward the maxillary sinus ostium from which it exits the sinus.

In some cases, in the infundibulum these thick secretions may reenter the maxillary sinus once again through an accessory ostium and the mucus may continue to circulate again and again in an endless circle. As long as the natural ostium is patent, this finding may not be significant. If, however, the maxillary ostium is blocked by disease (Fig. 2.35) or if nasal infection is present, this is one of the

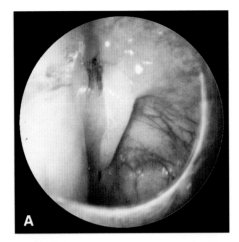

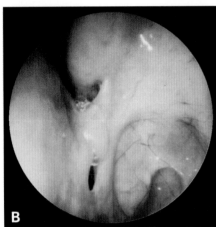

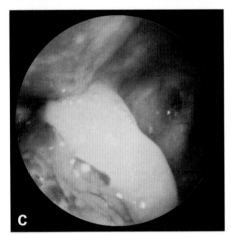

FIGURE 2.34 Viscous pathological mucus enters the maxillary sinus through an accessory ostium in a fontanelle (A) and following the natural mucociliary pathways, is transported toward the natural ostium where it leaves the sinus (B). In the infundibulum, the secretion reenters the maxillary sinus through the accessory ostium (C) and thus travels in a circle.

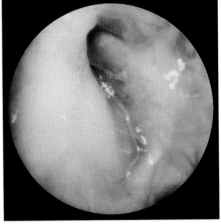

FIGURE 2.35 The natural ostium of this left maxillary sinus is blocked due to a prolapse of inflamed mucosa from the infundibulum.

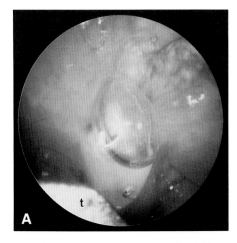

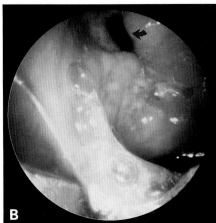

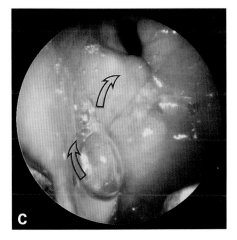

ways by which pathogens may be transported into the maxillary sinus from the nose. If the ostium is blocked, then the infected secretions cannot leave the sinus and maxillary sinusitis may result.

Sometimes during sinuscopy it is almost impossible to identify the maxillary sinus ostium, especially if the mucosa is swollen. When the patient performs the Valsalva maneuver (pinching his nose and blowing it), air usually bubbles into the maxillary sinus through its ostium thereby indicating its position. In many cases, when the patient attempts to blow his nose harder, he may force infected secretions back into the maxillary sinus from the ethmoidal prechambers. Figure 2.36 illustrates such a case. The maxillary ostium cannot be clearly identified. During the Valsalva maneuver some air bubbles indicate the position of the ostium. When the patient blew harder, viscous secretion was pressed back into the sinus where it slipped down to the sinus floor. After 2 to 3 minutes, the secretion was slowly transported toward the natural ostium, which it was unable to leave by because of its viscosity and the fact that the ostium was somewhat stenotic. There was anterior ethmoidal disease blocking the hiatus semilunaris. Every time the patient blew his nose, the secretion from the infundibulum and the ostial region was forced back into the maxillary sinus where it slipped to the floor and the cycle repeated. If in such a case, a secondary or superinfection occurs, then an acute maxillary sinusitis will result (Fig. 2.37).

FIGURE 2.36 A, Note the thick secretion blocking the maxillary sinus ostium. B, During the Valsalva maneuver, the mucus was forced back into the sinuses and slipped to the floor. C, This mucus was then transported back again toward the natural ostium as shown by the *arrows*. t = trocar sleeve.

FIGURE 2.37 Tomogram of the patient shown in Figure 2.36 indicated the need for maxillary sinuscopy on the right side. From the tomogram, it was not clear whether the disease in the right maxillary sinus was the result of mucosal swelling, secretion, cysts, or polyps. Note the disease in the middle meatus on both sides. At sinuscopy, the mucosa of the maxillary sinus appeared almost normal and the opacification seen in the radiograph was the result of retained highly viscous secretion. There was no indication for surgery to the maxillary sinus.

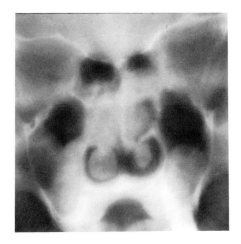

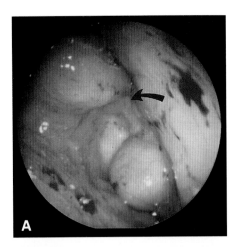

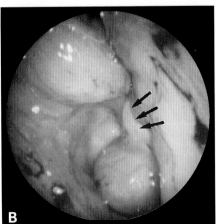

FIGURE 2.38 *A,* Note how the natural ostium of this right maxillary sinus seen after the evacuation of an empyema is totally blocked (*arrow*). *B,* When the patient performed the Valsalva maneuver, the pus was forced back out of the infundibulum into the sinus (*arrows*).

Figure 2.38 demonstrates such a case. An empyema and thickened secretion were removed from this maxillary sinus with an aspirator. The mucosa was edematously swollen and the ostium could not be identified. Air bubbles gave a tentative indication of where the ostium might be located. When the patient was asked to blow his nose, a stream of pus was pressed back into the maxillary sinus from out of the ethmoidal infundibulum. This depicts another mechanism by which pathogens can be transported back into the maxillary sinus via the natural ostium against the direction of mucociliary clearance.

Through the nasal valve, the major portion of the airstream is directed toward the entrance of the middle meatus and the head of the middle turbinate (Fig. 2.39). This is the area of greatest contact between the nasal mucosa and airborne irritants and pathogens. The secretion pathways of this area are such that particles deposited in this area can reach the larger sinuses. This appears to be the reason why the adenocarcinoma of the ethmoid that develops in hardwood woodworkers usually originates in the area of the anterior ethmoid, as this is where the carcinogens are deposited.

FIGURE 2.39 This is a schematic drawing of airflow through the nasal valve. Approximately 90 percent of the airflow is directed at the insertion and head of the middle turbinate and thus at the entrance of the middle meatus.

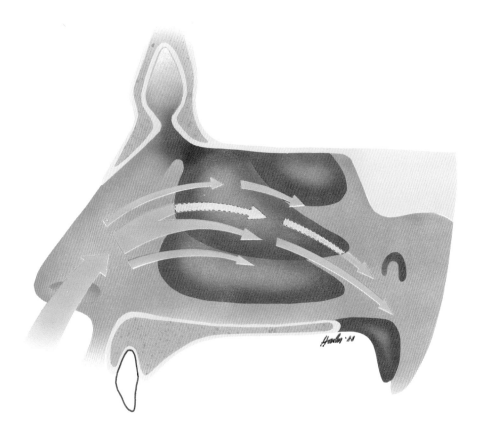

CONCLUSIONS

The frontal and maxillary sinuses are dependent sinuses, subordinate to their prechambers in the ethmoid and lateral nasal wall.

Drainage and ventilation of the larger sinuses are essential to the maintenance of normal function. The ventilation and drainage of the maxillary and the frontal sinuses pass through very narrow and complicated clefts before they reach the free middle meatus. These clefts, the ethmoidal infundibulum and the frontal recess respectively are parts of the anterior ethmoid. The larger sinuses therefore are dependent upon the health and proper functioning of these prechambers.

Those disorders that produce any additional stenosis of these very narrow key areas may result in the contact of opposing mucosal areas with mucus retention. If infected, smaller or larger areas of subacutely or chronically diseased mucosa may persist. Frequently these areas of intimate mucosal contact can be identified as the site of origin of polyps.

These areas may be clinically free of symptoms until the nasal cavity becomes infected. If the infection spreads into these key areas resulting in partial or complete obstruction of the prechambers or the ostia of the larger dependent sinuses, the clinical picture of an acute or chronically infected maxillary or frontal sinus follows. Despite the fact that the symptoms of infection in these larger sinuses are usually the clinically dominant symptoms, the underlying cause is generally not to be found in the larger sinuses themselves, but in the clefts of the anterior ethmoid in the lateral nasal wall.

Most of the inflammatory diseases of the frontal and maxillary sinuses are secondary diseases, i.e., rhinogenic and caused by infection within the nasal cavity and the anterior ethmoids. In more than 90 percent of our patients, the underlying cause could be identified as a lesion in the lateral nasal wall.

These were the most significant conclusions about the etiology and pathophysiology of sinusitis that resulted from Messerklinger's endoscopic studies of the early 1950s and 1960s. Messerklinger also noted that after a limited resection of disease with clearing of the key areas of the anterior ethmoid and reestablishment of drainage and ventilation via the natural pathways, even massive mucosal pathology in the dependent frontal and maxillary sinuses usually healed without direct intervention in these sinuses. Mucosal changes, which up to then had been regarded as "irreversible," returned to normal in a couple of weeks following what were usually minimal endoscopic procedures.

SUMMARY

1. Infections of the larger sinuses are usually rhinogenic, spreading from the nose through the compartments of the anterior ethmoid to the frontal and maxillary sinuses.

2. If sinusitis does not heal or recurs constantly, a focus of reinfection usually persists in one of the narrow clefts of the anterior ethmoids. These foci may interfere with nasal function and from these areas infection may spread locally to involve the prechambers and the larger sinuses.

3. This is true even for cases that were primarily of dentogenic, traumatic, or bloodborne origin, where the sinusitis kept recurring after the primary source of infection was cured.

4. The narrow or stenotic areas primarily involved are the ethmoidal infundibulum at the entrance to the maxillary sinus and the frontal recess at the entrance to the frontal sinus.

5. The frontal and maxillary sinuses are subordinate to the anterior ethmoid. They are ventilated and their mucus is drained into the nose via the anterior ethmoid. Their physiologic as well as pathologic condition is therefore dependent upon the health of the anterior ethmoid.

6. After the clearing of disease in the clefts of the anterior ethmoid and the reestablishment of ventilation and drainage via the physiologic routes, even massive changes in the dependent sinuses usually heal without the latter having been touched.

In order to establish a diagnosis and discover the underlying cause for a recurring chronic or sometimes an initial acute sinusitis, the area of the lateral nasal wall must be investigated for disease with the understanding that most of the pathology in the larger sinuses is secondary and reactive. The exceptions to these principles in our case material are rare. The primary exception to this rule is a true dentogenic sinusitis, which accounts for less than 2 percent of our patient population. Usually we see these patients only when their sinus problems persist and after dental treatment has cured the primary source of their disease. In these cases we usually find that a focus of infection has remained in one of the stenotic ethmoidal prechambers and requires further treatment.

Foreign bodies in a sinus, e.g., aberrant root-filling material, may provoke maxillary sinusitis by irritating the mucosa by its size, weight, and perhaps by its chemical composition, especially if the material is too large to be transported out of the ostium. Blood in one of the larger sinuses after trauma may become infected and thus lead to sinusitis. Mucus retention or cholesterol cysts may cause considerable problems and depending upon their location may affect the patency of the ostium, which in turn may promote sinusitis. Allergens may be deposited in one of the larger sinuses and cause a local reaction there. Usually, however, inhaled allergens are deposited at the entrance of the middle meatus and affect the ethmoidal clefts and prechambers of the maxillary and frontal sinuses first, so the principles mentioned above can be applied in these cases too.

Therefore we must concentrate our diagnostic efforts on those conditions that might produce stenosis of the narrow and delicate system of clefts and air cells of the middle nasal meatus and lateral nasal wall. We must also look for those factors, e.g., the many anatomic variations that may occur in these areas, which may interfere with normal nasal function and predispose a patient to recurring sinusitis.

Chapter 3

SPECIAL ENDOSCOPIC ANATOMY OF THE LATERAL NASAL WALL AND ETHMOIDAL SINUSES

Preface: A Historical Confusion

Names are needed that the learner may understand the mind of his master. But if he have many masters and they use the same name to denote different things he will become confused and the confusion will become the worse confounded if this name connotes something that is not there.

In anatomy especially must we be careful of our terms; for structure is the basis of all function and if we impart a wrong concept of the structure the student is like to go astray in his interpretation of its meaning.

In anatomy then a name must:

(1) Denote one thing only

(2) Be used by all to denote this thing.

Further, if it connotes any attribute:

(3) This attribute should always be present.

In the anatomy of the nose there are two terms which violate these principles, "infundibulum" and "hiatus semilunaris". It is of interest to note that neither is applied to a structure, but that each is used to designate an area or space. The word infundibulum is only applied to one space at a time; but is used by different authors to denote some four or five different regions of the nose. The term hiatus semilunaris is used either to denote a space beneath the middle turbinal, which space is a three dimensional cavity, or to denote the two dimensional area whereby this space opens into the middle meatus.

With neither is the space or area to which the term is given always of the shape that the name implies. Some of the parts to which the term infundibulum is applied are oft-times not like funnels, and whether it be a gap or a groove the hiatus semilunaris is only a demi-lune in once out of twice.*

*T. B. Layton, D.S.O., M.S. Prefatory letter, Catalogue of the Onodi Collection in the Museum of the Royal College of Surgeons of England, published for the Royal College of Surgeons of England by The Journal of Laryngology and Otology, London 1934.

As T. B. Layton demonstrated in 1934, in this "Prefatory letter to the catalogue of the Onodi collection" there was, and still is, considerable diversity and confusion among anatomists, rhinologists, and surgeons concerning the use and definition of the terms "hiatus semilunaris" and "infundibulum." In a historic review, Layton investigated the derivation of these two terms and showed that the term "hiatus semilunaris" goes back to Zuckerkandl. Zuckerkandl used the term "hiatus semilunaris" as we do today, to denote the *two-dimensional* cleft between the posterior margin of the uncinate process and the anterior surface of the ethmoid bulla. The *three-dimensional structure* that today we call the ethmoidal infundibulum was described by Zuckerkandl initially as a depression extending from the hiatus semilunaris anteriorly-inferiorly, and anterior-superiorly into the lateral nasal wall with the ostium of the maxillary sinus located on its floor posteriorly.

In 1870 Zuckerkandl attributed the origin of the term "infundibulum" to the Frenchman Boyer, even though Boyer did not actually describe the ethmoidal infundibulum, but rather the cleft that Killian later designated as the frontal recess, i.e., the prechamber to the frontal sinus in the ethmoid. This interpretation was later disputed. Zuckerkandl, who apparently misinterpreted Boyer, was not yet acquainted with the term "recessus frontalis." From the developmental point of view, the recessus frontalis refers to the anterior superior end of the definitive middle meatus, thus, a cleft in the anterior ethmoid.

Onodi referred to Killian and designated the recessus frontalis to be a space under the "operculum conchae mediae," i.e., the most superior and anterior part of the middle turbinate, containing the ostium of the frontal sinus superiorly. Grünwald, in his excellent anatomic studies, tried to clarify the anatomic nomenclature, even though he rejected the term "infundibulum." He coined the term "sinus lateralis" (synonyms: recessus suprabullaris, recessus bullaris, suprabullar cells, etc.), "hiatus semilunaris superior," "interlamellar cells," and others.

During subsequent years (1900 to 1925) a number of renowned authors coined terms for the clefts of the anterior ethmoid, although these designations were highly individualistic, with the result that three or more terms were used for the same structure. The infundibulum was described variously as frontal, maxillary, ethmoidal, or of the middle meatus. What was termed "recessus frontalis" by one author, was called the "ductus naso-frontalis" by another or the "recessus anterior meatus medii" by a third. The terms "hiatus semilunaris" and "ethmoid infundibulum" were used interchangeably and the recessus frontalis was called the "frontal infundibulum of the hiatus semilunaris." Although most early authors defined the hiatus semilunaris as a two-dimensional cleft, others described it as a three-dimensional space. This confusion continues even today.

The definitions of these clefts of the ethmoid were of limited significance for the radical surgery of the times, since during these procedures all bony septa of the ethmoid system were removed and the maxillary, frontal, and ethmoidal sinuses all were widely opened. It was only with the introduction of endoscopic microsurgery and endoscopic diagnosis that made a precise description and definition of these clefts of critical importance. It was also through the introduction of these new techniques that the key role of these clefts in the pathophysiology of the area was "rediscovered." Even today, there remains a problem in communication between different authors or surgical schools because the same structures are still referred to by different names.

The following description of the anatomy of the lateral nasal wall presents concepts and a nomenclature that is based upon the developmental history of the area and which has proven satisfactory for endoscopic diagnosis and therapy over several decades. We also wish to simplify the nomenclature confusion by presenting a unified system.

ETHMOID BONE

The ethmoid bone is a paired bony scaffold, which is held together by a horizontal plate (Fig. 3.1). This horizontal plate is the lamina cribrosa (cribriform plate), the name of which is derived from the multiple perforations that serve as conduits for the olfactory filaments. Between the two laminae cribrosae, there is anteriorly a superiorly pointing spur, the crista galli. Across from the crista medially along the entire length between the two laminae cribrosae and at right angles to them inferiorly is the perpendicular plate.

The initially confusing structure of the bony details, appropriately named the "ethmoidal labyrinth" that is attached to the lamina cribrosa makes up the bulk of the ethmoid. With some imagination, it can be likened to a box of matches, standing on one end. It can be further subdivided by bony septa and has the following characteristics.

The system has its own bony margins in only two directions. Laterally the lamina papyracea forms a thin bony divider from the orbit. In some cases, the lamina papyracea may have dehiscences, in which case the periosteum of the ethmoid and that of the orbit lie adjacent to each other. Such dehiscences provide a pathway in cases of disease in the ethmoid, through which the inflammatory process can spread to the orbit.

Medially, toward the nasal cavity, the ethmoid is bordered by the middle turbinate (the first ethmoidal turbinate) and by the superior turbinate (the second ethmoidal turbinate). Occasionally, there may also be an uppermost supreme turbinate (the third ethmoidal turbinate).

The ethmoid is open in all other directions. It can be "approached" anteriorly through the middle, superior, and if present, the supreme meatus. Posteriorly and inferiorly, the ethmoidal clefts open into the corresponding nasal passages and finally into the choanae. A part of the posterior cells of the posterior ethmoid borders the sphenoid sinus. This means that the anterior surface of the sphenoid constitutes the major component of the posterior wall of the posterior ethmoidal cells, which have no bony wall of their own even here.

The fact that the ethmoid *is open cranially* is extremely important. These open cells and clefts are effectively closed by the appropriate extensions of the frontal bone. The frontal bone extends with its foveolae ethmoidales across the top of the ethmoidal cells and clefts. The bony roof of the ethmoid is thus provided primarily by the frontal bone. This is of great significance for the behavior of fractures, the appearance of CSF fistulas and the possibility of iatrogenic injuries (see Chapters 11 and 13). The most anterior and superior clefts of the ethmoid assume a funnel shape, narrowing toward the frontal sinus ostium superiorly, because of the "superposition" of the frontal bone.

It should be obvious from the above description that the ethmoid can be intelligently described and understood only in relation to and embedded into the bony *and* connective tissue and mucous membrane structures in its immediate topographic vicinity.

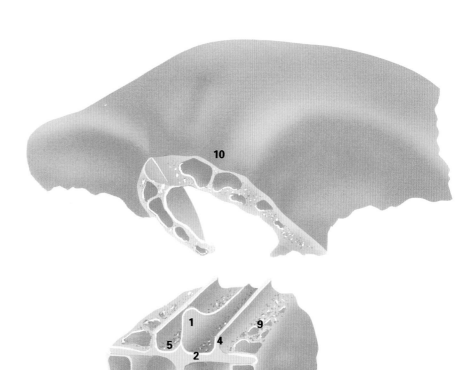

FIGURE 3.1   A schematic drawing of the ethmoid and frontal bones. 1 = crista galli; 2 = lamina cribrosa; 3 = septum nasi; 4 = lamina lateralis of lamina cribrosa; 5 = fossa olfactoria between 1, 2, and 4; 6 = lamina papyracea; 7 = concha media; 8 = concha superior; 9 = ethmoidal clefts and cells, open superiorly; and 10 = os frontale with foveolae ethmoidales.

BONY STRUCTURES OF THE LATERAL NASAL WALL

Embryology

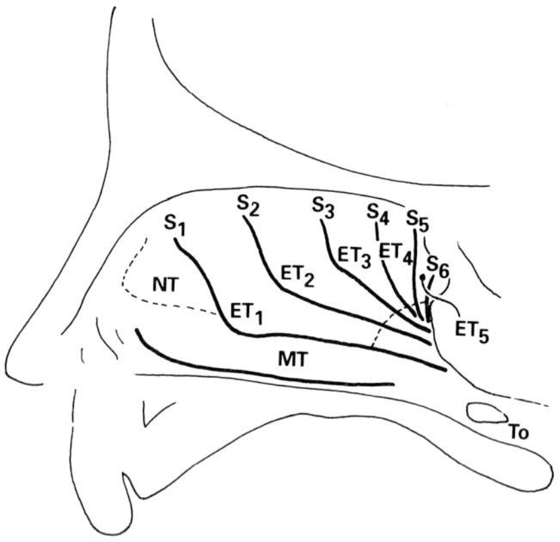

The complicated relationships of the lateral nasal wall can be better understood if the embryologic development of the turbinates and the ethmoid are first considered.

As shown by Zuckerkandl, Killian, Peter, and others, the ethmoidal turbinates originate from ridges in the lateral nasal wall of the fetus. In the 9th to 10th week, 6 major furrows develop that may be reduced by fusion to 3 or 4 (Fig. 3.2). These furrows are separated by ridges that have an anterior ascending portion (the ramus ascendens) and a posterior, inferior, and more horizontal portion (ramus descendens). In this, they begin to resemble the fully developed turbinates. Not all of these furrows and ridges persist during the further development of the fetus (Figs. 3.3 to 3.5). Entire ridges and furrows, or parts thereof, may fuse and disappear to finally result in the nasal turbinates of the adult.

FIGURE 3.2 A schematic drawing of the major turbinates and furrows in the human fetus in their original positional relationship. ET_1 to ET_5 = ethmoturbinals 1 to 5; MT = maxilloturbinal; NT = nasoturbinal; S_1 to S_6 = major furrows; and To = pharyngeal opening of the eustachian tube. (Modified from Killian and Peter.)

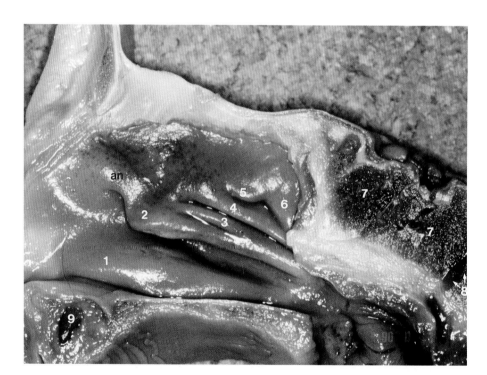

FIGURE 3.3 A view of the lateral nasal wall in a newborn. 1 = the inferior turbinate and 2 = the middle turbinate. The middle turbinate still shows the sharp crease at the transition from the descending part to the ascending part. This transition is almost at right angles. 3 = the longitudinal torus above a sagittal groove in the medial surface of the middle turbinate, which may occasionally persist in an adult. These probably originate from a fusion of the middle turbinate with an adjacent ethmoturbinal and/or an intermediate turbinate. 4 = the superior turbinate; 5 = the supreme turbinate; 6 = the probable remnants of the last ethmoturbinal in the sphenoethmoidal recess; 7 = the Bertini ossicles of the unpneumatized sphenoid; 8 = the spheno-occipital synchondrosis; 9 = a dental germ (upper incisor); and an = the agger nasi. (Dissection by Dr. Anderhuber, Graz.)

FIGURE 3.4 *A*, A coronal section through the lateral nasal wall, orbit, and maxilla of a newborn. The uncinate process can be seen clearly. Lateral to it the ethmoidal infundibulum can be seen. Note the small blister-like maxillary sinus, which has already developed from the infundibulum. 1 = uncinate process; 2 = maxillary sinus, developing (*arrows*) from the ethmoidal infundibulum; 3 = dental germ; cm = middle turbinate; ci = inferior turbinate; and s = septum. (Dissection by Dr. Anderhuber, Graz.) *B*, The development of the maxillary sinus from the ethmoidal infundibulum in the fetus and infant. This evolution explains why the ostium of the fully developed maxillary sinus is normally found on the floor of the infundibulum. i = ethmoidal infundibulum and s = septum. (Modified from Peter.)

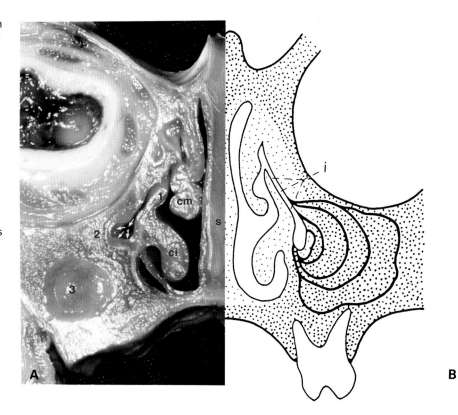

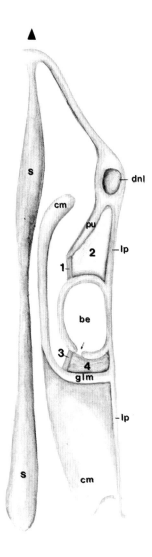

FIGURE 3.5 On this horizontal (axial) section through a right lateral nasal wall, the relationships of some of the compartments of the anterior ethmoid are shown in a simplified schematic form. The proportions of the individual parts are intentionally distorted and exaggerated. The purpose of this drawing is to illustrate the principles of the topographic relationships. The view is toward a lateral nasal wall from above. The section is almost parallel to the hard palate, just above the horizontal portion of the ground lamella of the middle turbinate. The ground lamella is thus shown in its ascending, middle portion. The ethmoidal bulla is attached laterally to the lamina papyracea. The uncinate process inserts into the lateral nasal wall, directly behind the nasolacrimal duct. One reaches the ethmoidal infundibulum through the inferior hiatus semilunaris. The sinus lateralis is reached through the superior hiatus semilunaris. Note that the ethmoidal bulla normally opens into the lateral sinus (*arrow*).

The position of the superior hiatus semilunaris is chosen somewhat arbitrarily. It can not be nearly as accurately shown anatomically as can the position of the inferior hiatus semilunaris. Depending on the shape and depth of the lateral sinus and on the distance between the middle turbinate and the ethmoidal bulla, the cleft of the superior hiatus semilunaris can be placed slightly more medially or laterally. To indicate this range of position, we have not shown the superior hiatus semilunaris precisely in the sagittal plane.

The *black triangle* indicates the tip of the nose; s = nasal septum; cm = concha media; glm = ground lamella; pu = uncinate process; dnl = nasolacrimal duct; lp = lamina papyracea; be = bulla ethmoidalis; 1 = inferior hiatus semilunaris; 2 = ethmoidal infundibulum; 3 = superior hiatus semilunaris; and 4 = sinus lateralis. (Drawing by M. Schröckenfuchs, M.D.)

The inferior turbinate, the maxilloturbinal, represents an individual bone that has nothing in common with the later, ethmoidal turbinates, the so-called ethmoturbinals. The first primary furrow of the lateral nasal wall is located between the first and second ethmoturbinals. The first ethmoturbinal regresses during later development and never develops into a permanent turbinate. The uncinate process must therefore be regarded as the descending portion of the first ethmoturbinal. The agger nasi is a remnant of the ascending portion of the first ethmoturbinal that is also referred to as the nasoturbinal.

The descending part of the first primary furrow, i.e., the depression between the first and second ethmoidal turbinate becomes the ethmoidal infundibulum. Its superiorly ascending part becomes the frontal recess. Continuing pneumatization of the frontal recess into the frontal bone finally results in the formation of the frontal sinus.

The roots of the confusing anatomy in the area of the frontal recess go back all the way to its embryologic development.

Additional furrows (frontal furrows) and the corresponding ridges (frontal ridges) between them evolve into elevations and depressions that ultimately may form anterior ethmoidal and infundibular cells. If these develop in the area of the frontal sinus ostium, their endoscopic differentiation may be very difficult and, in case of disease, impossible. Similar difficulties in differentiation may arise when not only the frontal recess, but also a frontal ethmoidal cell (bulla frontalis) develops simultaneously in the frontal bone. This can lead to the development of a "dual" frontal sinus. If they are similar in size, it may be impossible to determine which of these two is the true frontal sinus and which is the frontal ethmoidal cell.

The permanent middle turbinate develops from the second ethmoturbinal, the permanent superior turbinate develops from the third ethmoturbinal. The most superior (supreme) turbinate develops from the fusion of fourth and fifth ethmoturbinals. The permanent middle meatus and the hiatus semilunaris develop from the descending portion of the first primary furrow. The superior meatus develops from the second furrow and the uppermost meatus from the third primary furrow.

Looking at it from a developmental point of view, it becomes apparent that the bony structures of those formations on the medial wall of the ethmoid, known as the turbinates, are really only the ends of bony lamellae that traverse the entire ethmoid. They extend laterally to the lamina papyracea, superiorly to the lamina cribrosa and, between the ethmoidal foveolae, to the frontal bone.

If an attempt is made to reduce the ethmoidal labyrinth of an adult to the identifiable ground lamellae, the following picture emerges (Fig. 3.6).

The first, incompletely developed lamella is represented by the uncinate process. It may extend to the skull base and to the middle turbinate, but not necessarily. In its upper segment, it frequently turns laterally and extends to the lamina papyracea.

If the bulla lamella is intact and extends to the base of the skull, it separates the frontal recess from the more posteriorly located segments of the anterior ethmoid. If an intact closed bulla lamella extends far anteriorly, the frontal recess becomes very narrow. This lamella clearly has a decisive influence over the shape of the frontal recess. Pneumatization of the bulla lamella results in the formation of the ethmoidal bulla (the bulla ethmoidalis).

The third ground lamella corresponds to that of the middle turbinate. It is the most constant and complete lamella formation and separates the anterior and posterior ethmoidal labyrinths (see the section: Ground Lamella of the Middle Turbinate).

The fourth ground lamella is formed by the attachment of the superior turbinate, while the occasionally present, small supreme turbinate adds a fifth lamella.

The passages between these ground lamellae are designated as the interturbinal meatus.

FIGURE 3.6 This sagittal CT of a cadaver demonstrates the ground lamellae persisting in an adult. Note the hourglass-like contour of the floor of the frontal sinus, which narrows toward the frontal sinus ostium and widens again in the frontal recess (*dotted lines*). 1 = uncinate process; 2 = ethmoidal bulla; 3 = ground lamella of the middle turbinate; 4 = ground lamella of the superior turbinate; sf = sinus frontalis; osf = ostium sinus frontalis; osph = ostium sinus sphenoidalis; cm = concha media; and ci = concha inferior (the maxilloturbinal).

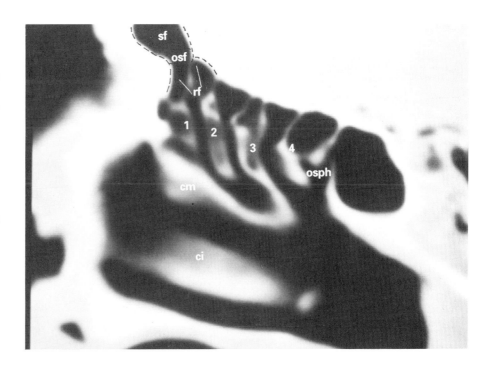

Further subdivision of the ethmoidal labyrinth results from the formation of more or less developed transverse septa in the interturbinal meatus. Occasionally there are only small incomplete ridges, but there may also be bony septa that divide the interturbinal meatus almost completely and form cells and cavities that communicate with the interturbinal meatus only through a small ostium.

This development of these transverse septa explains why, occasionally the ethmoidal infundibulum (as a remnant of the interturbinal meatus) may be further subdivided. In its most anterior part, this can lead to the development of recesses, as seen very clearly in the anatomic specimen in Figure 3.25. Initially these recesses are small, but they may become larger, so that we begin to refer to them as ''cells.'' These ''infundibular cells'' may complicate the anatomic situation, particularly in the passage from the uppermost part of the infundibulum to the frontal recess.

All this makes it clear that the number of cells in both the anterior and posterior ethmoidal labyrinth depends upon the development of the septa in the interturbinal meatus. In rare cases, if there are no septa at all, the ethmoidal labyrinth may consist of a single cell that corresponds to the original configuration of the interturbinal meatus.

Variations, disturbances, and anomalies in the formation of the ground lamellae and in the septation of the interturbinal meatus explain not only the variability in the number of cells in the anterior and posterior ethmoid, but also the variable ratio of the volume of these two areas. As is emphasized in the discussion of "Ground Lamella of the Middle Turbinate," the border between the anterior and posterior ethmoid may become severely obscured by invaginations of the cells. Posterior ethmoidal cells can displace the ground lamella far anteriorly and make it appear to lie within the anterior ethmoid. In contrast, anterior ethmoidal cells may in extreme cases extend to the anterior wall of the sphenoid sinus.

As Zuckerkandl, Hajek, and Killian have stated, the only certain point of reference for the topographic orientation of an ethmoidal cell is its ostium. Cells that open into the middle meatus belong to the anterior ethmoidal labyrinth and those that open into the superior meatus belong to the posterior ethmoidal labyrinth.

The expressions used occasionally in the past: "ethmoidal cells of the middle meatus" and "ethmoidal cells of the superior meatus" would be more accurate from a developmental and clinical perspective than the current designation of anterior and posterior ethmoidal sinuses. We want to avoid further confusion and thus refrain from suggesting changes in nomenclature. We retain the terms "anterior and posterior ethmoid," with the ground lamella of the middle turbinate as the border between them.

Uncinate Process

Looking at the lateral nasal wall of an anatomic preparation from the medial side, after resection of the vertical portion of the middle turbinate, two distinct bony structures can be seen (Fig. 3.7). These are the uncinate process and the ethmoidal bulla (bulla ethmoidalis).

The uncinate process is a thin, almost sagittally oriented bony leaflet that runs from an anterosuperior position posteroinferiorly. If one ignores the numerous fine bony spicules at its posterior free end and at its anteroinferior insertion, the uncinate process resembles a slightly bent hook or a boomerang. Its posterosuperior margin is sharp, concave, and lies largely parallel to the anterior surface of the ethmoidal bulla, which is located just behind it. The already mentioned, fine bony spicules at the posterior end of the uncinate process attach to the lamina perpendicularis of the palatine bone and inferiorly to the corresponding ethmoidal process of the inferior turbinate. The ascending, anterior convex margin of the uncinate process is in contact with the bony lateral nasal wall and can extend as far as the lacrimal bone. The uppermost segment of the uncinate process is no longer visible behind the insertion of the middle turbinate. This uppermost portion can extend to the base of the skull, or it may turn laterally (partially or completely) and insert into the lamina papyracea. It may also turn frontally and fuse with the insertion of the middle turbinate. There may be further divisions, inlet formation, or combinations of all of the above. A more detailed description is given as part of the discussion of the ethmoidal infundibulum.

In the bony skeleton, there are always defects between the uncinate process and the inferior turbinate that are covered with a dense connective tissue, which is a continuation of the periosteum, and by the mucous membranes. In the bony skeleton, these defects lead into the maxillary sinus, but should not be confused with its natural ostium. These are the structures that Zuckerkandl called the posterior and anterior nasal fontanelles. Since these fontanelles do not have a bony base, this part of the lateral nasal wall is known as its membranous area.

The concave, free posterior margin of the uncinate process is not fused with any other bony structure. Between it and the anterior surface of the bulla ethmoidalis, there is a sickle-shaped two-dimensional cleft, frequently only 1 to 2 mm wide, which Zuckerkandl called the hiatus semilunaris. Through it, the path leads anteriorly into a three-dimensional space lateral to the uncinate process, which is called the ethmoidal infundibulum.

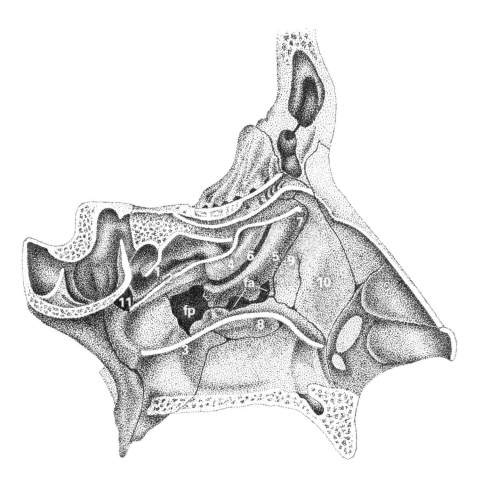

FIGURE 3.7   Bony structures of the lateral nasal wall. 1 = edge of resected superior turbinate; 2 = edge of resected middle turbinate; 3 = edge of resected inferior turbinate; 4 = ethmoidal bulla; 5 = uncinate process; 6 = hiatus semilunaris between the ethmoidal bulla and the uncinate process; 7 = agger nasi; 8 = inferior turbinate bone; 9 = lacrimal bone; 10 = processus frontalis of the maxilla; 11 = sphenopalatine foramen; fa = anterior (inferior) nasal fontanelle; and fp = posterior nasal fontanelle. (Modified from Pernkopf E. Atlas der topographischen und angewandten Anatomie des Menschen. 3rd Ed. Vol. 1. München: Urban & Schwarzenberg, 1987: Fig. 102.)

Ethmoidal Bulla and Lateral Sinus

The ethmoidal bulla is the most constant, and usually the largest air cell in the anterior ethmoid. It sits like a bleb, attached to the lamina papyracea, and is created by pneumatization of the bulla lamella. Occasionally, an ethmoidal bulla is poorly developed and it may even be totally absent. Zuckerkandl and Grünwald described a series in which the bulla lamella was not pneumatized in up to 40 percent of cases. For this reason, they named the bony bulge produced by the bulla lamella the "torus lateralis" (lateral bulge). In the series of ethmoids operated on by us, the incidence of minimal or no pneumatization was only 8 percent.

Depending upon the degree of its pneumatization, the bulla can fill the middle meatus like a balloon. Posteriorly, the ethmoidal bulla may fuse over a variable distance with the ground lamella of the middle turbinate. Superiorly, the bulla lamella can reach the roof of the ethmoid as a frontally oriented plate, and thus form the posterior wall of the frontal recess. This division may be vestigial or completely absent. In this case, there is a direct communication between the frontal recess and a pneumatized space located above and behind the bulla, the lateral sinus or sinus lateralis (Grünwald). Depending on its size, the lateral sinus is delimited by the roof of the ethmoidal bulla (below), the lamina papyracea (laterally), by the roof of the ethmoid (superiorly), and the middle turbinate (medially). Dorsally, the sinus lateralis can extend far posteriorly and inferiorly between the ethmoidal bulla and the ground lamella of the middle turbinate. If there is a complete separation of the sinus lateralis and the frontal recess because of a prominent bulla lamella, then the lateral sinus will open into the middle meatus only between the ethmoidal bulla and the middle turbinate. This cleft-like connection also has a sickle-shaped appearance in a specimen and was designated "hiatus semilunaris superior" by Grünwald.

Ground Lamella of the Middle Turbinate

The most anterior superior insertion of the middle turbinate is adjacent to the crista ethmoidalis of the maxilla, which produces an anterior bulge, known as the agger nasi. The posterior end of the middle turbinate is attached to the crista ethmoidalis of the perpendicular process of the palatine bone.

The intervening area of insertion of the middle turbinate can be divided into three parts (Fig. 3.8).

As can be seen clearly from the medial side, the anterior third of the middle turbinate is entirely vertical and inserts directly to the base of the skull, at the lateral edge of the lamina cribrosa. From here, the line of insertion turns laterally and reaches the lamina papyracea where it proceeds sharply inferiorly. When viewed from the medial side, we can see only the free vertical segment of the turbinate in this area. The bony plate of the ground lamella, located almost entirely in the frontal plane can be seen only after adequate dissection. In the last third of its insertion, the ground lamella of the middle turbinate takes a usually easily identifiable sharp turn toward the horizontal. This horizontal part of the ground lamella forms the roof of the posterior third of the middle meatus. The free medial vertical part of the turbinate tapers until the posterior end of the turbinate.

We can thus distinguish three sections of the insertion of the middle turbinate that lie in different planes.

The anterior third of the middle turbinate inserts vertically in a purely sagittal direction onto the lateral end of the lamina cribrosa, directly across from the lamina lateralis.

In the middle third, the middle turbinate is fixed to the lamina papyracea by its ground lamella, which here runs in an almost frontal plane.

In the posterior third, the now almost horizontal ground lamella forms the roof of the most posterior section of the middle meatus and is fixed to the lamina papyracea and/or to the medial wall of the maxillary sinus.

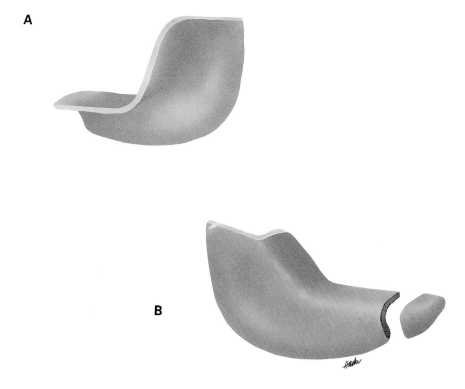

FIGURE 3.8 A schematic drawing of the ground lamella of the right middle turbinate. *A*, As seen from laterally and anteriorly. *B*, As seen from medially and posteriorly. The tip of the posterior turbinate end is shown "cut off" to demonstrate both the vertical and horizontal parts of the middle turbinate in the posterior third of the middle meatus. For details, see text.

This insertion along different planes: vertical, frontal, and horizontal, contributes significantly to the stability of the middle turbinate. It is therefore not surprising that after resection of the posterior two-thirds of the middle turbinate, as recommended by several surgical schools, the remainder of the anterior segment becomes unstable; it remains after all only fixed in one plane, namely the sagittovertical. Even in endoscopic procedures, for manipulations in the posterior ethmoid or sphenoid, perforations in the frontal course of the ground lamella of the middle turbinate should not be too sweeping, so that the stability of the entire structure is not compromised.

The middle section of the ground lamella is worthy of special consideration: this frontally situated attachment plate is not necessarily a smooth or level surface. Well pneumatized anterior ethmoidal cells can cause this plate to bulge dorsally and give it a posterosuperior orientation (Fig. 3.9). This is the case especially when the lateral sinus is fully developed. Under certain circumstances, such anterior ethmoidal cells can extend almost to the leading edge of the sphenoid sinus. Conversely, the cells of the posterior ethmoid can cause the midsection of the ground lamella to bulge anteriorly. Also, the superior nasal meatus can develop so far anteroinferiorly that it can either make the ground lamella of the middle turbinate bulge forward, or in some cases, grows into the bony lamella of the middle turbinate, producing a concha bullosa of the middle turbinate, which Grünwald described as "interlamellar cells."

In the presence of a number of the variations described above, it becomes readily apparent that the ground lamella of the middle turbinate can have an extremely variable appearance. In some cases, this may make identification intraoperatively, or by preoperative radiography, extremely difficult (see Chapter 7).

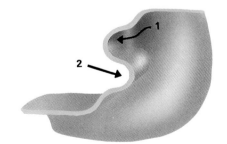

FIGURE 3.9 A schematic drawing of the ground lamella of the right middle turbinate as seen from laterally. Indentations of the ground lamella by anterior ethmoidal clefts (lateral sinus) (*1, arrow*) and by posterior ethmoidal cells (*2, arrow*) are demonstrated.

Posterior Ethmoid

The ground lamella of the middle turbinate is the border between the anterior and the posterior ethmoidal sinuses. All cells and clefts belonging to the posterior ethmoid open posteriorly and above the ground lamella in the superior (and occasionally the supreme) meatus. The number of cells and clefts that make up the posterior ethmoid varies between one and five. The volume of the posterior ethmoid depends largely on the structure and course of the ground lamella of the middle turbinate. The number of cells in the posterior ethmoid depends to a large extent upon whether the ground lamellae of the superior (and supreme) turbinate extend to the lamina papyracea and whether or not there are further subseptations present. Clinically this is of limited significance. The behavior of the most posterior cells of the posterior ethmoid, however, are of the greatest importance to the surgeon, since these can develop laterally along and even superiorly over the sphenoid sinus. This extensive development can extend so far that the most posterior point of a posterior ethmoidal cell can extend laterally 1.5 cm beyond the anterior wall of the sphenoid sinus. The sphenoid sinus may be bypassed to the same extent superiorly by ethmoidal cells. These cells, named after the Hungarian, Onodi cells, can stand in an intimate spatial relationship to the optic nerve (Fig. 3.10). The optic nerve may appear prominently on the lateral wall of

A

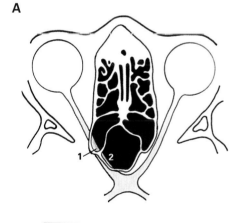

FIGURE 3.10 *A,* This schematic drawing shows the relationship of the optic nerve to the lateral wall of a posterior ethmoidal cell (Onodi cell, or sphenoethmoidal cell) and the sphenoid sinus. Note how far lateral to the anterior sphenoid sinus wall the Onodi cells may pneumatize. *B,* Detailed view. 1 = Optic nerve bulging into an Onodi cell; and 2 = Optic nerve bulging into the sphenoid sinus.

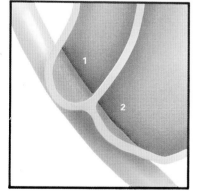

B

such an Onodi cell and may, in fact be surrounded by such cells. The internal carotid artery may also impinge on the lateral wall of the posterior ethmoidal cells (Fig. 3.11).

Under no circumstances should the surgeon assume that the anterior wall of the sphenoid sinus is always directly behind the most posterior point of the last posterior ethmoidal cell. In the presence of an Onodi cell the anterior wall of the sphenoid sinus does not run frontally, but occasionally in an acute angle from anteromedial to posterolateral.

If, during a surgical procedure, it becomes necessary to open the anterior wall of the sphenoid sinus by way of the anterior and posterior ethmoids, it is highly advisable to stay as far medially and inferiorly as possible. After perforation of the ground lamella, one should never make the mistake of dissecting posterolaterally along the lamina papyracea to seek the sphenoid sinus behind the last fringes of the Onodi cells. *This is the precise spot where the optic nerve is most likely to be injured.*

In endoscopic procedures, the Onodi cells frequently appear as pyramidal outgrowths of the posterior ethmoid in a posterolateral and/or superior direction, with the tip of the pyramid pointing posteriorly, away from the surgeon. This can be best seen with a 0 degree lens (see Fig. 3.11A).

The lamina papyracea forms the lateral wall of the posterior ethmoid. It is very thin in this area and may show dehiscences, through which orbital contents may prolapse into the posterior ethmoid (see Chapters 4 and 13). In some cases the yellow orbital fat can be identified shining through the lamina papyracea. In continuation of a prominent apex of the orbit, the bulge of the optic nerve can sometimes be seen on the lateral wall of the posterior ethmoid.

FIGURE 3.11 *A,* An Onodi cell in a right posterior ethmoid. Note the typically triangular or pyramid-shaped appearance with the tip of the pyramid pointing dorsolaterally. (0 degree lens, cadaveric dissection.) *B,* A schematic representation. 1 = optic nerve; 2 = carotid artery bulging into the posterior ethmoid and sphenoid sinus; 3 = resection line of the anterior wall of the sphenoid sinus; 4 = mucosa of the sphenoid sinus moved medially; 5 = lamina papyracea in the vicinity of the apex of the orbit; 6 = roof of the posterior ethmoid; 7 = spoon entering the sphenoid sinus; and 8 = pneumatized recess between 1 and 2.

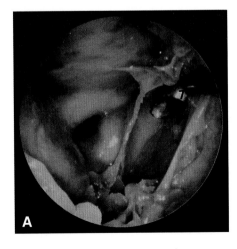

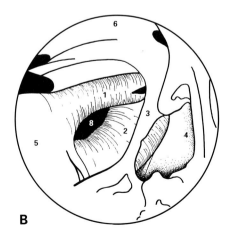

Sphenoid Sinus

The degree of pneumatization of the sphenoid sinus may vary considerably, even in the adult. As indicated in Chapter 4, if the cavities are symmetrical in the body of the sphenoid, they are divided sagittally by a septum almost exactly in the midline. In extreme cases, pneumatization may be so extensive that it involves not only the entire sphenoid, but also the clivus down to the foramen magnum, and extend laterally all the way to the foramen lacerum. Anteriorly, the pneumatization may involve the septum and anterolaterally the pneumatization may extend into the root of the pterygoid process. It is not uncommon for an extensively pneumatized sphenoid to be separated from the maxillary sinus only by a thin bony wall.

In cases of extensive pneumatization, the maxillary nerve (V_2) may bulge into the lateral wall of the sphenoid sinus. In extreme cases the nerve may be entirely surrounded by pneumatization. The canal of the vidian nerve may also bulge into this area from the floor of the sphenoid sinus (see Chapters 4 and 5).

The ostia of the sphenoid sinus are usually located in the sphenoethmoidal recess medial to the superior or supreme turbinate where they can usually be seen well with the endoscope. The shape of the ostia varies widely, they can be slit-like, oval, or round and there may be two ostia on one side. Occasionally it is possible to examine the interior of a sphenoid sinus through its natural ostium.

The floor of the sphenoid sinus is occasionally composed of ridges, covering the vidian nerve. The medial and the superior walls are usually smooth and the superior wall may balloon outward from pressure of the sella turcica (hypophysis).

Two bulges in the lateral wall of the sphenoid sinus are of considerable clinical significance. These are produced by the optic nerve and by the carotid artery. Depending on the degree of pneumatization, these two bulges may be barely noticeable or very obvious (Fig. 3.12). If the anterior clinoid process is also pneumatized, there may be a deep recess pointing laterally and superiorly between the optic nerve and the internal carotid artery.

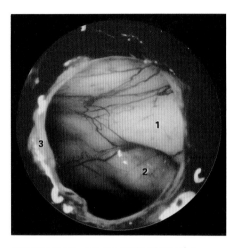

FIGURE 3.12 Endoscopic view of a normal left sphenoid sinus. (0 degree lens.) 1 = optic nerve; 2 = internal carotid artery; and 3 = margin of perforation in the anterior sphenoid wall.

The more superior bulge of the optic nerve extends from the front toward the back and usually gradually disappears toward the posterior wall. Occasionally the optic nerve runs along an arcuate course medially toward the optic chiasm, which then can be seen bulging into the lumen of the sphenoid sinus. The internal carotid artery lies adjacent to the sphenoid sinus during its passage through the cavernous sinus producing a variable bulge in the lateral wall of the sphenoid sinus (Figs. 3.12 to 3.14). In extreme cases this bulge may be prominent and the bulges of both carotid arteries may almost make contact in the midline. We have confirmed Kennedy's findings and found in almost 25 percent of all anatomic preparations that we examined, the bony canal covering the internal carotid artery was partially dehiscent (Fig. 3.14). In several cases, the artery was entirely uncovered (except by the periosteum and the mucosa of the sphenoid sinus) over an area of 10 × 6 mm. This incidence is greater than was previously suggested in the literature. A dehiscence of the bony wall covering the optic nerve was present in a lesser percentage of cases and in only 6 percent was the bone over the optic nerve "clinically dehiscent." By this we mean that the bone provided no resistance to a carefully probing instrument. In a patient, this could have caused damage to the nerve.

The direction of the septa that can be found in the sphenoid sinus is also important. It is not unusual to find additional septa along the median one, and occasionally two or three complete subseptations are encountered. Occasionally, the single septum may lie in an asymmetrical position and divide the sinus into one large and one small cavity. The course of the septum is not necessarily median. It frequently deviates laterally and superiorly in its posterior course and inserts into the bony bulges over the optic nerve or the internal carotid artery. Awareness of this is particularly important if the septa in a sphenoid sinus are scheduled to be perforated or removed (see Chapters 4 and 5).

As already mentioned previously, during the surgical procedure particular attention must be paid to the relationship of the sphenoid sinus to the cells of the posterior ethmoid. The most posterior point of an Onodi cell of the posterior ethmoid may extend up to 1.5 cm beyond the most anterior point of the anterior wall of the sphenoid sinus. This is particularly important if the sphenoid sinus is to be opened endoscopically, via the ethmoid. The anterior wall of the sphenoid sinus must never be sought behind the furthermost, "deepest," point of the posterior ethmoid. This is the precise point where the risk of injury to the optic nerve is the greatest (see Figs. 3.10 and 3.11).

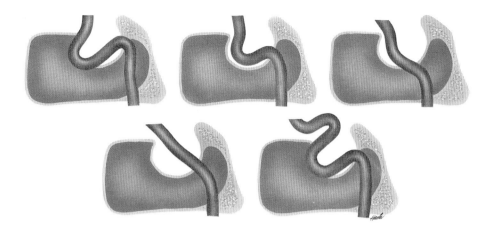

FIGURE 3.13 This schematic drawing shows variations in the course of the internal carotid artery in relation to the sphenoid sinus. The stretched versions are more likely to be encountered in younger individuals. These variations may result in different patterns of bulges of the internal carotid artery in the walls of the sphenoid sinus. (Modified from original by Dr. Kainz, Graz.)

FIGURE 3.14 A view into a left sphenoid sinus (cadaveric dissection). (0 degree lens.) 1 = optic nerve; 2 = bulge of the internal carotid artery with bone dehiscence in an area of 8 × 5 mm (*arrows*); and 3 = spoon (J-curette) palpating dehiscent carotid for demonstration.

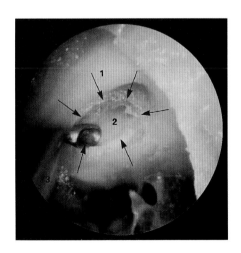

ROOF OF THE ETHMOID AND THE ANTERIOR ETHMOIDAL ARTERY

Since the ethmoid bone is open superiorly at least over its anterior two-thirds, the "roof" for these open cells and ethmoidal clefts is provided by the frontal bone. The frontal bone covers these open spaces with its foveolae ethmoidales. In this area, the frontal bone is both thicker and more dense than the adjacent bony ethmoid structures. This difference is greatest medially, in the transition from the thick bony lamellae of the frontal bone to the much thinner lamellae of the ethmoid. This occurs where the frontal bone abuts the primarily vertical lateral lamella of the lamina cribrosa (Fig. 3.1). This lateral lamella constitutes the lateral border of the olfactory fossa with the lamina cribrosa providing its floor. The lateral lamella of the lamina cribrosa is also the medial wall of the dome of the ethmoid. Its height and shape vary considerably from case to case. It is of critical clinical importance to remember that the highest point of the roof of the ethmoid may lie as much as 17 mm *above* the level of the lamina cribrosa.

Because the details of this segment of the roof of the ethmoid may vary so much in height, width, shape, and also from side to side, it is important that the surgeon have a thorough knowledge of the anatomy of this area prior to performing surgery. Only a good conventional or CT radiogram taken in the coronal plane can provide the surgeon with adequate information concerning a patient's individual conditions, variations, and potential hazards (Figs. 3.15 to 3.21).

The topographic relationships of the anterior ethmoidal artery are also of particular significance, since in its course from the orbit to the olfactory fossa, this vessel traverses three cavities: the orbit, the ethmoidal labyrinth, and the anterior cranial fossa. It is where the artery enters the anterior cranial fossa through the lateral lamella of the lamina cribrosa that the surgeon encounters the most critical area of the entire anterior ethmoid, and indeed of the entire anterior skull base. At this point, the lateral lamella of the lamina cribrosa presents the least resistance to a probing instrument, being only 1/10 as strong as the roof of the ethmoid.

FIGURE 3.15   This CT demonstrates the anatomy of the roof of the ethmoid. The thicker parts of the roof of the ethmoid, belonging to the frontal bone, can be distinguished from the thinner, medial wall of the ethmoid roof. The latter is formed by the lamina lateralis of the lamina cribrosa (*thin arrows* on the right side). Note on the left side, the anterior ethmoidal artery (*arrow*) passing through the lateral lamella of the cribriform plate. aea = anterior ethmoidal artery.

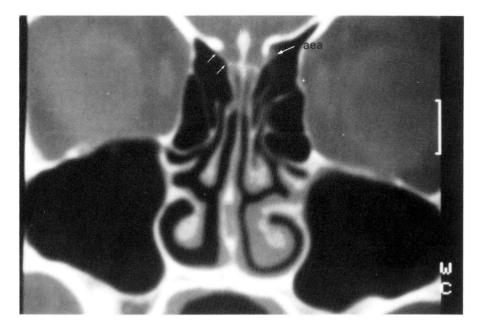

FIGURE 3.16   Note in this CT scan, the marked difference in the course of the roof of the ethmoid on the two sides. On the patient's right side the rise is a shallow slope. On the left side the rise is nearly vertical with an almost right angled turn into the roof of the ethmoid. Knowledge of these variations in the roof of the ethmoid preoperatively, is of the greatest clinical importance.

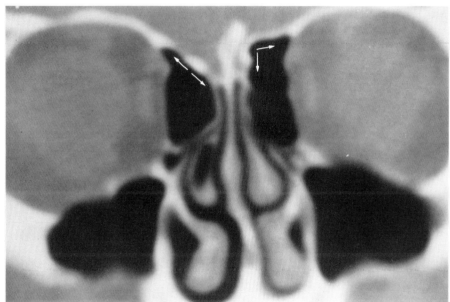

FIGURE 3.17   The low-lying roof of the ethmoid in an 8-year-old boy with cystic fibrosis. Note the distance between the lamina cribrosa and the roof of the orbit (*double arrow*). The *thin arrow* indicates lateral lamella of the lamina cribrosa.

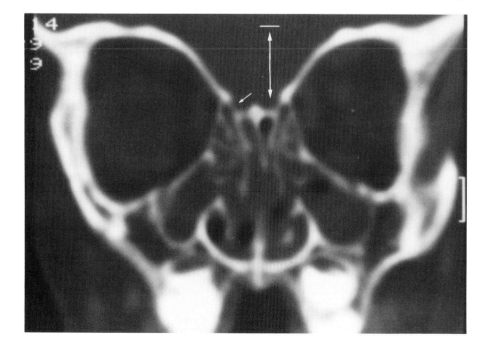

After its origin from the ophthalmic artery in the orbit, the anterior ethmoidal artery passes through the anterior ethmoidal foramen into the anterior ethmoid (Fig. 3.18). It crosses this structure surrounded only by a thin-walled bony channel (Fig. 3.19). In some cases, this ethmoidal canal is embedded in the roof of the ethmoid, particularly when this roof is low and rises only slightly above the level of the lamina cribrosa. In most cases, however, the canal is connected to the roof of the ethmoid by a bony mesentery, with an interspace of as much as 5 mm. The point of insertion of this ethmoidal canal, also known as orbitocranial canal, is usually directly behind the point where the roof of the ethmoid bends anterosuperiorly to form the posterior and superior border of the frontal recess. The first of the anterior ethmoidal cells reaching the lamina papyracea usually lies posterior to the canal. If there is no frontal sinus, the artery is usually located between the first and second of the ethmoidal cells that extend laterally to the lamina papyracea. In some texts these cells are referred to as the orbitoethmoidal cells. These points of reference can be seen only in an anatomic preparation, in the sagittal plane from the medial side. They are of little assistance in an endoscopic surgical procedure that must approach the roof of the ethmoid from the front and below.

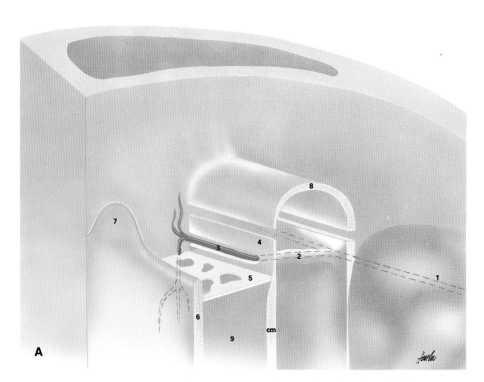

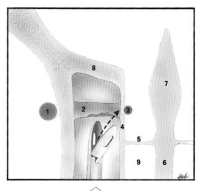

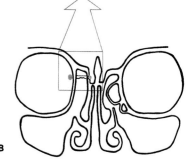

FIGURE 3.18 This is a schematic drawing of the course of the anterior ethmoidal artery. For details see text. The view is from medially behind and above toward the right anterior skull base. 1 = ophthalmic artery in the orbit; 2 = anterior ethmoidal artery in the bony canal traversing the ethmoid; 3 = anterior ethmoidal artery after penetration of the lateral lamella of the cribriform plate in the "ethmoidal sulcus"; 4 = lateral lamella of the cribriform plate; 5 = cribriform plate; 6 = septum nasi; 7 = crista galli; 8 = frontal bone (providing the roof for the ethmoid; and 9 = olfactory ridge of the common nasal meatus. B, An instrument is shown approaching the place of least resistance in the anterior skull base: the vicinity of the anterior ethmoidal artery in the ethmoidal sulcus.

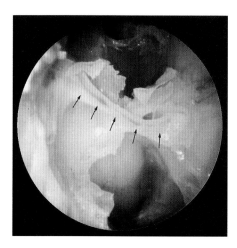

FIGURE 3.19 A left anterior ethmoid artery on its way from the orbit to the olfactory fossa through the ethmoid as seen with a 30 degree lens. The course of the artery in its bony canal (*arrows*) can be seen clearly, passing from right (the orbit) to left (the lateral lamella of the lamina cribrosa). The artery can be seen through the intact wall of its bony canal. The roof of the ethmoid can be seen behind the artery.

In order to identify the ethmoidal artery by this approach, it is best to follow the anterior surface of the ethmoidal bulla in the direction of the roof of the ethmoid. If this bulla lamella extends to the roof of the ethmoid, the ethmoidal artery can be found immediately adjacent to this point, usually 1 to 2 mm posteriorly. If the anterior bulla lamella does not extend to the roof of the ethmoid and if there is no complete bony separation between the frontal recess and the lateral sinus, the ethmoidal artery can be seen in the lateral sinus, depending on the configuration of this sinus. The artery can be seen here sometimes even during diagnostic endoscopy through a wide superior hiatus semilunaris, or more rarely from the frontal recess, without having to remove parts of the bulla.

After its occasionally sharply diagonal passage through the ethmoid, the anterior ethmoidal artery reaches the olfactory fossa in the anterior cranial fossa by breaking through the lateral lamella of the lamina cribrosa (the lateral wall of the olfactory fossa). At this point, the artery turns anteriorly in a groove of the lateral lamella, the so-called ethmoidal sulcus. At this point it gives off the anterior meningeal artery and finally reaches the nasal cavity through the cribroethmoidal foramen and the lamina cribrosa. In the nasal cavity it divides into the anterior nasal artery (superior, lateral, and medial branches), a posterior branch, and several small meningeal branches. This division into its terminal branches may take place before or after its passage through the lamina cribrosa.

The bony structures in the immediate vicinity of the anterior ethmoidal artery show remarkable variations in thickness. Those parts of the roof of the ethmoid formed by the frontal bone are much thicker and stronger than the lateral wall of the olfactory fossa formed by the lateral lamella of the lamina cribrosa (which equals the medial wall of the dome of the ethmoid). The frontal bone at the roof of the ethmoid has a mean thickness of 0.5 mm; the lateral lamina averages only 0.2 mm. In the ethmoidal sulcus, the thickness of the wall may be reduced to 0.05 mm. In this area, the bone is only 1/10 as strong as the roof of the ethmoid.

In a series of microdissections, Kainz established the length of the ethmoidal sulcus as 3 to 10 mm on the left and 3 to 16 mm on the right. The length of the ethmoidal canal varied from 4 to 13 mm on the left and from 5 to 15 mm on the right.

In 40 percent of cases, the canal showed bony dehiscences that resulted in a partially or completely open canal. The dehiscences were usually on the inferior side of the canal. There can also be significant differences between the two sides in the same person. On one side, the bony canal may be complete, whereas on the other side, the canal may be partially or completely open. In about 20 percent of the skulls that we studied, bony dehiscences were found on both sides.

The dura mater is attached only loosely to the skull. In the area of the olfactory fossa, however, the dura is not only thinner, but also firmly attached to the bone, particularly where the anterior ethmoidal artery, its branches, and the olfactory filaments pass through the lamina cribrosa. In the majority of cases, the anterior ethmoidal artery is intradural on its way through the olfactory fossa. In 29 of 40 skulls examined, the anterior ethmoidal artery was surrounded by dura from its entrance into the anterior ethmoidal canal all the way to the olfactory fossa. In eight cases, the artery entered the dura during its passage through the ethmoidal sulcus and in three cases, the artery was extradural along its entire course. In 75 percent of cases, the anterior ethmoidal artery was a single vessel on both sides. In 15 percent there were two branches and in one case, the anterior ethmoidal artery was absent. In this case, it was compensated for by an enlarged posterior ethmoidal artery. In this singular case, the anterior ethmoidal nerve was by itself in the orbitocranial canal. Apparently the ethmoidal arteries can compensate for each other's size, with a small anterior artery being accompanied by a larger posterior artery and vice versa.

Clinical and Surgical Significance

In all forms of endonasal surgery, and particularly after blunt cranial trauma, the anterior ethmoidal artery and its immediate surroundings represent the point of least resistance. Fractures, hemorrhages, dural lesions, and all their complications may occur in this area.

In blunt external trauma, fractures are most likely where there is a transition from thick bony segments to thinner ones. The lamina cribrosa and its lateral lamella are thus particularly prone to chip fractures. Because the dura is thin and attached firmly to the bone in this area, the anterior ethmoidal artery can be torn where it enters or leaves the olfactory fossa. Sharp bone fragments from the fracture site may puncture the dura and produce a persistent CSF fistula. The firm attachment of the dura may also lead to more extensive tears following blunt trauma also producing a CSF fistula.

Tiny lesions caused by bone splinters that are undetectable even by high-resolution CT may permit the entry of pathogens. In many cases, only repeated bouts of meningitis suggest the presence of such microlesions resulting from prior trauma that may have occurred years previously and to which the patient attached no importance. Using a fluorescein technique, these fistulae can usually be easily identified and located by endoscopy (see Chapter 11).

Since there may be dehiscences in the orbitocranial canal and also in the lamina cribrosa, the nasal mucosa may even normally lie in direct contact with the dura.

The olfactory filaments do not pass freely through the subarachnoid space, since they are surrounded by a perineurium from the olfactory bulb that corresponds to the leptomeninges. Subsequently they pass through the subdural space and the dura.

Injuries to the skull base with dural lesions and ensuing CSF fistulae in the area of the roof of the anterior ethmoid are most likely to occur when the lateral lamella of the lamina cribrosa is particularly high and thin. This also applies to direct (iatrogenic) trauma. The danger area is not the highest point of the roof of the ethmoid, which is formed by the frontal bone and is ten times as strong as the lateral lamella of the lamina cribrosa in the area of the ethmoidal sulcus. The weakest point of the entire anterior base of the skull is at the site where the anterior ethmoidal artery leaves the ethmoid and proceeds anteriorly in the ethmoidal sulcus of the olfactory fossa. The surgeon must exercise the greatest caution when working under the roof of the ethmoid in the vicinity of the anterior ethmoidal artery and when he turns his instrument medially. It is here that the extremely thin bone provides the least resistance to the instrument and that the danger of a perforation into the olfactory fossa and hence into the anterior cranial fossa is the greatest (see Fig. 3.18B).

The configuration of the olfactory fossa was classified into three types by Keros (Fig. 3.20). In Type I, the olfactory fossa is flat, the roof of the ethmoid is almost vertical and the lateral lamella of the lamina cribrosa is low. In Type II, the lateral lamella is higher, the course of the roof of the ethmoid is steeper and the olfactory fossa is deeper. In Type III, the roof of the ethmoid is considerably higher than the lamina cribrosa and the lateral lamella is particularly long and thin, and the olfactory fossa is correspondingly deep. Type III is the most dangerous one for the surgeon because of the likelihood of a perforation through the lateral lamella of the lamina cribrosa (see Figs. 3.18B and 3.20).

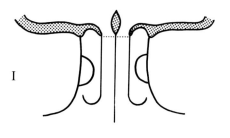

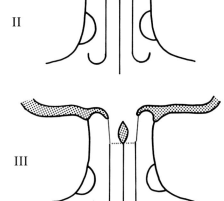

FIGURE 3.20 This schematic drawing shows the three different types of olfactory fossa according to Keros. Note the length increases of the lateral lamellae of the cribriform plate from Type I to Type III. (Modified from Dr. Kainz, Graz.)

Perforations through the lamina cribrosa proper can best be avoided by staying strictly lateral to the insertion of the middle turbinate. When manipulations at the roof of the ethmoid become necessary, every attempt should be made to identify the anterior ethmoidal artery (Fig. 3.21).

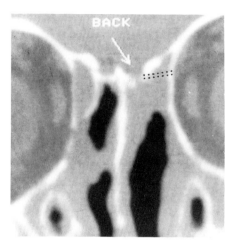

FIGURE 3.21   The CT of this patient shows an iatrogenic perforation of the roof of the ethmoid in the characteristic location (*arrow*), at the transition from the lateral lamella to the lamina cribrosa. The course of the anterior ethmoidal artery is indicated by a *dotted line*. In this patient, who had undergone microscopic endonasal surgery in another institution, the entire middle turbinate had been resected. This made anatomic orientation difficult and increased the risk of iatrogenic injury.

CLEFTS AND SPACES OF THE LATERAL NASAL WALL

The mucosal lining of the paranasal sinuses and the primary nasal cavity is not only functional, but also contributes to the shape of these areas. It is only after they are covered by mucous membrane, that the spaces and clefts of the ethmoid assume their definitive form and relationship to each other. Only after the maxillary sinus and the nasal passages are covered by mucous membrane do the fontanelles become membranous components of the lateral nasal wall, and the natural ostium of the maxillary sinus only assumes its definitive form after it is lined by mucosa.

The clefts and spaces of the lateral nasal wall that depend to a considerable degree on mucous membranes as far as their borders, extent, and pathophysiology are concerned are discussed.

Hiatus Semilunaris (the Inferior Hiatus Semilunaris of Grünwald)

The term "hiatus semilunaris" was coined by Zuckerkandl in 1880. He gave this name to the cleft *and* the depression that was seen from a medial view, between the free posterior margin of the uncinate process and the anterior surface of the ethmoidal bulla. In fact, this cleft does have the shape of a sickle, very much like a new moon.

In order to avoid the longstanding confusion in terminology between the hiatus semilunaris and the various interpretations of the different infundibula (ethmoidal, maxillary, frontal, etc.), in this text the term hiatus semilunaris is used to refer to a strictly *two-dimensional formation*, namely the sagittal cleft between the concave free posterior border of the uncinate process and the convex anterior surface of the ethmoidal bulla.

In this we largely follow Grünwald, even though he declined the term "ethmoidal infundibulum" and referred to the channel emerging from the hiatus semilunaris as the "canalis semilunaris." Our definition follows.

The hiatus semilunaris is a two-dimensional sagittally oriented formation that is bordered anteriorly by the concave posterior margin of the uncinate process and posteriorly by the convex anterior surface of the ethmoidal bulla. From the middle meatus, one can approach through this cleft, a channel or pocket directed anteroinferiorly and superolaterally, which is designated as the ethmoidal infundibulum (see below).

The hiatus semilunaris (inferior) is thus the "door" between the uncinate process and the ethmoidal bulla, through which we can reach the ethmoidal infundibulum.

This definition dispenses with all problems of interpretation, as to whether "hiatus semilunaris" means not only the cleft between the uncinate process and the ethmoidal bulla, but also the projection of this cleft, laterally as far as the lamina papyracea. In the latter case, a third dimension was attributed to the hiatus semilunaris in which the border to the true ethmoidal infundibulum was represented by an imaginary line, namely the projection of the free, posterior margin of the uncinate process onto the lamina papyracea. Such a definition lacks precision, particularly in the presence of pathologic processes and can give rise to further misunderstandings.

Grünwald describes a second hiatus semilunaris, the "superior hiatus semilunaris." By this he meant the cleft that appears between the ethmoidal bulla and the middle turbinate *when* there is a marked sinus lateralis posterior to and above the ethmoidal bulla. The hiatus semilunaris superior, then, is a sickle-shaped cleft, through which the lateral sinus can be probed, dorsomedial to the ethmoidal bulla. This cleft must not be mistaken for the turbinate sinus, which is a cleft in the sagittal plane, between a marked ethmoidal bulla and a laterally curved middle turbinate that surrounds the bulla. Analogously to the relationship between the hiatus semilunaris inferior and the ethmoidal bulla, one can say that the turbinate sinus proceeds superiorly and laterally through the hiatus semilunaris superior to the lateral sinus, if the latter is correspondingly pneumatized (Fig. 3.5).

Ethmoidal Infundibulum

In order to avoid any misunderstanding, in this text, the term "infundibulum" will only be used to refer to one specific space in the anterior ethmoid as described below. To clarify the topographic relationships, the term "infundibulum" is always accompanied by the adjective "ethmoidal."

The ethmoidal infundibulum is a cleft-like and, consequently, a three-dimensional space in the lateral wall of the nose, that belongs to the anterior ethmoid. The medial wall of this space is provided by the entire extent of the uncinate process and its mucosal covering. The major part of the lateral wall of the ethmoidal infundibulum is provided by the lamina papyracea of the orbit, with the frontal process of the maxilla and in rare cases the lacrimal bone providing the remainder of its lateral wall anterosuperiorly. The anterior border of the uncinate process fuses with these bones at a sharp angle and provides a bony connection inferiorly with the inferior turbinate. Bony defects in this area are covered by dense connective tissue (periosteum) and mucous membrane and are thus closed in the area of the anterior (inferior) nasal fontanelle. Through this line of attachment of the anterior margin of the uncinate process to the lateral nasal wall, the ethmoidal infundibulum ends blindly anteriorly in an acute angle. This is the reason the lumen of the ethmoidal infundibulum appears to be V-shaped in horizontal sections, e.g., an axial computed tomogram (Fig. 3.5).

If the middle turbinate is reflected superiorly in an anatomic preparation (Fig. 3.22), the structures previously described can be seen. The posterior free margin of the uncinate process, which bends slightly medially, is evident. The anterior insertion of the uncinate process can not be identified since it is covered by a layer of mucosa, which is continuous with that of the lateral nasal wall. Occasionally a slight depression (sulcus) can be seen along the line where the uncinate process arises from the lateral nasal wall.

Between the anterior wall of the ethmoidal bulla and the free posterior margin of the uncinate process, we find the two-dimensional hiatus semilunaris. Through this hiatus, anteriorly, inferiorly, and superiorly, a cleft-like hollow space, the ethmoidal infundibulum, which ends anteriorly in a sharp angle (corresponding to the line of attachment of the uncinate process) can be entered. Medially this space is bordered along its entire length by the uncinate process with its mucosal lining. The lateral wall is primarily composed of the lamina papyracea of the orbit, with some participation by the frontal process of the maxilla and by the lacrimal bone. Further inferiorly and posteriorly, the lateral wall of the ethmoidal infundibulum is formed by the mucosa-covered connective tissue components of the posterior fontanelle.

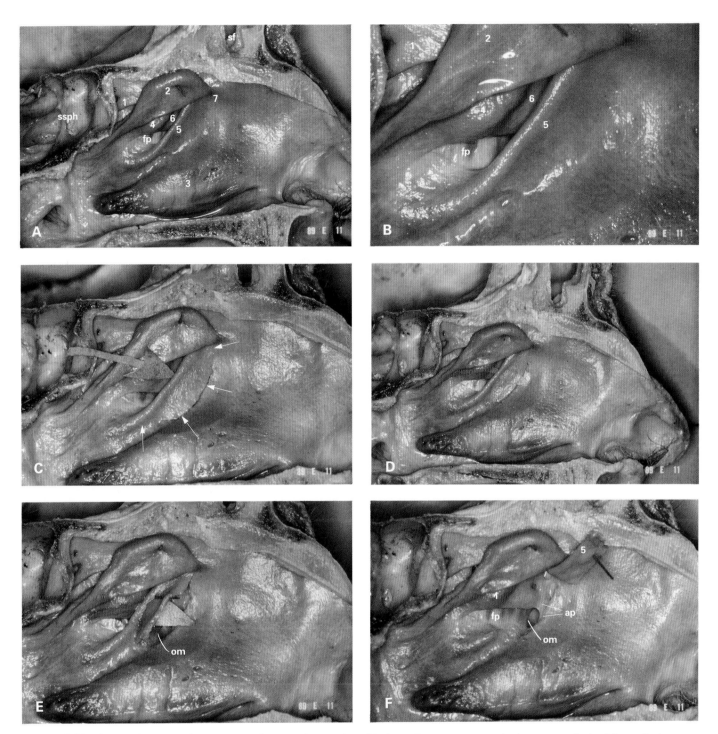

FIGURE 3.22 Cadaveric anatomic preparation displaying the ethmoidal infundibulum in the lateral nasal wall. The middle turbinate has been reflected superiorly for demonstration purposes. *A*, An overview. Key for *A* to *F*: 1 = superior turbinate; 2 = middle turbinate; 3 = inferior turbinate; 4 = ethmoidal bulla; 5 = uncinate process; 6 = hiatus semilunaris; 7 = agger nasi; sf = frontal sinus; ssph = sphenoid sinus; fp = posterior nasal fontanelle; om = maxillary sinus ostium; and fa = anterior nasal fontanelle. *B*, Close-up view. *C*, An incision through the anterior attachment of the uncinate process is indicated by the *small arrows*. The *red arrow* shows the way into the ethmoidal infundibulum. *D*, The *red arrow* is shown appearing through the anterior attachment of the uncinate process (out of the anterior blind end of the ethmoidal infundibulum. *E*, The hidden position of the maxillary sinus ostium at the floor of the middle to posterior third of the ethmoidal infundibulum is shown. *F*, The uncinate process has been resected inferiorly and folded upward, displaying the lateral wall of the ethmoidal infundibulum.

The posterior border of the ethmoidal infundibulum is, in large part, the anterior surface of the bulla ethmoidalis, from where the infundibulum opens into the middle meatus, through the hiatus semilunaris. Depending on the structure of the uncinate process, in its most superior portion the relationship of the ethmoidal infundibulum to the skull base and to the frontal recess may vary (see below).

A markedly schematic "cast" of the ethmoidal infundibulum would have the shape of an orange segment, with the difference that the wide side is posterior, i.e., on the concave side, and that the convex side is the thin edge. The hiatus semilunaris can be taken for the "door" through which the space of the ethmoidal infundibulum can be entered from the posteromedial side.

It must be noted that in most cases it is not possible to look into the maxillary ostium by looking into the middle meatus. The ostia seen with the endoscope in the middle meatus are almost always accessory ostia, either in the anterior or posterior fontanelle. Figure 3.22 shows clearly how the natural ostium of the maxillary sinus is hidden deep in the ethmoidal infundibulum.

Figure 3.22 demonstrates how a probe can be passed through the hiatus semilunaris behind the uncinate process and become visible again at the line of insertion of the latter. The insertion of the uncinate process was transected during the dissection. The part of the probe not visible is in the ethmoidal infundibulum. Only when the uncinate process is displaced medially and posteriorly (see Fig. 3.22F) can the position and size of the natural ostium of the maxillary sinus be seen. The natural ostium can usually be found at the transition from the middle to the posterior segment of the ethmoidal infundibulum, at its floor. These relationships become clear when the uncinate process is severed from its inferior insertion and folded superiorly (see Fig. 3.22F).

This preparation demonstrates the extent to which the natural ostium of the maxillary sinus and therefore the maxillary sinus itself depends on the condition of the ethmoidal infundibulum, the hiatus semilunaris, and adjacent middle meatus.

Inflammatory processes in any of these areas can easily extend to the adjacent areas and involve the hiatus semilunaris and the ethmoidal infundibulum. These areas may be partially or completely obstructed and thus produce poor ventilation and retention of secretions in the maxillary sinus.

Superiorly, the configuration of the ethmoidal infundibulum and therefore its relationship to the frontal recess depends largely on the behavior of the uncinate process. As shown in Figure 3.23 type I, if the uncinate process bends laterally in its uppermost portion and inserts on the lamina papyracea, the ethmoidal infundibulum is closed superiorly by a blind pouch called the recessus terminalis (terminal

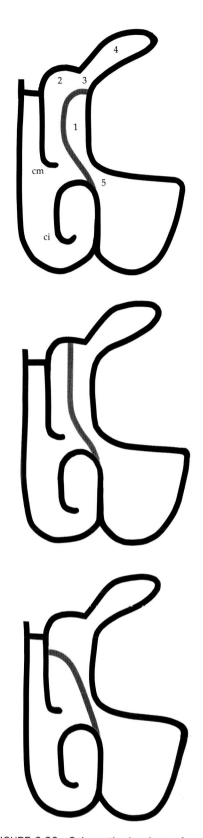

FIGURE 3.23 Schematic drawings of uncinate process variations (in *red*) show their impact on the relationship of the frontal recess and the ethmoidal infundibulum. 1 = ethmoidal infundibulum; 2 = frontal recess; 3 = frontal sinus ostium; 4 = frontal sinus; 5 = maxillary sinus ostium; cm = concha media; and ci = concha inferior.

recess). In this case the ethmoidal infundibulum and the frontal recess are separated from each other so that the frontal recess opens into the middle meatus medial to the ethmoidal infundibulum between the uncinate process and the middle turbinate. In this case the route of drainage and ventilation of the frontal sinus run medial to the ethmoidal infundibulum.

The uncinate process can also extend directly superiorly and either extend to the roof of the ethmoid or gradually taper anteriorly. It can also turn medially and fuse with the middle turbinate. In these last two situations, the frontal recess and the frontal sinus open directly into the ethmoidal infundibulum. This is, of course, also important in the spread of an inflammatory process.

If the ethmoidal infundibulum has a recessus terminalis, the separation from the frontal recess makes involvement of the latter less likely. Similarly, a disease in the frontal recess is not as likely to spread to the ethmoidal infundibulum and thus involve the maxillary sinus secondarily.

So far the structure of the ethmoidal infundibulum has been presented in a schematic form. In patients numerous variations occur.

The superior bony end of the uncinate process may be divided into three branches, which reach the base of the skull, the lamina papyracea, and the middle turbinate. Depending on the development of these branches, septations or inlets may be formed. The mucous membrane lining may produce partial or complete septation of the terminal recess and the formation of an additional blind pouch at the base of the skull or at the middle turbinate. In Figure 3.22 a number of clearly visible slight indentations can be seen in the lateral wall of the ethmoidal infundibulum when the uncinate process is deflected upward. These can expand anteriorly in varying numbers and sizes and evolve into the so-called infundibular cells. If such a cell develops anteriorly and superiorly, it can extend as far as the lacrimal bone and may be designated as an ethmolacrimal cell. The agger nasi may become pneumatized from the frontal recess (see below). Agger nasi cells also have the lacrimal bone as their lateral wall. If both forms of cells are present simultaneously, it may be difficult, if not impossible to sort them out accurately through the endoscope. This is particularly true when the cells are diseased.

Finally, the uncinate process itself may become pneumatized and cause a significant narrowing of the ethmoidal infundibulum and of the middle meatus.

Posteriorly, the ethmoidal infundibulum tapers parallel to the tapering of the uncinate process. Depending on the form of the uncinate process, the entire length of the ethmoidal infundibulum may reach 4 cm. Its greatest depth (measured vertically against the free posterior margin of the uncinate process) may be as much as 12 mm and its greatest width (free margin of the uncinate process to the lamina papyracea) 5 to 6 mm. The latter occurs primarily when the uncinate process is bent medially or is doubled back anteriorly.

It is important for the surgeon to remember that the ethmoidal infundibulum may be shallow, i.e., the uncinate process during its entire length is never further than 1 to 1.5 mm away from the lamina papyracea. The ethmoidal infundibulum may be practically atelectatic when anatomic variations (paradoxically bent middle meatus, concha bullosa) or pathologic processes compress the uncinate process against the lateral nasal wall.

Frontal Recess

The confusion surrounding the name and description of the space that, following Killian, we call the frontal recess of the anterior ethmoid is even greater than the multiplicity and variety of names that have been associated with the ethmoidal infundibulum. The frontal recess has been called: the "nasal part of the frontal sinus," the "frontal infundibulum," the "nasofrontal duct" and it has even been confused with the ethmoidal infundibulum.

We follow Killian's terminology for good reason: from a developmental point of view, this space is the superior continuation of the ascending branch of the first primary, interturbinal furrow, i.e., the groove between the first and second ethmoidal turbinates. The descending branch of this first furrow becomes the ethmoidal infundibulum and indicates the close topographic relationship between the two structures (see Fig. 3.22). The frontal sinus originates from the anterior pneumatization of the frontal recess into the frontal bone.

The term "nasofrontal duct" suggests a tubular bony structure that in reality exists only in the rarest of cases as a connecting link between the anterior ethmoid and the frontal sinus. The ostium of the frontal sinus is formed only when the frontal bone becomes attached to the ethmoid and when the immediate margins of the ostium of the frontal sinus are provided by parts of the ethmoid. If we examine a sagittal section of an anatomic preparation and look at the transition from the frontal sinus to the ethmoid (Fig. 3.24), we can see that the medial part of the floor of the frontal sinus is shaped like a funnel with the narrow end directed toward the ostium. Inferior to the ostium, in the area of the ethmoid there is another funnel-shaped space that widens from its narrowest point at the frontal ostium in a sagittal direction. In a sagittal section, therefore, there is an hourglass shaped structure, of which the narrowest part (the waist) is located at the frontal ostium and the lower part of which is designated as the frontal recess. Its limits, shape, and width are largely determined by the neighboring structures (Figs. 3.24 and 3.25).

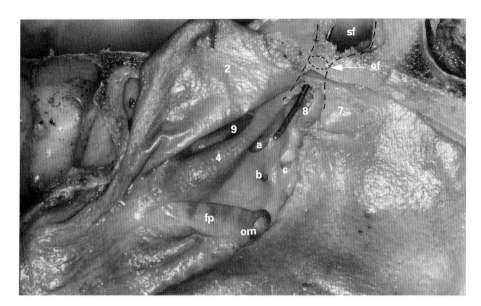

FIGURE 3.24 An anatomic preparation showing the frontal recess after total resection of the uncinate. A probe has been passed from the frontal sinus into the frontal recess. The *dotted line* demonstrates the hourglass shape of the frontal recess toward the sinus ostium and floor. A small agger nasi cell is present, pneumatized from the frontal recess. In this case, the frontal recess passes directly into the ethmoidal infundibulum (Figure 3.23 Type II and III). Also clearly visible in this case is the lateral sinus between the bulla and ground lamella of the middle turbinate. The semilunar cleft through which the lateral sinus can be entered from medially and inferiorly is the hiatus semilunaris superior. 2 = middle turbinate; 4 = ethmoidal bulla; 7 = agger nasi; 8 = frontal recess; 9 = lateral sinus; a, b, and c = indentations and small recesses in the lateral wall of the infundibulum; sf = frontal sinus; of = area of the frontal sinus ostium; fp = posterior nasal fontanelle; and om = maxillary sinus ostium.

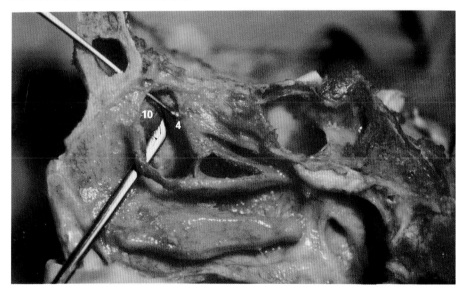

FIGURE 3.25 Here, the uncinate process forms a superior blind end (recessus terminalis), indicated by the hidden tip of the upbiting Blakesley forceps. The frontal recess opens medially of the infundibulum ethmoidale, between the uncinate process (laterally) and the middle turbinate (medially) (Probe). The middle turbinate has been fenestrated for demonstration; it contained two cells (concha bullosa), the anterior of which opened into the frontal recess, the posterior into the middle meatus. In both this and the previous figure, the ground lamella of the ethmoidal bulla reaches the skull base, thus somewhat narrowing the frontal recess and separating it from the lateral sinus. 4 = ethmoidal bulla and 10 = recessus terminalis.

Its medial border is almost always the lateral surface of the most anterior portion of the middle turbinate. It is only when the uncinate process is markedly bent medially and also fused with the insertion of the middle turbinate that its most anterior superior part serves in a small area as the medial wall of the recess. The lamina papyracea forms a large part of the lateral wall with its most anterosuperior extensions. If the ethmoidal infundibulum has a terminal recess, the uncinate process forms part of the lateral wall and also contributes to the floor of the frontal recess in its most anterior aspects. The roof is made up of those parts of the frontal bone that formed the roof of the ethmoid with their ethmoidal foveolae. On the way anteriorly they bend slightly superiorly from their horizontal orientation and ultimately become the posterior wall of the frontal sinus.

The frontal ostium is usually found in the most anterosuperior part of the frontal recess.

The posterior wall of the frontal recess can be a single entity, if the ground lamella of the ethmoidal bulla ascends in continuity and along its entire width to the roof of the ethmoid. In this case it separates the frontal recess from the lateral sinus, if there is one. Since the bulla lamella is frequently only incomplete and reaches the roof of the ethmoid only with some branches or not at all, the frontal recess may communicate widely posteriorly with a space above (and occasionally behind) the bulla ethmoidalis, namely the lateral sinus. Some rudimentary frontal ridges may exist in the frontal recess as smaller or larger, mostly transverse, bony ridges. They extend from the roof of the ethmoid in the frontal plane, downward and may also serve as the posterior wall of the frontal recess.

Depending on the position of the uncinate process, the frontal recess opens into the middle meatus, medial to the uncinate process and between this structure and the middle turbinate, or directly into the ethmoidal infundibulum. These latter arrangements are consistent with the developmental history of the area.

The state of the bulla lamella can affect the configuration of the frontal recess to a great extent. If it extends far forward and if the bulla is well developed, the frontal recess is narrowed. If there is additionally, marked pneumatization of the agger nasi and there are also additional frontal ethmoidal cells, the frontal recess may be narrowed to a small passage or to a tubular lumen. It is this situation that must have given rise to the term ''nasofrontal duct.'' But even if there is such a tubular configuration, it must be remembered, that this is *not* an independent bony structure, but a recess between other, independent bony structures (Fig. 3.26).

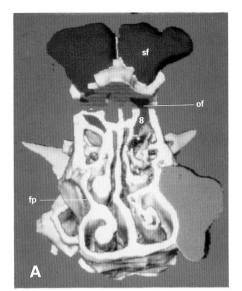
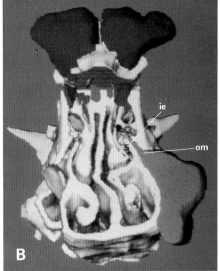
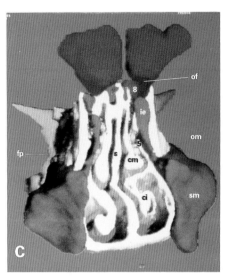

FIGURE 3.26 *A* to *C,* Three-dimensional computed tomographic reconstruction of the anterior ethmoid depicting the relationship of the frontal recess and ethmoidal infundibulum. Air in the frontal sinus and recess is shown as *purple*; air in the maxillary sinus and ethmoidal infundibulum is shown as *brown.* 5 = uncinate process; 8 = frontal recess; sf = frontal sinus; of = frontal sinus ostium; fp = posterior nasal fontanelle; ie = ethmoidal infundibulum; om = maxillary sinus ostium ; s = septum; cm = concha media; ci = concha inferior; and sm = maxillary sinus. (Courtesy of SJ Zinreich and DW Kennedy, Baltimore, MD)

The anatomic situation can be further complicated by the fact that most anterior ethmoidal cells develop from the frontal recess. Thus the pneumatization of the agger nasi may begin here. The middle turbinate can also become pneumatized from this source. Cells develop (not uncommonly) into the frontal bone, alongside the frontal sinus. These were called "the bulla frontalis" by Zuckerkandl. This variation may range from a bare suggestion of a bulge of the frontal recess into the floor of the frontal sinus to the formation of two or more approximately equally large cells on one side of the frontal bone. All these cells open into the frontal recess. In some cases it may become impossible to determine which of the cells is the true frontal sinus and which is the bulla frontalis.

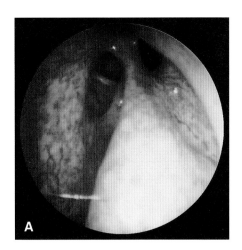

It therefore makes no sense from the perspective of the endoscopic diagnostician or surgeon to try to give a name or anatomic-topographic designation to every recess or inlet that can be seen with a 30 or 70 degree lens under the insertion of the middle turbinate (Fig. 3.27). Yet this attempt is made all the time. The subjective criteria used in the discussion of every cell, inlet, or recess vary enormously. The relationships of the uncinate process are too uncertain, particularly when there are pathologic mucous membrane changes or polyps present, and can only be really identified following careful

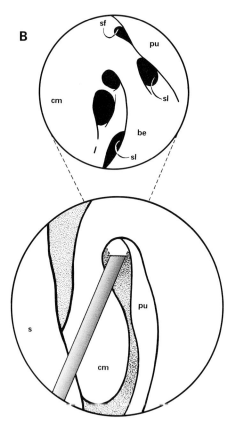

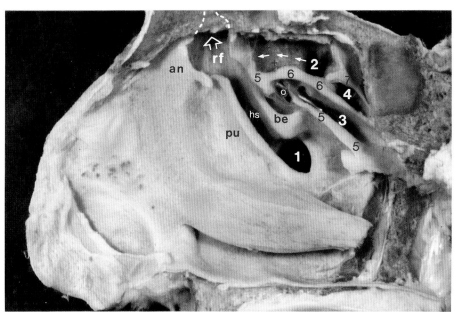

FIGURE 3.27 A, Endoscopic view into a frontal recess on a left side. (30 degree lens). B, Schematic diagram of the approach to the frontal recess and the view through the endoscope seen in A. sf = frontal sinus; sl = lateral sinus; pu = uncinate process; be = ethmoidal bulla; cm = concha media; and s = septum.

FIGURE 3.28 A dissection of a right lateral nasal wall, showing the frontal recess opening directly into the ethmoidal infundibulum, lateral to the uncinate process. The *outlined arrow* points to the ostium of the frontal sinus. The *dotted lines* indicate the cranial contour of the frontal recess as far as the ostium of the frontal sinus, which lies just at the edge of the illustration. A small cell has developed from the frontal recess into the agger nasi. The medial wall of the sinus lateralis (+) corresponds to the ground lamella of the middle turbinate, bulging far posteriorly. This posterior bulge was caused by a well developed sinus lateralis. During the dissection, it was opened from the medial side (*o*) and a sound was placed into the superior meatus from the sinus lateralis through a dehiscence in the ground lamella. 1 = large accessory ostium in the posterior fontanelle; 2 = posterior ethmoidal cell, extending anteriorly, medial to the sinus lateralis (*white arrows*); 3 = superior meatus; 4 = supreme meatus; 5 = line of resection of the middle turbinate; 6 = superior turbinate (lower margin of the resection: a view into the posterior ethmoid is possible through the window, 2); 7 = supreme turbinate; an = agger nasi; rf = frontal recess; hs = hiatus semilunaris (inferior); be = ethmoidal bulla; and pu = uncinate process. (Courtesy of Prof. Messerklinger, Graz.)

surgical dissection (Fig. 3.28). It is rare, and happens only when the access is very broad, that a direct view into the frontal sinus can be obtained and that this sinus can be differentiated from extensive frontal cell formation with supraorbital extension. Without a good CT scan (see Fig. 3.26), the various access routes to the frontal sinus can be identified endoscopically only in the ideal case and when there is no pathology in the ethmoid. In cases of disease, probability and clinical experience may occasionally allow more or less accurate conclusions, but absolute certainty can be obtained only after careful surgical dissection.

Sinus Lateralis (Lateral Sinus)

The space designated by Grünwald as the sinus lateralis is not a constant feature. When extensively pneumatized, it may extend above and beyond the ethmoidal bulla. Its borders include the lamina papyracea laterally, the roof of the ethmoid superiorly, the ground lamella of the middle turbinate posteriorly, and anteriorly and inferiorly, the roof and posterior wall of the ethmoidal bulla. When the sinus lateralis is well pneumatized, the ethmoidal bulla usually opens into it.

If the ground lamella of the ethmoidal bulla extends only partially or not at all to the roof of the ethmoid, the sinus lateralis may continue anteriorly into the frontal recess. The sinus lateralis can be reached through the superior hiatus semilunaris, medially between the ethmoidal bulla and the middle turbinate. This space, also termed "recessus suprabullaris" by Hajek, is usually referred to in the French literature as a suprabullar cell (susbullar cell—Mouret). We do not consider the term "cell" as a particularly good one for this space, since it is really only a cleft between the roof of the ethmoid, ground lamella, and bulla and has only a surface communication with the middle meatus through the hiatus semilunaris and anteriorly with the frontal recess.

This also demonstrates one of the primary problems in the nomenclature of the ethmoid area. Even the smallest inlets or depressions were repeatedly designated as independent "cells," particularly in the area of the frontal recess and were given different names by different authors. This makes any comparison extremely difficult since practically nobody gives or uses the same term for the same structure. We wish to emphasize again that we do not see any useful purpose in further subclassifying all the clefts and spaces that originate in the frontal recess or open into it. All the possible variations can be derived from the indicated interrelationships between the uncinate process and the ethmoidal bulla and the bulla lamella and the sinus lateralis.

Chapter 4

RADIOLOGY

W. Kopp, M.D.* and H. Stammberger, M.D.

There are four different imaging techniques available for the evaluation of the paranasal sinuses:

1. General (plain film) sinus radiographs,
2. Conventional tomography,
3. Computed tomography (CT scan), and
4. Magnetic resonance imaging (MRI).

CONVENTIONAL SINUS X-RAY TECHNIQUES

Routine or plain sinus X ray films are usually taken in four different projections:

1. Caldwell's view,
2. Water's view,
3. lateral view, and
4. axial view.

In plain radiographs, all radiodense structures located between the X-ray tube and the film overlie each other and are thus all projected onto the film. By choosing various projection angles, this "overlay" effect can be reduced or (at least) minimized.

* Department of Radiology, University School of Medicine, Graz, Austria.

This technique unfortunately allows only an evaluation of the larger paranasal sinuses. The delicate bony structures and the mucosal changes in the area of the ethmoid and especially of the lateral nasal wall cannot be adequately visualized (Fig. 4.1). Because the endoscopic surgeon is not as concerned with the secondary changes in the frontal and maxillary sinuses, but instead is interested primarily in the details and extent of the changes in the prechambers to these larger sinuses and the structures of the adjacent lateral nasal wall, more specialized radiologic techniques must be used to demonstrate more accurately the anatomic and pathologic changes affecting these areas (Fig. 4.2).

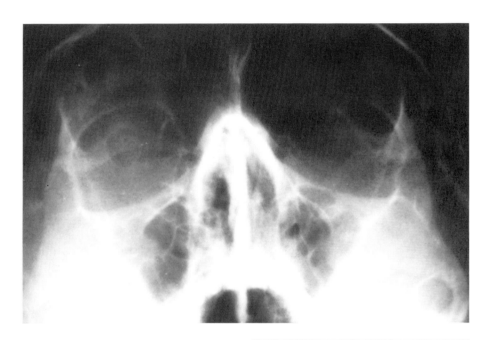

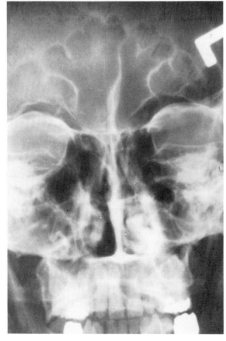

FIGURE 4.1 Routine plain radiographs of the paranasal sinuses. While this type of X-ray survey is suitable for identifying the presence or absence of gross disease in the ethmoid air cells and major paranasal sinuses, plain films are not accurate enough for the delineation of the under-lying anatomic variations.

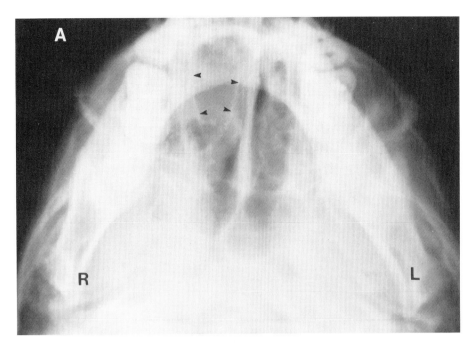

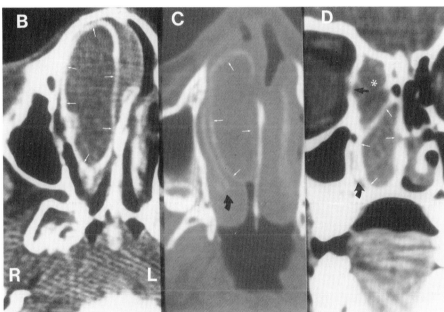

FIGURE 4.2 These are radiographs of an 8-year-old boy who presented with acute right orbital cellulitis caused by mucoceles in a giant concha bullosa and in the ipsilateral ethmoid sinus. *A*, This submentovertical plain radiograph demonstrates an opacification of the right ethmoid sinus (*R*). The bony perimeter of the large radiopaque concha bullosa is identified (*arrow heads*). In the axial (*B, C*) and coronal (*D*) CT sections, the unusually large concha bullosa of the right middle turbinate can be seen clearly. The outline of the concha bullosa is indicated (*white arrows*). The interior of the concha bullosa contains a mucocele. Note in *C* and *D* how the inferior turbinate is displaced laterally (*curved black arrow*). *D*, In the coronal section, a second mucocele (*asterisk*) can be seen in the anterior ethmoid. This anterior ethmoid mucocele has already eroded through a circumscribed area of the lamina papyracea (*straight black arrow*). (Courtesy of SJ Zinreich and DW Kennedy, Baltimore.)

CONVENTIONAL TOMOGRAPHY

Tomography allows details in selected planes of the body to be accentuated by blurring structures anterior and posterior to the plane of the picture. In a plain radiograph, these blurred structures would be superimposed on the area of interest. This blurring effect is obtained by moving two of the three components required for conventional plain radiography (the X-ray tube, the patient, and the X-ray film) while the third component remains stationary (Fig. 4.3). In conventional tomography, the X-ray tube and film usually move while the patient remains immobile. The movements of these two components are coordinated so that the details of the chosen plane are always projected on to the same area of the X-ray film and are consequently "in focus." In contrast to computed tomography, which actually selects single individual planes to project, conventional tomography projects all of the planes onto the film, with the selected plane being accentuated because it is the only plane that is truly in focus on the film.

Those structures anterior or posterior to this plane, depending on their density, size, structure, and distance, are depicted as a blurred shadow. The summation of these blurred shadows results in an almost unstructured background against which the structures of the plane in focus are clearly contrasted.

The plane of examination can be changed by moving the patient away from or towards the fixed rotation point. A definite slice thickness such as that available with computed tomography cannot be obtained with conventional tomography because the blurring effect increases continuously as the distance from the plane of investigation increases. The slice thickness that can be obtained with conventional tomography depends primarily upon the rotation angle. The greater the extent of the movement of the X-ray tube and the film, the thinner the slice will be.

There are two major types of tomography that vary according to the type of blurring.

Linear Tomography (Linear Blurring)

In linear (rectilinear) tomography, the X-ray tube and the film move parallel to the plane of investigation (Fig. 4.3A and B). This technique is not suitable for examination of the paranasal sinuses because the blurring effect masks the details of the ethmoidal structures and thus provides only limited information about the areas of greatest interest to the endoscopic surgeon.

There are several different types of multidirectional (pluridirectional) tomography available (Fig. 4.3 C and D). The difference between these types and the rectilinear types is related to the type of movement that can be produced by the equipment including: circular, elliptical, spiral, and hypocycloidal. Multidirectional tomography can provide excellent pictures and very detailed information about the ethmoid sinuses. The techniques of endoscopic diagnosis of sinus disease and functional endoscopic sinus surgery were developed using hypocycloidal polytomograms.

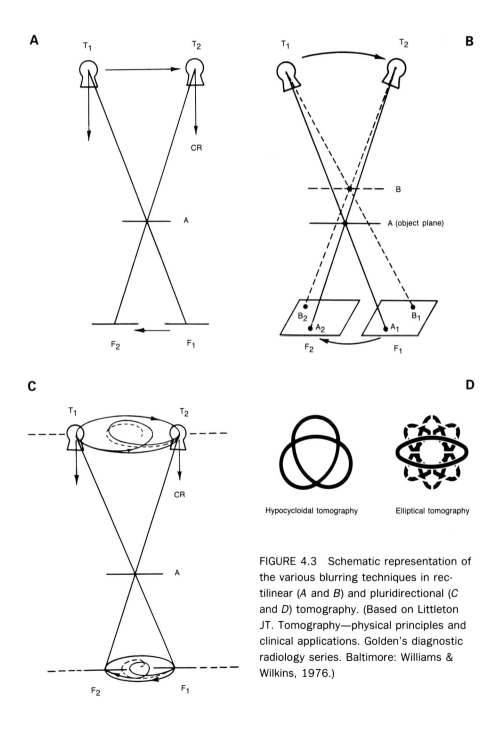

FIGURE 4.3 Schematic representation of the various blurring techniques in rectilinear (*A* and *B*) and pluridirectional (*C* and *D*) tomography. (Based on Littleton JT. Tomography—physical principles and clinical applications. Golden's diagnostic radiology series. Baltimore: Williams & Wilkins, 1976.)

Technique of Conventional Tomography

The sinuses can be tomogrammed in the frontal (coronal), lateral, and axial planes. The frontal or coronal plane is the best plane for endoscopic purposes as it corresponds to the way in which the structures present to the surgeon as he approaches the lateral nasal wall with the endoscope. In addition, the frontal plane allows the best comparison between the two sides of those structures of prime interest, i.e., the ethmoidal infundibulum, the frontal recess, the uncinate process, and the ground lamella because these structures are primarily located in the coronal plane. The preferred plane of investigation is vertical to the infraorbitomeatal (IOM) line. Tomographic X-ray films are taken at 5-mm intervals from the frontal to the sphenoid sinus (Table 4.1).

Slice Thickness

The thickness of the slice can be varied. However, for the anterior ethmoid, the slice should never be more than 5 mm thick so that no pathologic or anatomic changes are missed.

Positioning of the Patient

The patient should lie horizontally on his back (supine) with the legs being supported behind the knees or prone. The head must not be hyperextended and it should be fixed to avoid blurring artifacts from involuntary movements. It is important to place water sacks against the dorsolateral neck area to compensate for the X-ray density (Fig. 4.4).

The exposure time depends upon the technical requirements of the equipment and may also vary from patient to patient. For these reasons, the exposure time must be individually chosen.

TABLE 4.1 Parameters for Multidirectional Tomography

Patient position: supine (or prone), head fixed
Investigation plane: frontal preferred
Slice thickness: 5 mm
Area to be studied: from frontal to sphenoid sinus
Technique: multidirectional (hypocycloidal preferred)
Special hints: water sacks should be applied to the neck for density compensation

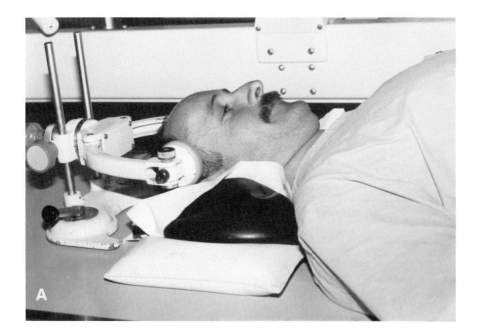

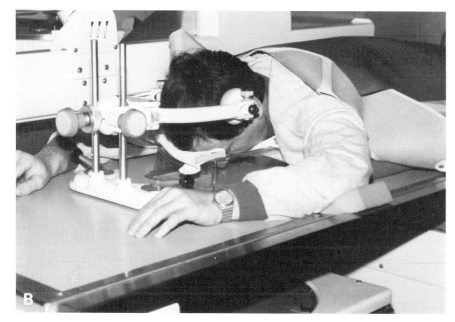

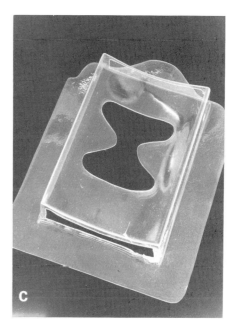

FIGURE 4.4 *A*, The supine position used for polycyclic, conventional tomography. The head is fixed in a special head holder. Note the water sacks placed on each side of the nape of the neck to equalize the density. *B*, The prone position for conventional tomography. In this position, the dose of radiation to the lens of the eye is significantly reduced. The patient's head rests in a special hard plastic shell that supports the forehead, chin, and cheek, while allowing normal breathing. The contact areas of the jaw and forehead are padded with foam rubber. *C*, The plastic support system used in the prone position.

COMPUTED TOMOGRAPHY

When compared to conventional X-ray techniques, computerized tomography (CT Scan) provides a superior and more versatile picture because there are no overlapping structures, and the information taken with each slice is stored in a computer as digital information, which can be electronically manipulated after the actual scanning has been completed (Fig. 4.5).

The principle of computerized tomography (CT) is presented here in a simplified form. An X-ray tube that moves around the longitudinal axis of the patient sends X-rays through the body from a number of different projections. Electronic detectors (which replace the traditional film), measure the strength of the X-rays after they have traversed the body.

With CT, the entire body is not examined, instead each exposure is limited to one single plane that is as a rule located perpendicular to the longitudinal axis of the body (when it was first invented, this technique was only performed in the axial plane and thus it was called computerized axial tomography or CAT scanning). The exposures and their measurements by the detectors are repeated in various positions and directions so that all of the formal elements of the plane are traversed by Röntgen rays more than once.

Because of this large number of projections, there is an absorption value (raw data) for each point of the cross section of the body. From these raw data, the density distribution of the plane under study is reconstituted into an image by a computerized mathematical formula or algorithm. The result of this computation exists in the computer as a series of coordinates of image points (picture elements) designated as a numerical matrix. Currently matrices with 256 × 256 and 512 × 512 pixels (picture elements) are used. Every plane is now divided theoretically into a mosaic of small volume elements (voxels), the surface area of which corresponds to the pixel and the height to the thickness of the chosen plane. The number assigned to the individual pixel corresponds to the density of that particular voxel. Because of the great density resolution capacity of computerized tomography, 4,000 levels of density can be distinguished.

The measure of density is the Hounsfield unit (HU), which was introduced by Hounsfield, the designer of the first CT unit. The Hounsfield scale encompasses densities from −1,000 to +3,000 and includes all clinically relevant tissues.

In order to show the CT image, the density values are represented as varying shades of gray and depicted on an electronic viewer. The human eye can distinguish only about 30 shades of gray. Consequently, the human eye will see approximately 100 adjacent density values as only a single shade of gray. This means that the human eye would be unable to differentiate structures in those areas in which the tissues differ by only a few Hounsfield units. To overcome this problem, the raw data within the computer is electronically manipulated by a technique called the electronic window technique. The electronic window selects a specific section of the spectrum of absorption values. All of the density values lying in the particular "window" selected are shown as shades of gray, while those density values lying outside the window are shown as black or white. By selecting the center point and range of the window, those structures of interest to the examiner can be displayed as visually distinguishable shades of gray.

FIGURE 4.5 A CT survey film showing the location of the individual cuts for coronal sections. The patient's head is maximally extended and angled so that the sections can be taken almost at right angles to the infraorbitomeatal line (IOM). The study extends from the frontal sinus anteriorly to the sphenoid sinus posteriorly.

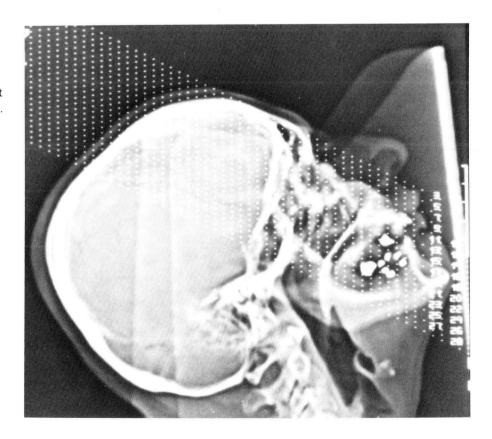

Technique of Computed Tomographic Examination of the Paranasal Sinuses

Plane of Investigation

As with conventional tomography, CT scans of the paranasal sinuses should be taken in the direct coronal plane, i.e., perpendicular to the IOM. The scans should extend from the frontal to the sphenoid sinus (see Fig. 4.5). The plane of examination is determined by angling the gantry and the patient's head parallel to the required plane. The newer generations of CT scanners allow a gantry angulation of up to 25 degrees and consequently even patients who have limited hyper-extension of the head can usually be scanned in the direct coronal plane. It should be noted, however, that the raw data obtained can be electronically manipulated so that any desired plane can be reconstructed in the computer after the scan has been completed.

Slice Thickness

The slice thickness should be set at 4 mm, although in cases in which extra detail is required a slice thickness of 2 mm may be used.

Slice Overlapping

If the radiologist only wishes to show the coronal plane (and not attempt a reconstruction of the other planes), then the scan is taken with each 4 mm slice bordering directly on the following slice. If the radiologist plans to create a computerized reconstruction of the other planes, i.e., sagittal or axial, then thinner or overlapping slices should be chosen to provide enough "information" for a reconstruction of good quality. Overlapping of the scans is accomplished when the table moves in increments less than the specified slice thickness, i.e., if the slice thickness is 4 mm, then the table would move in 3 mm increments. This results in the slices overlapping each other by one millimeter. This overlapping helps to minimize the "staircase phenomenon" (Fig. 4.6), which is seen in many reconstructions.

Positioning of the Patient

Ideally, the patient should be placed in the prone position with the head maximally hyperextended (see Fig. 4.5). The angulation of the gantry is chosen once the patient's head has been hyperextended as far as possible. If for example, in an elderly patient, hyperextension of the neck is not possible, then axial cuts can be taken from the frontal sinus to the hard palate and the coronal views reconstructed by the computer. In this event, overlapping slices should be taken as mentioned above (Table 4.2).

FIGURE 4.6 The typical "staircase" phenomenon occurs when a coronal reconstruction is prepared from nonoverlapping sections as seen in the lower right and middle left of this illustration. The patient was a 70-year-old female with adenocystic carcinoma of the left ethmoid and maxilla with invasion of the orbits.

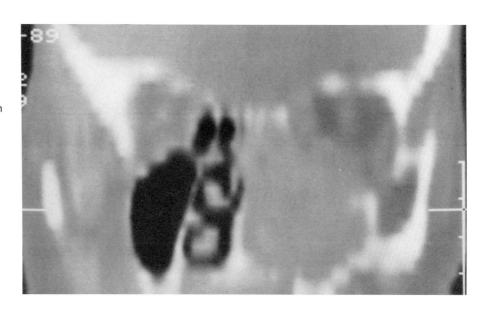

TABLE 4.2 CT Settings for Examination of the Sinuses*

Patient positioning: prone, head hyperextended	Slice thickness: 4 mm
	Table movement: 3 mm increments
Plane of investigation: direct coronal (or axial with coronal reconstruction)	Scan time: 5–7 seconds
	Window: +1,500 to 2,000 HU
Depth of scan: from the frontal to the sphenoid sinus	Center: −150 HU
	125 kV
Gantry angulation: perpendicular to the IOM	450 mAs
Matrix: 512×512	Zoom factor: 4–6

* As recommended by SJ Zinreich.

Choosing the Right Parameters

The correct parameters or settings depend upon the scanner used. The radiation level is usually set at 125 kV and 450 mAs with a scan time of 5 to 7 seconds. The zoom or magnification factor should be large enough to show all the details of the region on interest. An increase in the zoom factor corresponds to an increase in magnification, thereby allowing a much better resolution of detail.

Window Settings

The correct window settings are of critical importance for the examination and evaluation of the delicate mucosal and bony structures of the sinuses (Fig. 4.7). The best results are usually achieved with a relatively wide window (a width of between 1,500 to 2,000) and with a negative center of −150 Hounsfield units (Figs. 4.7 A and C). If a narrower window is used, the delicate bony septa and mucosal structures of the ethmoid region are usually not visible (Figs. 4.7 B and D).

Artifacts

Even when there are pronounced artifacts from dental fillings in the direct coronal cuts, these artifacts usually do not prevent the necessary information being obtained (Fig. 4.8 A and B). In most cases, a direct coronal scan, even one in which there are artifacts from dental fillings, will provide more accurate information than a good coronal reconstruction prepared from an axial scan.

FIGURE 4.7 *A*, With the correct window settings (window at + 2,000, center at − 150), the fine details of the anatomy of the ethmoids can be clearly seen. *B*, If narrower windows are used (in this case a window of 480, center 100) (windows which are better for showing bone), the fine soft tissue details of the ethmoids will not be visible. The selection of an incorrect window setting is a particularly serious error when subtle changes must be identified. In *C*, (W = 2,208, C = − 151) the soft tissue opacity in the ethmoidal air cells associated with the obvious maxillary sinus opacity can be seen. In *D*, which is the same section as *C*, viewed with a bone window setting (W = 350, C = 50) the ethmoidal disease cannot be identified because the wrong window settings were used. With incorrectly chosen windows, a large part of the cell walls, the septa and the mucous membrane lining of the ethmoid are not discernible, and only the massive secondary mucous membrane changes in the maxillary sinus can be seen.

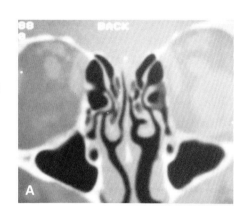 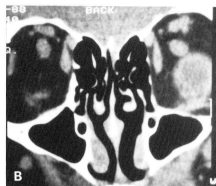

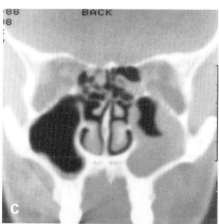 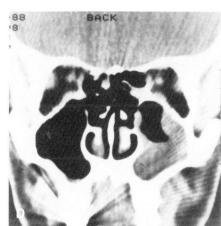

FIGURE 4.8 *A* and *B*, Even massive artifacts, e.g., dental fillings should not affect the radiologist's ability to evaluate the paranasal sinuses, if the appropriate window settings are selected.

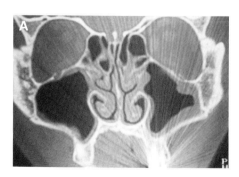 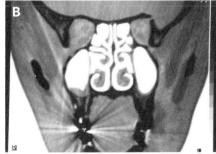

RADIATION EXPOSURE

The different tissues and organs of the body have variable sensitivities to irradiation. The most sensitive tissues or "critical" organs are the gonads, the bone marrow, and the lens of the eye.

The unit in which the amount of radiation absorbed by tissue is measured is called the Gray (Gy). One Gray is equal to one Joule per kilogram and corresponds to 100 rad. The critical dose of radiation for the lens of the eye is reported to be between 2 and 4 Gray (200 to 400 rad) if the dose is applied in a single or in a minimally fractionated dose. If the dose is more highly fractionated, i.e., given over longer intervals, then the critical dose rises to 10 Gray (1,000 rad). The lens is more sensitive to radiation in children and adolescents, and in this group these doses should never be exceeded.

In conventional tomography, the radiation dose to the lens depends basically upon the exposure parameters and the blurring technique used as well as the positioning of the patient. With multidirectional tomography, e.g., hypocycloidal tomography, there is a higher level of irradiation due to the longer exposure time (higher mAs) than is present with linear or circular tomography. The amount of radiation to the lens can be decreased by the use of amplifying foils and by positioning the patient in the prone position (see Fig. 4.4 B). When we use this technique for conventional tomography, the level of irradiation to the lens is approximately that of computerized tomography. During frontal tomography, the lens is exposed to 0.2 to 0.3 mGy (20 to 30 mrad) *per cut*. This adds up to a total irradiation of 2.5 to 3.5 mGy (250 to 350 mrad) for a frontal tomogram with 12 cuts or slices.

In the supine position, frontal tomography exposes the lens to a greater level of irradiation, 5 to 13 mGy (0.5 to 1.3 rad) per cut. Thus in such an examination with 12 cuts, the total exposure to the lens rises to between 60 and 150 mGy (6 to 15 rad). Even with this greater radiation dose of up to 15 rad, there is still a wide safety margin from the critical dose of 200 to 400 rad.

In contrast to conventional tomography where the lens is exposed to some radiation during each cut, in computerized tomography the lens is exposed to radiation only in those cuts which pass directly or tangentially through it. Any overlapping of the cuts in CT thus increases the exposure of the lens. One CT cut through the lens produces an exposure of about 4 mGy (420 mrad). With a 4 mm slice thickness, the lens will be exposed in two to three cuts only in the direct coronal plane. The overall exposure of the lens to radiation therefore varies between 1.2 to 9 rad (12 to 90 mGy). In contrast, a single general X-ray will expose the lens to 1.3 to 2 mGy (0.130 to 0.200 rad).

The amount of radiation to which the gonads are exposed during radiologic investigation of the sinuses is the result of scattered radiation. The dose depends on the distance of the area of investigation from the gonads and can be minimized by careful protection with lead foils and by exact focusing. The gonadal exposure in conventional tomography of the sinuses averages 0.6 mrad per cut for a total of 7.2 mrad when twelve cuts are taken. There is much less scattered radiation with computed tomography, and the resulting gonadal exposure is usually less than 5 mrad. This amount of radiation can be compared favorably to the 100 mrad of radiation to which the gonads are exposed each year from ''natural'' cosmic and terrestrial radiation.

MAGNETIC RESONANCE IMAGING

In magnetic resonance imaging (MRI), rapidly changing magnetic fields are used instead of ionizing radiation so that there is no radiation exposure to the body.

MRI studies permit a good visualization of the anatomic relationships and pathologic changes in the ear, nose, and throat (ENT) area (Fig. 4.9). One disadvantage of this technique is that it is unable to provide a direct image of the bony structures. Pure bony structures such as the lamellae of the ethmoid bone do not generate a signal in any of the MR sequences. For this reason, CT and standard tomography are much more suitable methods to show bony abnormalities and structural details. An additional advantage of MRI is that it is possible to take direct sagittal views.

On the basis of the differential signals given by different tissues, the MRI technique allows a precise assessment of the extent of a tumor and a particularly accurate differentiation between tumor tissue, inflammatory changes, and retained secretions (see Fig. 4.9A and B). Since swollen and hyperemic nasal mucosa also give a stronger signal, inflammatory changes of the nasal mucosa can be well demonstrated. In some instances, however, these inflammatory changes of the nasal mucosa can not be distinguished from a simple thickening of the mucosa such as may appear as part of the normal nasal cycle. Zinreich and his co-workers have demonstrated the mucosal changes of the nasal cycle using magnetic resonance imaging. We know today that the recurrent mucosal engorgement seen in the nasal cycle primarily affects the mucosa of the turbinates and of the ethmoid bone. The mucosa of the maxillary, frontal, and ethmoid sinuses is rarely affected by the nasal cycle.

FIGURE 4.9 *A*, This is a T1-weighted magnetic resonance image of an extensive paranasal sinus tumor (adenocystic carcinoma). *B*, In the T2-weighted magnetic resonance image, the tumor mass (*T*) can be more clearly distinguished from mucosal swelling and retained secretions (*arrows*) both of which are more signal intensive.

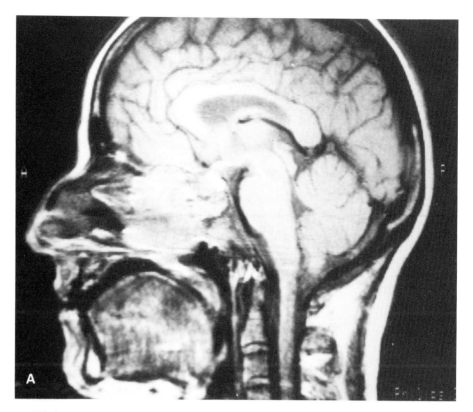

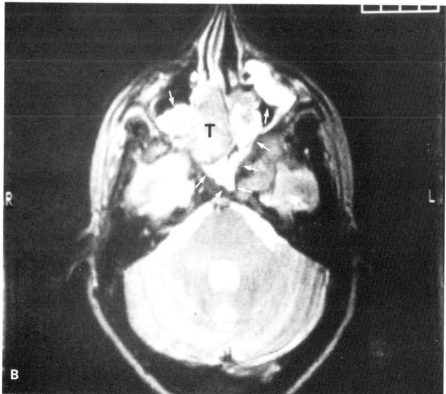

MRI is very useful in identifying mycotic infections of the paranasal sinuses (Fig. 4.10). While infected secretions and inflamed mucous membranes, e.g., in the maxillary sinus, give off an increased signal (become lighter) when changing from a T1 to a T2 weighted image, mycotic masses appearing in a maxillary sinus empyema appear optically empty when changing from T1 to T2. As shown in Figure 4.10A, there is a total opacification of the maxillary sinus in the T1 weighted image. When switched to a T2 weighted image, the intensity of the signal increases only peripherally, while it is almost non-existent in the center (Fig. 4.10B). This nonvisualized area corresponds to a mycotic mass that is surrounded by an empyema (more intensive T2 signal) in a maxillary sinus that is lined by an inflamed mucosa (more intensive T2 signal). This characteristic of mycotic masses, which can be seen regularly in *Aspergillus fumigatus* mycoses, is apparently due to the deposition of paramagnetically acting metallic salts in the mycotic masses (see Chapter 11).

Because of its more accurate depiction of the fine bony structures, CT is presently the superior method for the evaluation of anatomic variations and inflammatory changes in the ENT area. Nevertheless, the rapid evolution and development of the MRI technique, especially in the area of three-dimensional reconstruction, certainly assures this technique an important role in the future. To date there is no evidence of any long-term deleterious effects of MRI.

FIGURE 4.10 *A, Aspergillus* mycosis in the right maxillary sinus. In the T1-weighted MRI there are almost homogenous shadows with a suspicious central "nucleus." *B,* In the T2-weighted MRI there is an increased signal intensity in the marginal mucosal swellings and retained secretions. The "nucleus" appears to be blank.

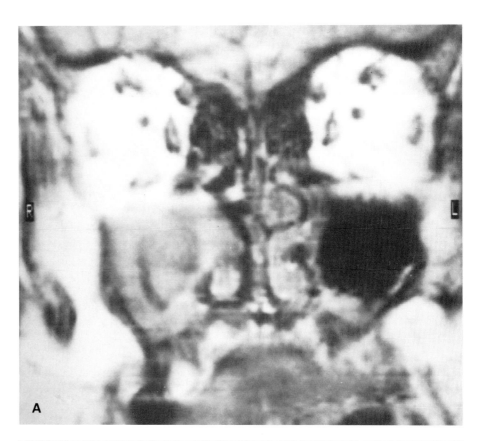

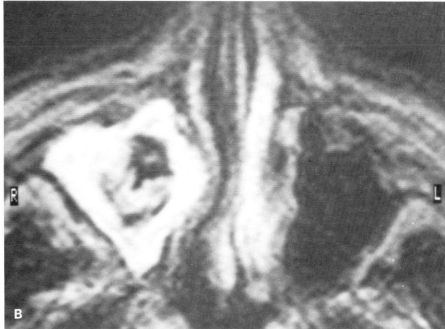

CONVENTIONAL VERSUS COMPUTED TOMOGRAPHY

A comparison of the advantages and disadvantages of conventional and computed tomography must take into consideration not only the resolution and quality of the images produced, but also such factors as the level of radiation exposure, as well as the costs and availability of the necessary equipment. Resolution and contrast are the two most important factors in the production of a high quality X-ray image. Computed tomography provides a much higher level of contrast than conventional tomography due to the ability of CT to more accurately resolve the various structural densities.

It is sometimes difficult with conventional tomography to differentiate between the minor opacifications produced by mucosal swelling and the artifacts that result from the blurring process. With CT this problem is less pronounced, although it still exists. With CT, a minor opacification may appear where the cut passes directly or tangentially through the septum or mucosa of a cell. In both cases, the significance of these minor opacifications can only be established by carefully studying the cuts anterior and posterior to the slice in question (Fig. 4.11).

When there are massive inflammatory changes or soft tissue masses that almost obliterate the paranasal sinuses and decalcify the thin bony lamellae, conventional tomography is unlikely to be of value as it does not detect minor bony abnormalities (Fig. 4.12). When the decalcification is more extensive, the minimal differences in density between the bone and the surrounding soft tissue structures usually render the bony septa invisible in conventional tomography (Fig. 4.13). Conventional tomography is also usually unable to differentiate between inflammatory changes and malignant infiltration with bony destruction.

The superior resolution of CT allows a much better visualization of the bony structures and a better discrimination between inflammatory and neoplastic changes in these cases (see Fig. 4.12A and 4.13B).

FIGURE 4.11 This pair of tomographs shows an example of the type of artifact that can appear in both conventional and computed tomography. In both pictures there appears to be a shadow in the anterior ethmoid. This shadow arose from the left uncinate process that is rotated from the sagittal plane into the frontal plane (a medial rotation of the uncinate process which is an anatomic variation) and thus is hit by both the tomogram/CT sections tangentially. *A*, This is a conventional tomogram. In this tomogram, the rotated uncinate process (*arrow*) extends medially to the lateral lamella of the concha bullosa, with which it fuses. Superiorly, the uncinate process extends at this point to the base of the skull. On the right side, it maintains its sagittal orientation and is in contact superiorly with the concha bullosa on this side. *B*, A similar situation on a CT scan. On the left side, the uncinate process on the left side is rotated in the frontal plane and is therefore tangentially cut by the CT section. Medially, the upper half of the uncinate process is fused with a thin lateral lamella of the concha bullosa (*small arrows*). On the right side, the uncinate process is in its normal sagittal orientation and terminates superiorly just below the base of the skull (*open arrow*).

pu = uncinate process.

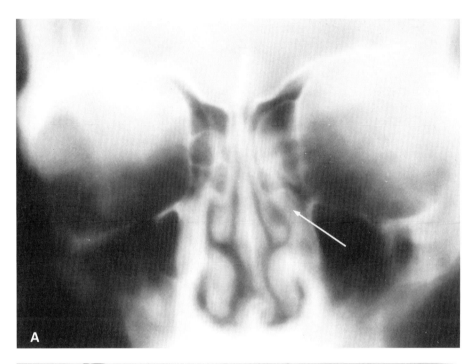

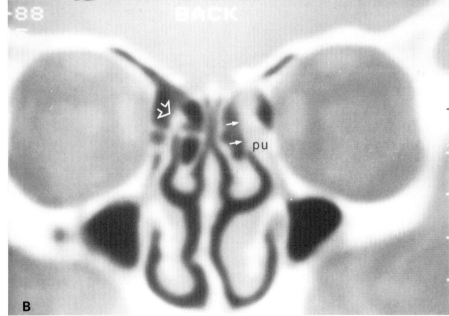

FIGURE 4.12 *A*, This is a CT scan of a patient with recurrent polyposis who has undergone numerous surgical procedures including a partial resection of the middle turbinate. The remaining bony structures can be seen within the mass of polyps and scar tissue. On the left side, the *open arrow* points to a suspected bony defect that was evidently made in the lamina papyracea during one of the earlier procedures. The defect in the lamina papyracea appears to be closed by scar tissue. *B*, This is a conventional tomogram of a similar patient. In contrast to the CT, the differences in density are not nearly as obvious. The still existent, delicate bony structures of the ethmoid can barely be discerned on the left side. On the right it can no longer be determined whether bony landmarks are still present in the soft tissue mass. A surgically relevant finding is the unusually deeply located ethmoid roof (*arrows*).

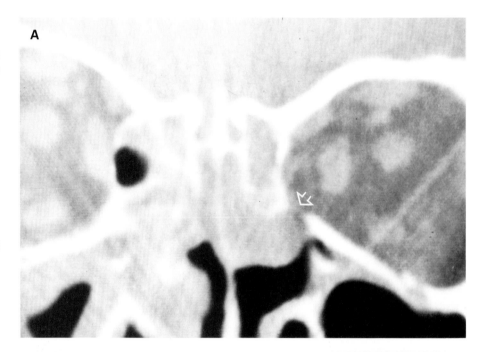

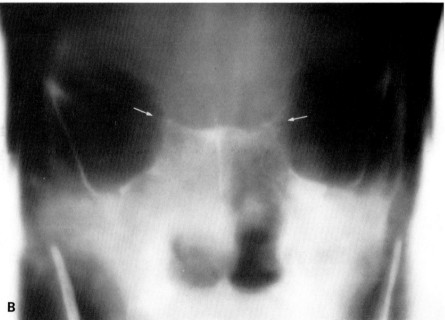

FIGURE 4.13 A comparison of sections from a conventional tomogram (*A*) with those from a CT scan (*B*) in a patient with multiple hemangiomas extending from the orbit through the lamina papyracea of the right eye intracranially and from there into the ethmoid. The superiority of the CT scan is obvious. Even without contrast material the displacement of and the penetration through the lamina papyracea and roof of the ethmoid are much more clearly shown than in the conventional tomogram.

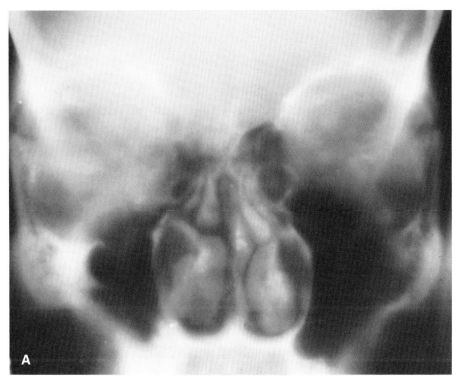

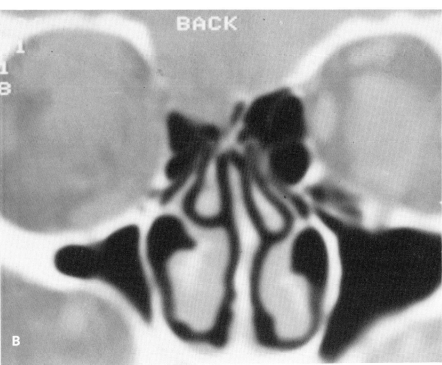

Another advantage of CT is the additional information that can be extracted from the picture. Distances and angles from and between various structures can be measured directly in each plane (Fig. 4.14), as can be densities of the different structures. Secondary reconstructions in various planes can be computed from the stored raw data without any further radiation exposure to the patient. Unfortunately, these reconstructions are usually of lower quality and resolution than the primary or direct cuts and they are usually not suitable for the identification of minor mucosal changes or bony defects. Direct sagittal cuts can only be obtained with conventional tomography or MRI.

There is less radiation exposure with CT than with conventional tomography. Patient comfort is one of the main advantages of conventional tomography. This may be a significant advantage for elderly patients who are unable to produce (and hold for 10 to 15 minutes) the hyperextension of the head required for CT.

The costs of CT are higher than conventional tomography in many countries, due to the high cost of the scanner and the service fees. When both techniques are available, CT is the modality of choice as it is superior in the majority of cases. Hypocycloidal tomography can still produce satisfactory images and provide the physician with useful information. Linear tomography should be considered obsolete.

Advanced CT modalities such as high resolution CT (HRCT) are only rarely required for the evaluation of inflammatory processes. We use HRCT when attempting to identify small bony defects in the roof of the ethmoid, e.g., after previous ethmoid surgery or when attempting to identify the source of a cerebrospinal fluid leak.

If possible, conventional tomography and CT should *not* be performed when the patient's nose and sinuses are acutely infected because the soft tissue swelling resulting from active inflammation prevents the important basic pathologic changes in the key areas of the lateral nasal wall from being visualized. The surgeon needs the best information possible about the underlying causes if he is to plan a functional endoscopic approach with the aim of minimally invasive surgery.

FIGURE 4.14 *A,* This film shows how distances can be measured on a CT pilot film. In this patient, the distance from the nasal spine to the anterior wall of the sphenoid sinus (*1*) is 5.3 cm and to the ostium of the frontal sinus (*2*) is 4.5 cm. The corresponding angles from the horizontal are 31 and 76 degrees. *B,* In this patient, the distance from the nasal spine to the anterior wall of the sphenoid sinus (*1*) is 5.2 cm and from the nasal spine to the frontal ostium (*2*) is 4.5 cm. Since the angles in this instance were measured with the patient supine, the angles between the plane of the image and the horizontal plane are 27 degrees for distance (*1*) and − 8 degrees for distance (*2*).

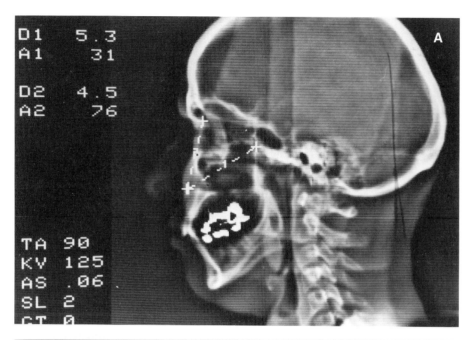

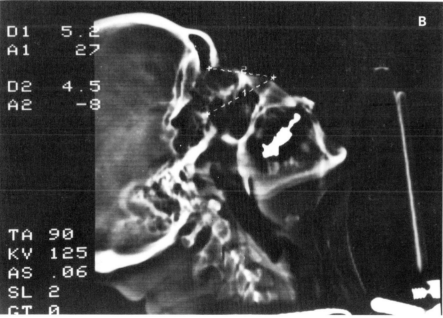

Three-Dimensional Reconstructions

The development and application of modern computers has dramatically changed imaging technology. It is now feasible to reconstruct three-dimensional models from the raw CT data and display them on a screen (Fig. 4.15). This three-dimensional reconstruction technique makes it possible to create and view three-dimensional representations of a head from any direction and any rotational angle (and also to make the reconstruction spatially "transparent"). This allows fascinating insights from any desired angle. Details of anatomic structures and spatial relationships can be represented and highlighted in the area of the paranasal sinuses, through a variety of color coding (Figs. 4.15 A and B). With this technique, pathologic processes can be shown and a surgical approach with extraction of the lesion from the surrounding normal tissues can be simulated on the television screen. This enables the surgeon to obtain an excellent understanding of the size and relationships of the lesion and the possibilities of reconstructing the defect. This same computer program also permits planning of the necessary reconstructive steps (Fig. 4.15D). One such example is the utilization of exogenous "replacement components," designed accurately with computer assistance, to repair defects created by a partial resection of the mandible or to fill a calvarial defect.

To date, three-dimensional (3-D) reconstruction techniques have little to offer in the area of functional nasal endoscopy with the exception of the study of anatomic relationships. While the costs of the equipment for 3-D reconstruction are currently prohibitive, it is anticipated that over time this type of computer will become much less expensive and more widely available. Attempts to aid surgery with real-time 3D-reconstructions on the monitor, guided by a sensor on the tip of the instrument in use, are still in their infancy.

FIGURE 4.15 *A*, This three-dimensional reconstruction of the paranasal sinuses was made from the CT data of an actual patient. The computer technology is so sophisticated that the areas of little interest can be blocked out on the screen. In this image, the frontal bone and parts of the maxilla are blocked out and their lumen is color-coded. This permits an excellent spatial representation of the infundibulum that forms a clear terminal recess on the left side as well as the frontal recess. On the right side, the ostium of the maxillary sinus can be seen hidden in the depth of the infundibulum. On this side there is an accessory maxillary sinus ostium in the posterior fontanelle. The frontal sinus, frontal recess and infundibulum are color-coded to make their spatial visualization easier. oa = accessory ostium in the posterior fontanelle of the right maxillary sinus; om = ostium of the maxillary sinus; rf = frontal recess; rt = recessus terminalis; and i = infundibulum. *B*, The reconstruction can be rotated in all planes on the screen. *C*, Any segment of the paranasal sinus system can be "excised" on the screen. This is demonstrated in this photograph in which a horizontal "cut" has been made by the computer through the glabella and a vertical "cut" through the infundibulum. This maneuver clearly shows the relationship between the infundibulum and the frontal recess. oa = accessory ostium. *D*, Current research is directed toward developing instruments and probes that can be connected to the CT data stored in the computer and that can show the surgeon all the anatomic structures in the vicinity of his surgical instruments in real time. In this way the precise position of the instruments may be determined. This reconstruction shows the results of a study performed with a model skull. It is difficult to predict how soon these techniques will be available or their cost-effectiveness for endoscopic sinus surgery. In view of the exponential growth in technology, it may be assumed that these and even more improved techniques will probably be available to all practitioners within a few years. (Courtesy of SJ Zinreich and DW Kennedy, Baltimore.)

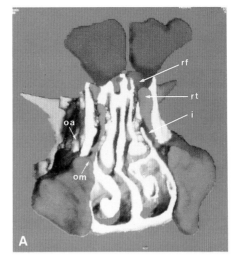

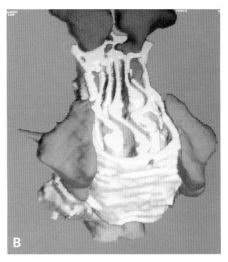

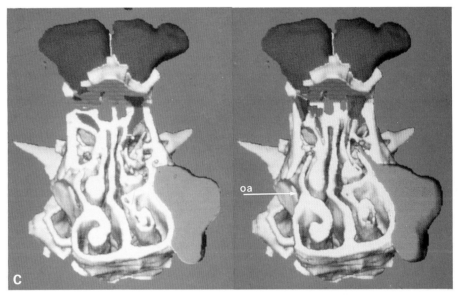

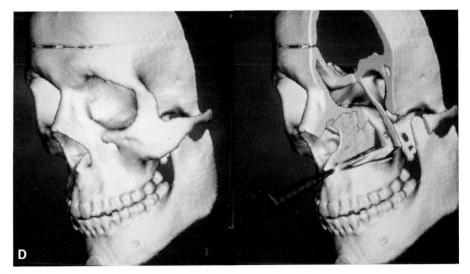

RADIOLOGIC ANATOMY

Only the principal features of normal CT anatomy, as shown in the coronal view, are described in this section. The most common variations of the normal anatomy are discussed and some of these variations are shown in the illustrations. A detailed description of the numerous and clinically important variations of the anatomy of the ethmoid is presented in Chapters 3 and 5. Since not all of the anatomic structures of interest are found in "ideal" configuration in one single patient, we have taken illustrations from several patients to demonstrate the key anatomic features.

If the supraorbital ridge is prominent and the frontal sinus well developed, the frontal sinus is occasionally seen anterior to the root of the nose. In this event, the soft tissue of the eyelids and nose can also be seen in the same cut (Fig. 4.16). In the next two sections (Fig. 4.17 and 4.18), using a 4-mm separation between sections, the frontal sinus is seen in its full extent without necessarily showing its ostium. The principal septum of the frontal sinus is not always located in the midline and there may be a number of additional incomplete septa.

It should be remembered that not every air space in the frontal bone is necessarily part of the frontal sinus. An anterior ethmoid air cell can expand into the frontal bone from the recessus frontalis and appear as a "frontal bone bulla" (bulla frontalis, see Fig. 4.16) either in addition to the frontal sinus or (then usually located near the midline) as the only air cell in the frontal bone.

The frontal recess appears further posterior. Depending on the direction of the view, an hourglass-shaped narrowing of the frontal recess can be recognized toward the entrance to the frontal sinus. The narrowest part of the hourglass-shape usually corresponds to the ostium of the frontal sinus (see Fig. 4.18).

FIGURE 4.16 Coronal CT section at the level of the glabella. The frontal sinus is fully developed. Delicate septations, originating from the anterior wall of the frontal sinus are clearly visible. 1 = frontal sinus and 2 = frontal bone "bulla."

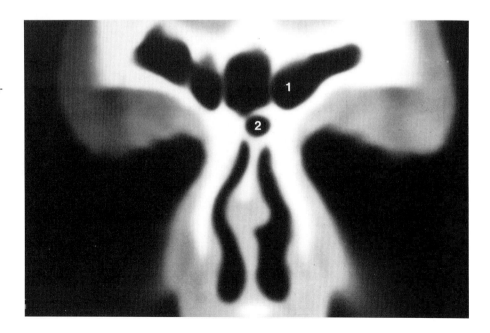

FIGURE 4.17 This cut is 4 mm posterior to the previous section. The agger nasi cells are visible for the first time. The most anterior part of the insertion of the inferior turbinate can be seen. The soft tissues of the upper eyelid, the cornea and the lens are also visible. 2 = frontal bone "bulla"; 3 = agger nasi cells; ci = inferior turbinate; and c = cornea and lens.

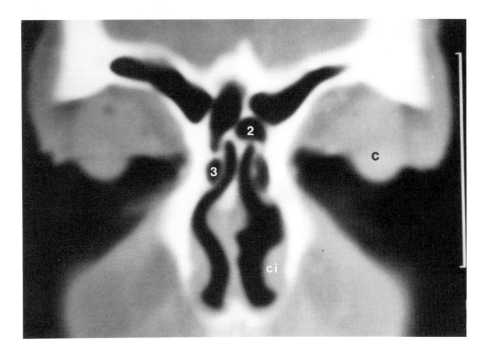

FIGURE 4.18 A section 4 mm further posterior. The transition from the frontal sinus to the frontal recess can be seen. The *arrows* mark the hourglass narrowing in the area of the frontal sinus ostium on the left side. The lacrimal fossa and the nasolacrimal duct are tangentially cut. The inferior turbinate is now well developed, while the middle turbinate is not yet visible. 1 = frontal sinus; 3 = agger nasi cells; 4 = lacrimal fossa; 5 = naso-lacrimal duct; 6 = frontal recess; 7 = septal tubercle; and 8 = first cut across the anterior wall of the maxillary sinus.

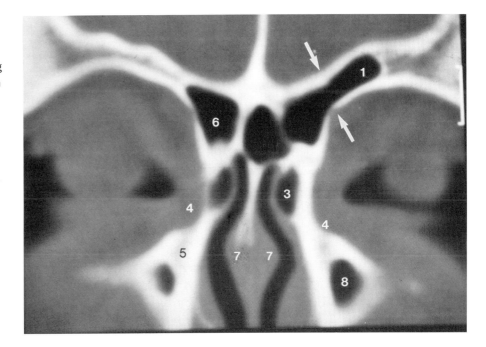

Once inside the skull, the beginning of the crista galli can be seen (Fig. 4.19). The crista galli may be quite small, but it may also be large and may contain air. Occasionally the route of pneumatization of the crista galli can be followed in CT image series (see Fig. 4.32) from the frontal sinus or from the recessus frontalis. If the crista galli is extensively pneumatized from the frontal recess, this fact must be considered should it become necessary to open the frontal recess. In these cases the path to the frontal sinus is almost always further laterally, leading superiorly and anteriorly.

If the agger nasi is pneumatized (see Fig. 4.19), then, depending on the degree of pneumatization, these agger nasi cells may be visible prior to the first section that cuts through the frontal recess. Agger

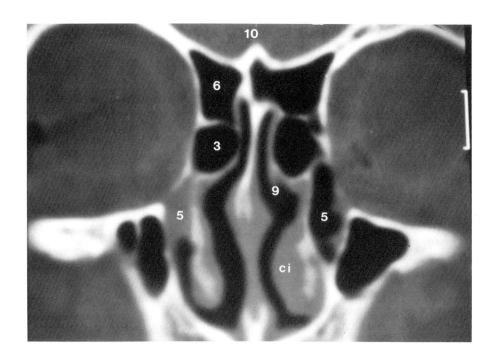

FIGURE 4.19 The frontal recess and agger nasi cells are fully displayed. The agger nasi cells are very well pneumatized bilaterally in this patient. A thin bony septum separates the agger nasi cell from the frontal recess, which extends further superiorly and anteriorly. Dorsally, this septum gradually fades, since the agger nasi cells are pneumatized from the frontal recess in this patient. On the left, the most anterior part of the insertion of the middle turbinate arises from the lateral wall of the nose. In this case, the pneumatization of the agger nasi cell extends as far as the in- sertion of the middle turbinate. The nasolacrimal duct is shown bilaterally along its entire vertical length. On the right the section appears to cut through its opening in the inferior meatus. On the left there is air in the nasolacrimal duct. At the base of the skull, the crista galli begins to appear. Its most anterior part appears to be slightly pneumatized from the direction of the frontal recess. 3 = agger nasi cells; 5 = nasolacrimal duct; 6 = frontal recess; 9 = middle turbinate; 10 = crista galli; and ci = inferior turbinate.

nasi cells can usually be easily identified by the presence of pneumatization of the lateral nasal wall *before* the most anterior part of the attachment of the middle turbinate appears in the picture. This makes it easy to distinguish an agger nasi cell from an unusually large bulla ethmoidalis. The lacrimal fossa (see Fig. 4.19) is located lateral to the agger nasi cells, separated only by the thin and frequently dehiscent lacrimal bone. From the lacrimal fossa, the course of the nasolacrimal duct can be followed in the next one or two cuts (Figs. 4.19 and 4.20). The nasolacrimal duct opens into the inferior nasal meatus in the plica lacrimalis (Hasner's valve). It is not unusual to see air in the nasolacrimal duct.

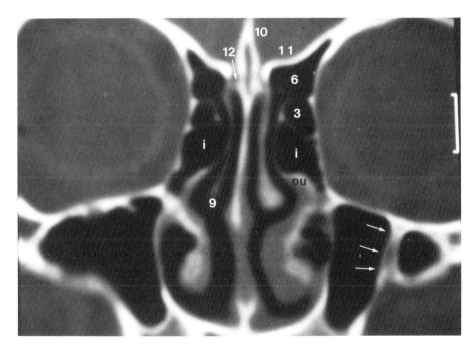

FIGURE 4.20 In this section, the uncinate process is identified as such for the first time. Medially it delimits an unusually deep infundibulum that is closed superiorly by an agger nasi cell, which slowly decreases in size. In this section, the ostium of the maxillary sinus is not yet visible. It is evident that in this patient the frontal recess does not open directly into the infundibulum, but instead drains medial to the infundibulum into the middle meatus between the uncinate process and the middle turbinate. The crista galli is well developed. The roof of the anterior ethmoid consisting here of the frontal bone is well marked. The olfactory fossa can also be identified. In the left maxillary sinus is a hump in the facial wall caused by the slightly inferior course of the infraorbital nerve (*arrows*). 3 = agger nasi cell; 6 = frontal recess; 9 = middle turbinate; 10 = crista galli; 11 = anterior ethmoid; 12 = olfactory fossa; i = infundibulum; and pu = uncinate process.

One section further posterior (Fig. 4.21) shows, medial to the agger nasi cell, the middle turbinate with its attachment to the roof of the ethmoid. The crista galli is now well differentiated and depending on the height of the roof of the ethmoid, the olfactory fossa is well developed. The superior, usually very thin and almost horizontal bony layer that separates the agger nasi cell from the anterosuperiorly (towards the ostium of the frontal sinus) oriented frontal recess disappears from the picture, since the agger nasi, pneumatized from the frontal recess, merges into it in the more posterior views.

The uncinate process develops from the point at which the inferior turbinate bone attaches to the medial wall of the maxillary sinus. The uncinate process has its major vertical ascent in the anterior sections and it is here that it appears to be the longest. The lumen of the ethmoidal infundibulum may be seen between the uncinate process and the medial wall of the orbit. Depending upon the position of the uncinate process (see Fig. 4.25 and 4.33), the ethmoidal infundibulum may either proceed cranially into the frontal recess or it may form a blind pouch, the recessus terminalis (terminal recess). A terminal recess is found when the uncinate process deviates cranially and laterally and inserts into the lamina papyracea. When this happens, the frontal recess opens medially to the uncinate process, opening between the uncinate process and the middle turbinate. The ostium of the maxillary sinus is not usually seen in the first section that goes through the infundibulum, since it is usually located at the floor of the infundibulum at the junction of the middle and posterior thirds of the infundibulum.

FIGURE 4.21 In this section, the middle turbinate shows slight pneumatization on the left side, which originates from the frontal recess (6, arrow). This is the first section showing the bulla ethmoidalis and the fully developed infundibulum (row of arrows). The uncinate process is minimally pneumatized. The black arrows on the right side point to the ostium of the maxillary sinus. In the left maxillary sinus an arrow points to the course of the infraorbital nerve in the roof of the sinus. 6 = frontal recess; be = bulla ethmoidalis; i = infundibulum; pu = uncinate process; and om = ostium of the maxillary sinus.

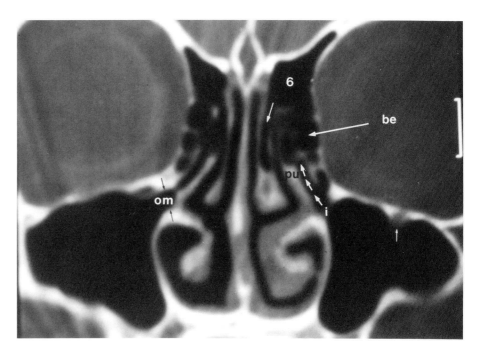

The next section (Fig. 4.22) usually shows the ethmoidal bulla and its relationship to the uncinate process. The cleft between the anterior surface of the bulla and the posterior free edge of the uncinate process is the semilunar hiatus. The hiatus semilunaris appears as a two-dimensional structure, like a door through which the three-dimensional ethmoidal infundibulum may be reached (see Chapter 3). In the next sections, (Fig. 4.23 and 4.24) the uncinate process appears to become shorter and shorter, a natural result of sectioning. When the sections are taken in the coronal plane, the hook shaped uncinate process is seen anteriorly in its greater vertical extent and posteriorly in its shortest one (Fig. 4.25). A section precisely through the ostium of the maxillary sinus demonstrates these anatomic relationships very well. The ostium of the maxillary sinus can be seen at the extreme lower "end" in the floor of the infundibulum. The infundibulum itself is located between the lamina papyracea laterally and the uncinate process medially. The infundibulum opens medially into the middle meatus of the nose through the hiatus semilunaris.

The small "septa" that are frequently seen vertically on the anterior wall of the maxillary sinus represent the infraorbital nerve, progressing from the roof of the maxillary sinus anteriorly and inferiorly to the facial wall of the sinus and causing the formation of a bony ridge. On coronal sections, this ridge appears as a more or less pronounced septum.

Depending upon the extent of pneumatization of the bulla, its lumen now appears. Occasionally the lumen seems to be septate, which may cause difficulty in differentiating between a true septation and a Haller's cell protruding from the floor of the orbit.

FIGURE 4.22   The infundibulum can be easily identified between the lamina papyracea and the uncinate process. The hiatus semilunaris on the left side is outlined by a pair of *parallel black lines* for identification. The *row of white arrows* shows the path from the ostium of the maxillary sinus through the infundibulum and the hiatus semilunaris, into the middle meatus. The bulla ethmoidalis is fully displayed. In this patient, the middle turbinate attaches to the skull precisely in the angle between the horizontal running lamina cribrosa and the vertical running lateral lamina of the lamina cribrosa. The transition of the extremely thin lateral lamina into the substantially thicker roof of the ethmoid (frontal bone) is striking. 13 = lamina cribrosa; 14 = lateral lamina of the lamina cribrosa; and be = bulla ethmoidalis.

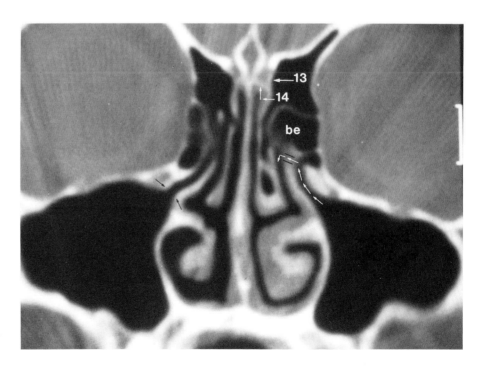

The olfactory fossa is fully developed in Figure 4.23, and the thin cribriform plate is now clearly recognizable. Below the cribriform plate is the origin of the middle turbinate and extending cranially, the extension of the lamina lateralis of the cribriform plate can be seen. The superior part of the roof of the ethmoid is formed not by the ethmoid bone but by the frontal bone and its ethmoid foveolae (see Chapter 3). The frontal bone covers the roof of the ethmoid superiorly and laterally, thereby making the roof of the ethmoid substantially thicker than the lamina cribrosa and its lateral lamella. This can be seen clearly radiologically.

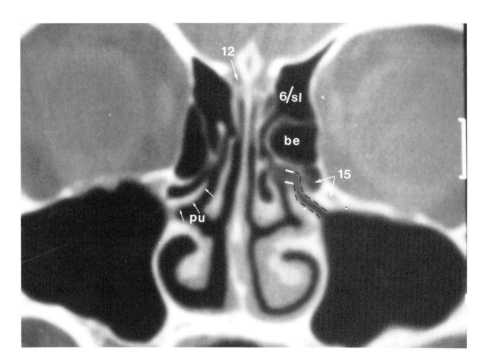

FIGURE 4.23 The uncinate process runs in the sagittal direction in this section and hence seems shorter (*arrows*). The infundibulum is outlined by a *broken black line* on the left side for easier identification. The opening of the infundibulum into the middle meatus, through the hiatus semilunaris is indicated by the *white lines*. The infundibulum is slightly narrowed from the lateral side by small cells. These correspond either to the septations of a large bulla ethmoidalis or to freestanding Haller's cells. The middle turbinate is still attached to the skull. Above the bulla, the frontal recess becomes an extended lateral sinus. The olfactory fossa is shown in its greatest extent. The olfactory fossa is "framed" by the lateral lamina of the lamina cribrosa, the lamina cribrosa itself and the crista galli. 6 = frontal recess; 12 = crista galli; 15 = Haller's cells or septations of a large bulla ethmoidalis; sl = lateral sinus; be = bulla ethmoidalis; and pu = uncinate process.

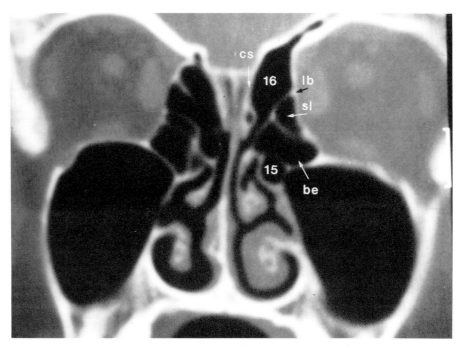

FIGURE 4.24   The insertion of the middle turbinate has separated from the roof of the ethmoid and extended laterally to the lamina papyracea of the orbit to join "*basal lamella*" (lamina basalis). The superior turbinate (concha superior) becomes visible with its insertion with the skull. Between the superior turbinate and the basal lamella the superior meatus and later the cells of the posterior ethmoid become visible. In this section, a distinct supraorbital recess is visible on the left side. 15 = Haller's cells or septations of a large bulla ethmoidalis; 16 = superior meatus; cs = concha superior; lb = lamina basalis; sl = lateral sinus; and be = bulla ethmoidalis.

The frontal recess may either disappear gradually posteriorly or it may terminate at the lamella of the bulla at the point where the bulla reaches the skull. If the lamella of the bulla is incomplete or missing in its uppermost part, the frontal recess passes into a variably pneumatized space above the ethmoidal bulla called the lateral sinus. Depending on its pneumatization, the lateral sinus may extend between the roof of the bulla (below), the lamina papyracea (laterally), and the roof of the ethmoid (above) posteriorly and inferiorly. The posterior-superior border of the lateral sinus is the basal lamella of the middle turbinate. The lateral sinus may open into the middle meatus of the nose medially between the bulla and the middle turbinate through the "superior semilunar hiatus" (Grünwald).

If the middle turbinate is pneumatized, its pneumatization usually originates from the frontal recess. Middle turbinates may also be pneumatized from the lateral sinus or directly from the middle nasal meatus.

FIGURE 4.25 This schematic drawing illustrates the relationships of the uncinate process in coronal sections from front to back. In *section a-a*: the uncinate process is shown in its greatest vertical extent. In this case it forms a recessus terminalis, since cranially the uncinate process bends laterally and inserts into the lamina papyracea of the orbit. For this reason the infundibulum appears to be closed on all sides in this section. The ostium of the maxillary sinus is not yet shown, since the section is clearly anterior to the ostium. The *arrow* indicates the direction of drainage from the frontal recess in this case. In *section b-b*: the fully developed infundibulum is shown. The uncinate process is still shown primarily in its vertical course and hence it appears to be very elongated. Between the bulla ethmoidalis and the uncinate process, the narrow cleft of the hiatus semilunaris appears (*double arrows*). It is through this cleft that the infundibulum is reached (the position of the ostium of the maxillary sinus is indicated by the *dashed circle*). In *section c-c*: the uncinate process slowly fades posteriorly and the infundibulum becomes very shallow. Eventually, accessory ostia appear in the area of the posterior nasal fontanelles. The *double arrow* points to the fading hiatus semilunaris. In this section, the middle turbinate appears to have two insertions. The vertical insertion corresponds to its transition into the superior turbinate and the lateral insertion bending laterally toward the lamina papyracea corresponds to the true basal (ground) lamella. In *section d-d*: the infundibulum and the hiatus semilunaris have now almost completely disappeared. The bulla can be seen at its extreme posterior end. The middle and the superior turbinates have now separated. The isolated insertion of the superior turbinate at the skull can be seen just as clearly as the basal lamella of the middle turbinate. In this section, the basal lamella points straight laterally. i = infundibulum and be = bulla ethmoidalis.

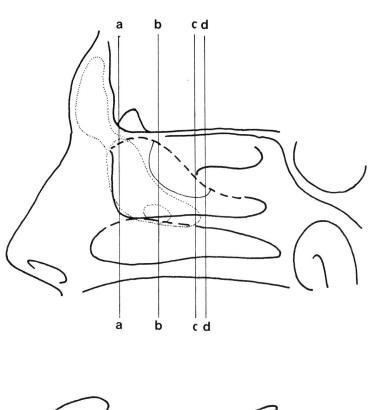

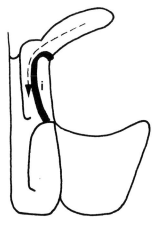

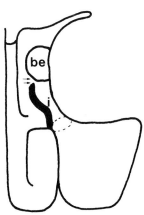

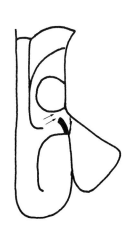

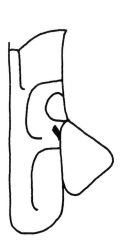

a – a   b – b   c – c   d – d

The diagram in Figure 4.26 and the sections shown in Figures 4.28 and 4.29 show the transition from the anterior to the posterior ethmoid. The uncinate process melds into the lateral wall of the nose and the posterior nasal fontanelle appears as its extension. At this point an accessory ostium is frequently present and can readily be identified radiologically.

The bony base of the middle turbinate separates (Fig. 4.27) from the roof of the ethmoid at this point and swings laterally to insert on the lamina papyracea. The apparent split or dual attachment of the base of the middle turbinate with the skull and lateral wall of the nose appears in the picture because the superior turbinate bone has not separated entirely from the middle turbinate in the section in which it first appears. This space implies an anterior "blind pouch" of the superior nasal meatus. If the pneumatization of the meatus extends further anteriorly and inferiorly into the middle turbinate, then the concha bullosa that Grünwald has designated as an "interlaminary cell" is formed.

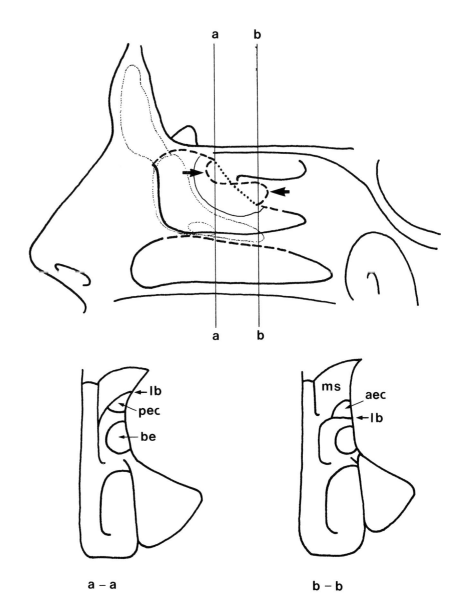

FIGURE 4.26 This is a schematic representation of the changes in the basal (ground) lamella. The basal lamella may be hemmed in dorsally by the cells of the anterior ethmoid, the lateral sinus, and also by the ethmoidal bulla itself. Additionally, the cells of the posterior ethmoid and the superior meatus may hem it in anteriorly (arrows). These relationships may produce a complicated picture on coronal sections. In section a-a: the superior meatus has developed into a blind pouch between the basal lamella and the vertical insertion of the middle turbinate. In addition, a posterior ethmoidal cell has grown through the basal lamella anteriorly. In section b-b: an anterior ethmoidal cell has grown through the basal lamella posteriorly. The superior turbinate has separated clearly from the middle turbinate and the superior meatus is fully developed. lb = basal lamella; pec = posterior ethmoidal cell; be = bulla ethmoidalis; ms = superior meatus; and aec = anterior ethmoidal cell.

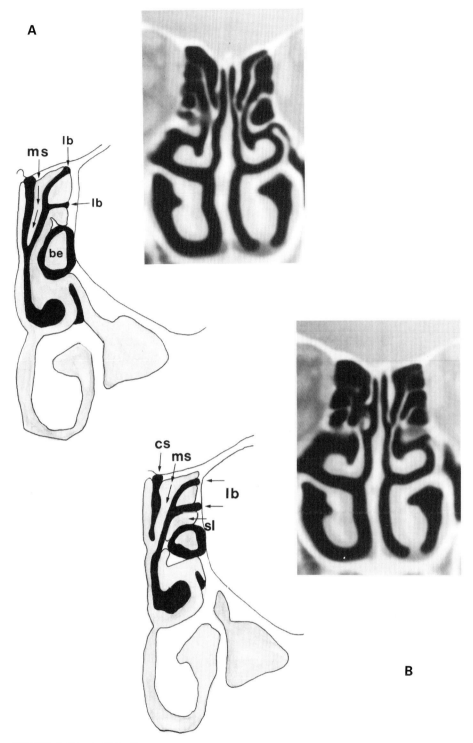

FIGURE 4.27   *A*, This CT scan shows the transition of the middle turbinate to the superior turbinate. Here the middle turbinate appears to have two insertions. One is vertical and extends to the base of the skull, and the other is directed, at a slant, laterally and superiorly and inserts in the lamina papyracea. This configuration arises because the anterior end of the superior meatus grows into the insertion of the middle turbinate and thus the superior meatus develops a blind pouch. The laterally directed lamella is the basal lamella of the middle turbinate. *B*, In this section which is 4 mm further posterior, the basal lamella has separated from the superior turbinate. The superior meatus, the basal lamella, and the lateral sinus can be clearly distinguished. An incidental finding was that the patient has no uncinate process on the right side. ms = superior meatus; lb = basal lamella; be = bulla ethmoidalis; cs = concha superior; and sl = lateral sinus.

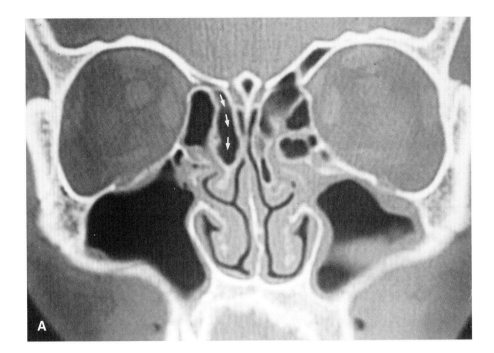

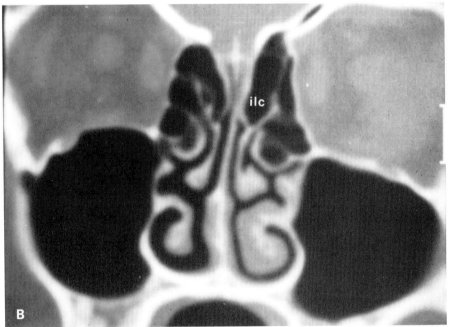

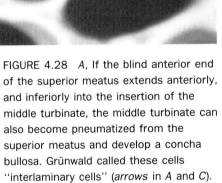

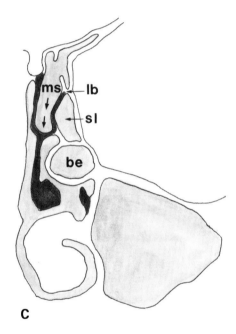

FIGURE 4.28 *A*, If the blind anterior end of the superior meatus extends anteriorly, and inferiorly into the insertion of the middle turbinate, the middle turbinate can also become pneumatized from the superior meatus and develop a concha bullosa. Grünwald called these cells "interlaminary cells" (*arrows* in *A* and *C*). *B*, The insertion of the middle turbinate on the left side of this CT scan contains a large interlaminary cell which resulted from pneumatization of the middle turbinate from the superior meatus. *C*, This is a schematic drawing of *B*. ilc = interlaminary cell; ms = anterior blind end of the superior meatus; lb = basal lamina; sl = lateral sinus; and be = bulla ethmoidalis.

In Figures 4.27, 4.28, and 4.29 the middle turbinate is easily recognizable as such and the line of attachment of the middle turbinate, the "ground lamella" runs in a frontal and horizontal plane (in the section). Depending on the degree of pneumatization of the maxillary sinus, the ground lamella may be attached to the medial wall of the maxillary sinus in the posterior third of its course where it forms the roof of the middle nasal meatus.

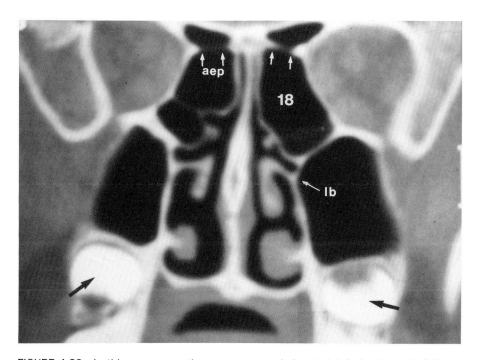

FIGURE 4.29 In this case, a section through the posterior ethmoid shows supraorbital pneumatization. It is unusual that the posterior ethmoid artery is located bilaterally in a small osseous channel, several millimeters below the roof of the ethmoid. Ordinarily the posterior ethmoid artery is located right in the roof of the ethmoid. The *black arrows* point to the not yet erupted third molars in the maxilla. aep = posterior ethmoid artery; lb = basal lamella of the middle turbinate; and 18 = posterior ethmoid sinus.

Between the basal lamella of the middle turbinate, curved laterally (Fig. 4.30), and the superior turbinate, first the superior nasal meatus and, in further sections, the cells of the posterior ethmoid appear. These cells usually appear wider than the anterior ethmoidal cells. The course of the roof of the ethmoid becomes flatter and is frequently almost horizontal just before it reaches the sphenoid. It is not unusual, however, to find extensive supraorbital pneumatization in the posterior ethmoid, which may even be more extensive than supraorbital pneumatization of the anterior ethmoid, where it most frequently originates from the lateral sinus or the recessus frontalis.

Figure 4.31 shows the sphenoid sinus. It should be noted that the most posterior cells of the posterior ethmoid may extend far laterally and, under certain circumstances, the posterior cells may even extend above the body of the sphenoid. These cells are the "Onodi cells," which may abut the optic nerve.

FIGURE 4.30 This CT scan shows the normal relationships in the posterior ethmoid. The almost horizontal course of the basal lamella of the middle turbinate can be seen. The basal lamella inserts into the lamina papyracea on the left and in the medial wall of the maxillary sinus on the right. Above the basal lamella is the superior meatus. Above this, the cells of the posterior ethmoid can be seen flanked medially by the superior turbinate. ms = superior meatus.

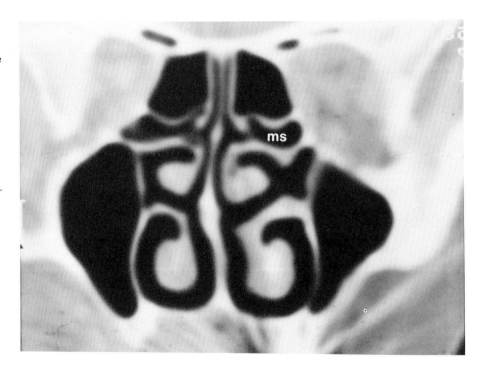

FIGURE 4.31 *A,* This is a CT cut through a sphenoid sinus that is generally somewhat small and which has a midline intersinus septum. The clinoid processes are not pneumatized. The choanae are shown below. The posterior end of the inferior and middle turbinates can still be seen. The pterygoid process appears laterally. *B,* This is a section through an extensively pneumatized sphenoid sinus (polycyclic tomography). On the bottom the root of the pterygoid process can be seen. Directly above it is the prominent canal of the vidian nerve and in the lateral wall the foramen rotundum and the bilaterally quite prominent internal carotid artery can be seen. The bones over its anterior bulge appear to be dehiscent. There is an extensively pneumatized anterior clinoid process (*thin arrows*) between the optic nerve and the internal carotid artery. 19 = pterygoid process; 20 = vidian nerve canal; 21 = internal carotid artery; 22 = optic nerve; and fr = foramen rotundum.

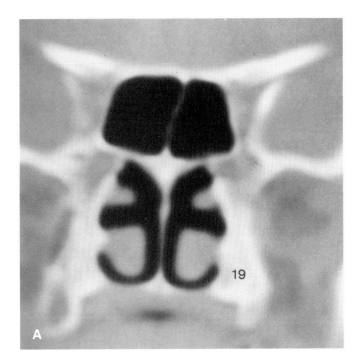

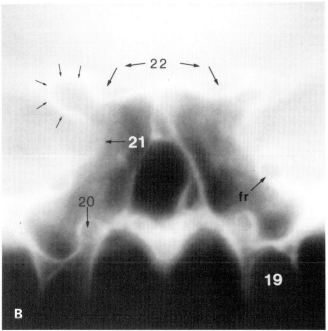

Occasionally pneumatization of the most posterior portions of the septum can be seen to originate from the sphenoid sinus.

The sphenoid sinus may be pneumatized to a variable degree. In extreme cases, the pneumatization may extend far into the anterior clinoid process, around the optic nerve, the foramen rotundum, the vidian canal and, inferiorly, to the attachment of the pterygoid process. If the pneumatization extends far anteriorly, direct contact with the maxilloethmoidal recess of the maxillary sinus may occur (see Fig. 4.44).

Of primary interest in the sphenoid sinus is the behavior of the bony layer over the internal carotid artery, which in up to 25 percent of cases, appears to be clinically dehiscent (see Chapter 3). The carotid artery in its course through the cavernous sinus may bulge far medially into the sphenoid sinus. Especially if there is a simultaneous pneumatization of the anterior clinoid process, a deep, posterolaterally oriented recess may be formed between the ridge of the internal carotid and the ridge of the optic nerve. Below the ridge of the carotid, the course of the second branch of the trigeminal nerve can be seen in the foramen rotundum. The vidian canal runs along the base of the pterygoid process.

Occasionally, the optic nerve causes only a slight bulge in the superior-lateral wall of the sphenoid sinus and in some cases, the optic nerve may pass through the sphenoid sinus covered only by a very thin bony layer. These anatomic variations obviously increase substantially the surgical risks. (See also Chapter 13.)

Normally, the sphenoid sinus has only one septum, which separates the right and left sides. In many cases however, the septum is *not* located in the midline, but proceeds laterally in its posterior segments to insert itself, in some cases directly, at the thin bony ridge of the internal carotid artery. This situation also is of surgical importance when for example the bony septum must be resected due to extensive pathology within the sphenoid. If the course of the intersinus septum is as lateral as described above, great care must be taken so that the bone over the internal carotid artery is not fractured causing arterial injury (see Figs. 4.40 and 4.41).

The course of the septum of the sphenoid sinus and the presence of the Onodi cells can be demonstrated more clearly in axial CT sections. In coronal sections, particularly in the first few sections that cut through the sphenoid sinus, "subseptations" may frequently be erroneously suggested, since in addition to the sphenoid sinus, sections of the posterior ethmoid (Onodi cells) may also be shown.

Sections even further posteriorly may show the meeting of the optic nerves in the optic chiasm as well as the sella turcica.

Important Anatomic Variants

Only a few examples of anatomic variants are presented here (Figs. 4.32 to 4.45) as most of the variants, particularly the clinically significant ones, are found in the corresponding specific chapters.

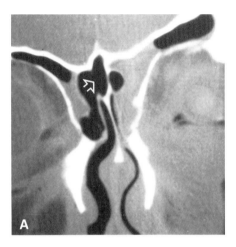 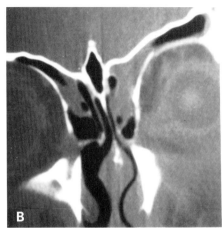

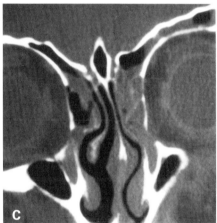

FIGURE 4.32   These scans show the pneumatization of a crista galli from the right frontal recess. In *A*, the wide communicating channel between the frontal recess and the crista galli can be clearly seen (*arrow*). The frontal recess also pneumatizes the agger nasi on this side. One section posteriorly, *B*, the pneumatization extends superiorly and dorsally into the crista galli. One section further posteriorly, *C*, the crista galli does not seem to have any connection to the anterior ethmoid. The middle turbinate on the right side is now fully developed.

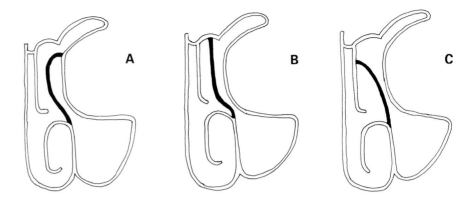

FIGURE 4.33   This is a schematic representation of the principal variations in the course of the uncinate process. *A,* the uncinate process is bent laterally on top and inserts in the lamina papyracea. This closes the infundibulum superiorly and forms a terminal recess (recessus terminalis). In this event, the frontal recess (and thus the frontal sinus) opens medial to the uncinate process, between it and the middle turbinate. *B,* the uncinate process runs straight superiorly and reaches the skull along its entire length, or only along one part of it. In this case the frontal recess drains directly into the ethmoidal infundibulum. When the uncinate process has this configuration, it may become a bony ridge at the underside of the skull. The uncinate process then separates the most superior parts of the frontal recess from the lateral sinus (if present), just above the bulla. When the uncinate process follows this course there is frequently a narrow, occasionally closed, blind pouch between the middle turbinate and the uncinate process. *C,* the uncinate process turns medially and fuses with the middle turbinate. Occasionally this fusion extends dorsally to the lamella of the bulla. Such a fusion with the middle turbinate (or the lateral lamella of a concha bullosa) is seen most frequently when the uncinate process turns medially into the frontal plane.

FIGURE 4.34 On the basis of a single section, it is sometimes difficult to determine whether the ethmoid cells growing into the floor of the orbit represent true Haller's cells or simply protrusions of an ethmoidal bulla.

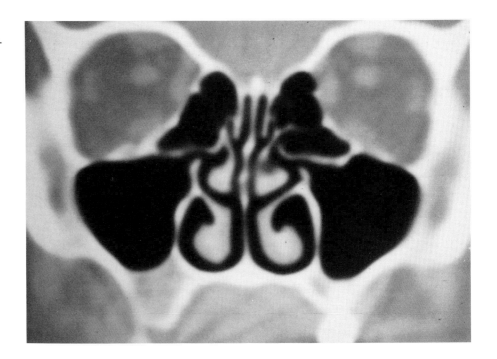

FIGURE 4.35 This is a section through the transition from the anterior to the posterior ethmoid. There are accessory maxillary sinus ostia (*arrows*) in the posterior fontanelles on both sides of the nose. In spite of this, there is pathology in the maxillary sinus (with disease of the anterior ethmoid, not shown in this scan). This is evidence that ventilation of the maxillary sinus through a nonphysiologic location is not alone sufficient to prevent disease. oa = accessory ostium.

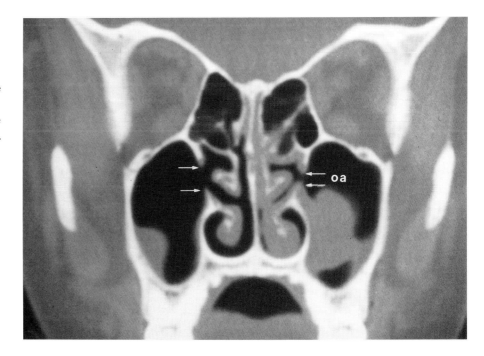

FIGURE 4.36 This section is through the anterior wall of the sphenoid sinus (*arrows*). The vomer is slightly pneumatized from the sphenoid. The posterior ends of the inferior and middle turbinates can be clearly seen, and the end of the superior turbinate is just barely visible.

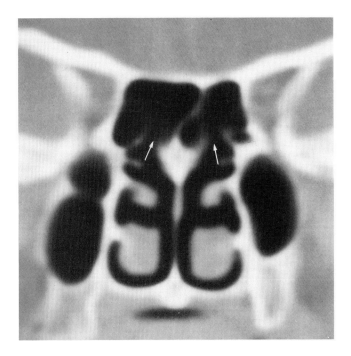

FIGURE 4.37 In this horizontal CT section, the *arrows* point to the natural ostia of the sphenoid sinus. Note how the pneumatization of the most posterior ethmoid cells extends far laterally and their topographic proximity to the optic nerve.

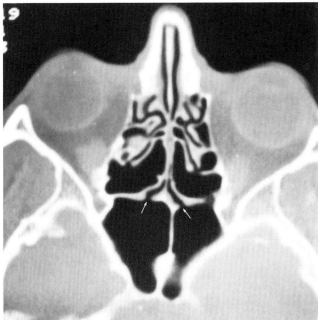

FIGURE 4.38   *A*, Extensive pneumatization of the vomer that clearly originates
in this case from *B*, the left sphenoid sinus (*arrow*). Note the extensively pneumatized clinoid process.

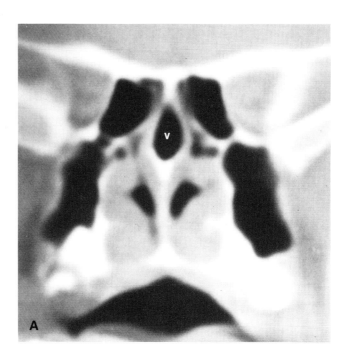

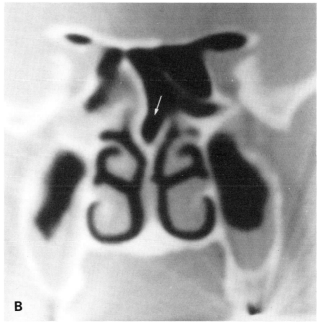

FIGURE 4.39 This is an example of an extensively pneumatized sphenoid sinus that extends far laterally into the skull and inferiorly into the pterygopalatine fossa.

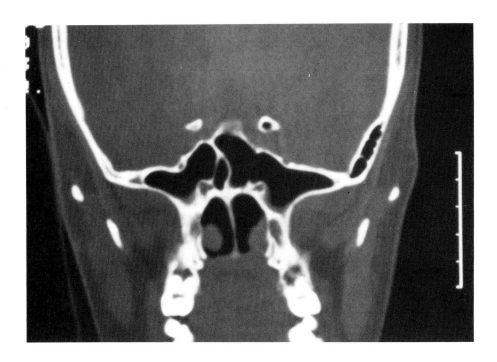

FIGURE 4.40 When a sphenoid sinus is as extensively pneumatized as seen in Figure 4.39, the internal carotid artery may traverse the lumen of the sphenoid sinus almost without any bony covering. On the right side a sphenoid sinus septum crosses laterally and inserts just above the internal carotid artery.
aci = internal carotid artery.

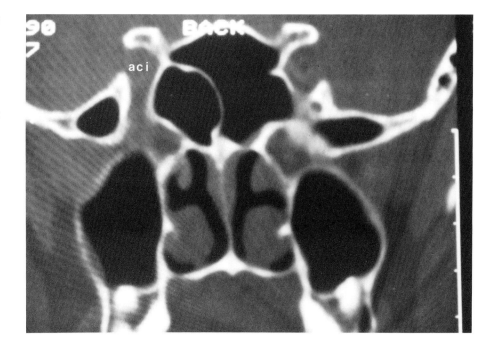

FIGURE 4.41 This patient was scheduled for surgery for a mucocele of the sphenoid sinus (*white arrows*). There is a thick bony septum that is attached directly to the wall of the internal carotid (*black arrows*). These findings are of paramount importance in determining the correct side of surgical approach.

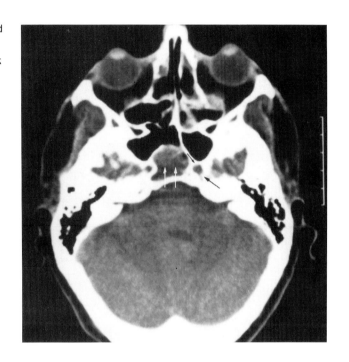

FIGURE 4.42 In this patient, the sphenoid septum produces a marked asymmetry, with the left sphenoid sinus being substantially smaller than the right. Below the roof of the sphenoid sinus, the septum divides and inserts bilaterally on the bony bulges covering the optic nerves (*arrows*).

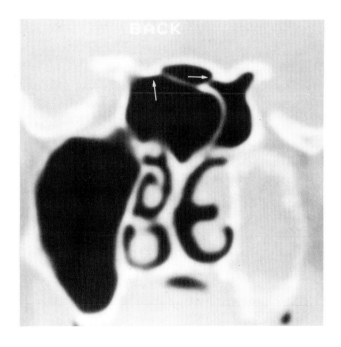

FIGURE 4.43 In this axial CT scan, the most posterior cells of the posterior ethmoid are particularly well pneumatized and extend laterally beyond the sphenoid. This results in very close proximity to the optic nerve. When such "Onodi cells" are present, the surgeon must be very careful to open the sphenoid sinus as far medially (adjacent to the septum) and as inferiorly as possible. The *arrows* indicate the direction from which the optic nerve is most prone to injury during the endoscopic sinus surgical procedures.

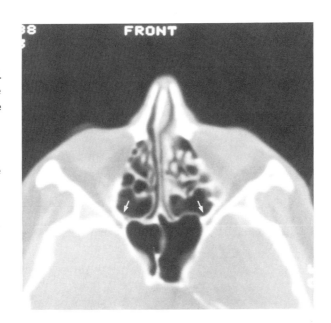

FIGURE 4.44 In this axial scan there has been an unusually extensive pneumatization of the sphenoid. The sphenoid sinus extends anteriorly and inferiorly and is in contact with the most posterior, medial part of the maxillary sinus. Note the asymmetry of the sphenoid sinus septum. sm = maxillary sinus.

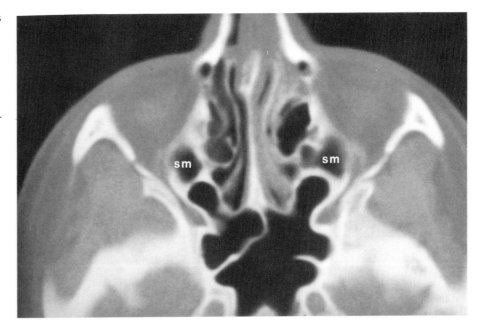

FIGURE 4.45 *A*, This axial CT section cuts a few millimeters below the lamina cribrosa. The anterior ethmoid is diseased. The difficulty with this section is that in sections that cut through the lamina cribrosa, or just cranial to it, the olfactory bulb and the structures of the olfactory fossa have the same density as inflammatory mucous membrane changes and thus these important structures cannot be distinguished from inflammatory changes with any degree of certainty. In isolated mucous membrane swellings in the olfactory region of the nose, the margins of the olfactory region can also not be determined with any precision in this type of section. *B*, In this case, there was a meningoencephalocele of the right anterior ethmoid that had penetrated the right cranial cavity through the frontal recess. A definitive diagnosis was only made on the basis of the coronal sections. fo = olfactory fossa; ro = rima olfactoria; and mec = meningoencephalocele.

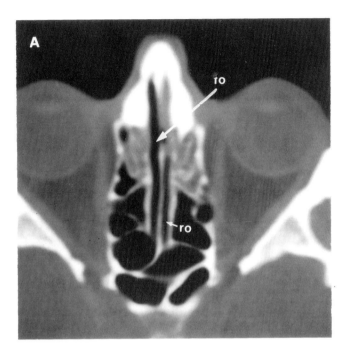

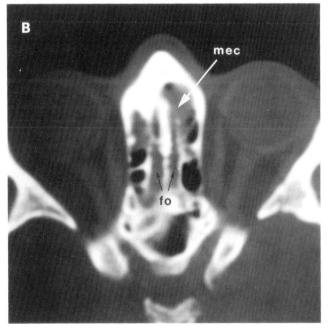

Preoperative Considerations

In a review of the tomograms or CT scans immediately prior to surgery, the surgeon should direct his or her attention to the following areas depending on the suspected pathology and the surgical procedure planned:

What is the condition of the ethmoid infundibulum?

- Is it almost atelectatic?
- Is the uncinate process immediately adjacent to the lamina papyracea or is the infundibulum wide?
- At what angle does the uncinate process stand to the lamina papyracea?
- Will I be able to resect the uncinate process directly at its anterior attach-

ment, or is there a real risk of injuring the orbit by carrying the knife too far laterally because of the narrowness of the infundibulum?

- Would it be safer in the given case to resect the uncinate process "in strips" from its free posterior margin anteriorly?

What are the relationships of the uncinate process superiorly, particularly to the frontal recess?

- Is there a recessus terminalis?
- Can I see whether the frontal recess opens medially or laterally into the uncinate process?

- What is the position of the frontal sinus?
- Is it symmetrical?

Is the ethmoidal bulla small or large?

- Is it pneumatized?
- Is there a lateral sinus?
- What is the relationship of the medial wall of the orbit to the middle turbinate?

- Can it be distinguished, does it bulge unusually strongly against the ethmoid?
- Are there bony defects from a previous operation?

Are there abnormalities in the course of the roof of the ethmoid?

- Can the bony margins be identified precisely?
- To what extent does the roof of the ethmoid project over the cribriform plate?
- Is the olfactory fossa shallow or deep?

- Do the ethmoidal cells extend supraorbitally?
- Are the right and left sides symmetrical?

What is the relationship of the posterior ethmoid to the sphenoid sinus?

- Are there Onodi cells?

- Is the optic nerve involved with them?

To what extent is the sphenoid pneumatized?

- Are the internal carotid artery and the optic nerve prominent and is there a suspicion that their bony cover may be dehiscent?
- Is the clinoid process well pneumatized, i.e., should I expect a

deep recess between the carotid artery and the optic nerve?
- What is the course of the sphenoid septa?
- Are there bony attachments over the carotid and the optic nerve?

If the patient had previous surgery:

- What was removed?
- Can I identify the middle turbinate or its remnants?
- Is there evidence of a bony defect or

scar formation in the lamina papyracea, the periorbita and/or the roof of the ethmoid, the dura and cribriform plate?

The surgeon should make it a habit to look at these points on the preoperative X-ray tomographs in the form of a regular "checklist."

Chapter 5

ENDOSCOPIC AND RADIOLOGIC DIAGNOSIS

In our institution, diagnostic nasal endoscopy is a routine component of the clinical evaluation of every patient with evident or suspected disease of the nose and paranasal sinuses. The endoscope helps the examiner recognize changes that may remain hidden from the naked eye or even from inspection with the microscope. As a result of the endoscopic examination, provisional diagnoses may be made, confirmed, expanded, or revised. The endoscopic examination also assists the otolaryngologist in deciding whether local and/or systemic drug therapy may be promising or whether surgical intervention is indicated. The decision to investigate the patient further with tomography or CT scan is usually based on a combination of the history and the endoscopic findings.

A primary acute sinusitis is not normally an indication for a CT scan. However, if there is evidence of complications such as periorbital abscess or worse, of incipient intracerebral complications, and antibiotic therapy does not provide prompt and definite improvement, tomography should be performed prior to surgical intervention. It is a general rule that every patient scheduled for an endoscopic surgical procedure *must* have a preoperative CT scan or tomogram. While this adds a significant cost factor, in our view it is mandatory, not only for medicolegal reasons (see Chapter 13). In a patient with a history of chronic or recurrent sinusitis over a period of months, or even years, that keeps flaring up despite a variety of medical therapies, tomography should be performed, if diagnostic endoscopy reveals changes in the lateral wall of the nose that might only be improved by surgery. Since a number of diseases of the lateral wall of the nose can not always be recognized and identified by endoscopy, we perform tomography even when the endoscopic findings are unremarkable, provided that the history and physical examination suggest the presence of some disease in the area of the ethmoid sinuses.

CT scans or tomograms should be done in cases where the patient has a history of recurrent frontal or maxillary sinusitis treated repeatedly by conservative means and where numerous X-rays showed opacification of the involved sinus. Tomography can frequently demonstrate predisposing anatomic variations or disease in key sites that can then be treated by a targeted, minimally invasive endoscopic procedure.

The tomogram or CT scan should be scheduled so that, if possible, it falls into a relatively disease-free period. Our intent is not to demonstrate diffusely swollen mucous membranes, retention of secretions, or even to diagnose an empyema in one of the larger paranasal sinuses, but rather to document the underlying changes in the anterior ethmoid as clearly and accurately as possible. It is particularly important in cases of chronic or recurrent sinusitis that the patient's infection be treated with local and systemic medical therapy and "improved" as much as possible prior to radiologic investigation. We have repeatedly observed that in patients who had their tomograms performed during a period of maximal symptoms, even the most massive changes in the maxillary sinus, which appeared radiologically as completely opaque, were markedly improved in a very short period of time by minor changes in ventilation and drainage resulting from preoperative medical therapy. Maxillary sinus endoscopy frequently shows perfectly normal conditions even when 10 days earlier tomography showed marked soft tissue swelling, cyst formation, or even total opacification of the maxillary sinus. These findings suggest that mucosal changes in the maxillary sinus are not only highly reversible, but that mucosal pathology can appear very rapidly and may revert to normal with equal speed, and that one should not establish the need for surgery on the radiographic appearance of a maxillary sinus alone.

If the patient needs surgery again, e.g., for a recurrent polyposis, and if the pathologic changes are evident on endoscopy, we do not routinely require a repeat tomogram or CT scan. Obviously the previous films must be available to the surgeon: with these in hand, the surgeon can orient on any anatomic variation, particularly of the roof of the ethmoid, and, along with the operative report of the first operation, form a mental picture of the previous surgical procedure. In these cases it is sufficient to order a survey film to evaluate the secondary changes in the frontal and maxillary sinuses.

The situation is different when either the nasal endoscopic examination reveals no visible pathology, if there are complications, or if the patient has undergone the previous operation in another hospital. In these cases a new tomogram or CT scan is ordered.

Tomography and CT scans are also very helpful in instructing and advising the patient. With the serial images, it is usually possible to explain the pathophysiologic relationships, even to a lay person and it is relatively easy to explain the proposed surgical procedure. In addition, by showing the obvious proximity of the orbits, the skull base, etc. these images are useful to demonstrate the potential dangers of both the disease itself and the operative procedure.

PREPARATION FOR DIAGNOSTIC ENDOSCOPY

The nasal mucosa is sprayed with a mixture of topical anesthetic and mild vasoconstrictor in equal parts (we use 2 percent Pontocaine and oxymetazoline hydrochloride). The examiner waits for a few minutes to allow vasoconstriction and anesthesia to take effect before commencing the examination. For the first examination, we prefer to use a mild vasoconstrictor rather than adrenaline, since these mild vasoconstrictors do not alter the color and the surface structure of the mucosa as much and these features may be of diagnostic significance.

Surface anesthesia can also be achieved with other substances such as cocaine in liquid or flake form. If cocaine flakes are used, they are usually put in place with a nasal cotton tipped applicator. The flakes should be applied primarily at those sites to be exposed to the greatest pressure by the endoscope, the aspirator, or any other instrument that may be used during the procedure. These locations include any septal deviation, the base and free edge of the middle turbinate, and the entrance of the middle meatus. The floor of the nose and the nasal septum to be in contact with the endoscope on its way to the nasopharynx as well as the sphenoethmoidal recess should also be anesthetized.

For the examination, the physician sits at the patient's right. The patient is in the supine position facing the examiner. We prefer this position to the sitting position because the patient is more relaxed and because the head, while moveable, is well supported in two planes. This minimizes the risk of mucosal injury due to an unintentional or reflex movement of the head.

Table 5.1 displays the basic instruments required for a diagnostic endoscopic examination. The maxillary sinus trocar is included, although maxillary sinus endoscopy is *not a routine component* of the diagnostic endoscopic procedure (see the section: Endoscopy of the Maxillary Sinus).

TABLE 5.1   Basic Instruments for Diagnostic Nasal Endoscopy

Nasal Endoscopes
Essential
   30 degree lens, 4 mm with handle
Useful additional lenses
   30 degree lens, 2.7 mm
   70 degree lens, 2.7 or 4 mm

Instruments
1 Freer elevator
1 flexible sound
1 assortment of suction tips
  (rigid and soft)
1 maxillary sinus trocar with sheath
1 biopsy forceps

Technique of Diagnostic Endoscopy

The endoscopic examination of the nasal cavity and the lateral wall of the nose is usually accomplished in three steps.

1. The first step consists of an inspection of the nasal vestibule, the nasopharynx, and the inferior nasal meatus.
2. This is followed by an examination of the sphenoethmoidal recess and the superior nasal meatus.
3. Examination of the middle meatus.

The best instrument for diagnostic nasal endoscopy is the 4 mm external diameter 30 degree nasal endoscope. This endoscope has enough direct forward vision to permit introduction in the direction of the main axis and thus avoid injury to the mucous membranes. It also has just enough of a viewing angle to permit a good view of the meatus of the nose and a general survey of the nasopharynx. If the passages are very narrow, a 2.7 mm endoscope may be used with a 30 degree or 70 degree lens angle.

As long as there is no need for additional instrumentation (e.g., an aspirator or biopsy forceps) the endoscope can be guided with both hands. If a second instrument is required, the hand position illustrated in Figure 5.1 should be used: the endoscope is held between thumb and forefinger of the left hand, which rests lightly on the cheek and bridge of the nose of the patient (Fig. 5.2).

Before use, the endoscope must be treated to prevent fogging of the lens. The lens should be warmed and briefly dipped into an antifog solution, e.g., Ultrastop. A small glass cup holds the antifog solution (Fig. 5.3). A small piece of cotton placed in the cup prevents injury to the endoscope as it is carefully dipped into the solution.

A thin film of antifog solution must remain on the lens in order to assure freedom from fogging.

When the endoscope is introduced, the examiner must take care to avoid injury to the mucous membranes, making every effort to keep the lens away from the mucous membranes throughout the entire procedure. Accumulations of mucus and other secretions can usually be easily bypassed or removed by suction. If mucous secretions come into contact with the lens, withdrawing the endoscope slightly may permit the mucus to slide off the lens. It is not always necessary to completely remove the endoscope from the nose and wipe the lens.

FIGURE 5.1 This schematic drawing illustrates the proper technique for holding the endoscope with the patient in the supine position.

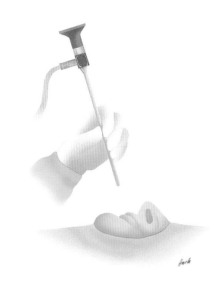

FIGURE 5.2 The correct technique for holding the endoscope and the suction tip during diagnostic endoscopy.

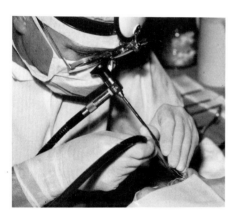

FIGURE 5.3 The acrylic container with antifog solution.

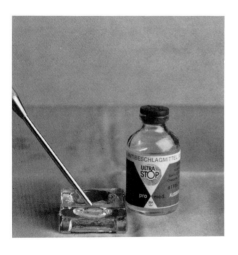

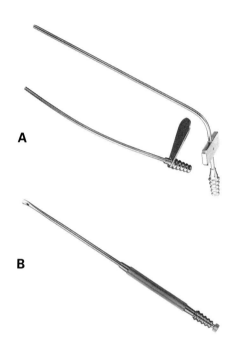

FIGURE 5.4 *A*, Curved and angled nasal suction tips. *B*, Freer elevator with integrated suction channel.

Prior to commencing the examination, the physician and the patient should agree on a signal that the patient can give, should he feel a sneeze or a cough coming on. This signal allows the examiner to withdraw the endoscope and any other instruments quickly from the nose so that injuries due to involuntary sneezing and coughing can be avoided.

Endoscopic examination of the nose should be performed in a systematic manner. The first look provides a general survey and orientation within the nose. The examiner should first look in the direction of the middle meatus, without actually approaching it too closely. This provides an excellent overview of the nose and allows recognition of anatomic or pathologic abnormalities, e.g., a deviation of the nasal septum, ridges and spicules can be evaluated as to their size and location. The appearance, color, and state of engorgement of the nasal mucous membranes should be noted as well as the presence of any abnormal mucus or purulent material. The width and patency of the nasal vestibule should be noted.

The foamy "secretions" frequently encountered in the narrow spaces of the nose following the application of the topical anesthetic spray should be removed with an aspirator, introduced parallel to the endoscope. For this we use the same nasal aspirators that are used during endoscopic sinus surgical procedures (Fig. 5.4). A disposable polyethylene catheter may be used for cleaning the nasal cavities.

In the next step of the examination, the nasopharynx is reached by passing the endoscope through the nasal cavity. Depending on the anatomic configuration of the nasal cavities, this can usually be achieved without difficulty by advancing the endoscope below the inferior turbinate. If there is not enough room between the inferior turbinate and the nasal septum, the endoscope is advanced along the floor of the inferior meatus. The ostium of the eustachian tube can be used as a landmark in the nasopharynx (Fig. 5.5). Its function can also be readily observed when the patient swallows on command. At this point, abnormalities in the transportation of secretions may be seen, e.g., pathologic secretions that lie centrally over the orifice of the eustachian tube or that remain attached in Rosenmüller's fossa (Fig. 5.6). A slight medial rotation of the endoscope allows an inspection of the posterior wall of the nasopharynx and the roof of the palate with the 30 degree lens. In the nasopharynx, the examiner can assess the shape, size, and inflammation of the adenoidal tissues, or see the scars where this tissue had been removed. Occasionally a small slit or round opening is seen that enters into a small depression or even into a slightly superiorly directed passage. This is the remnant of Rathke's pouch. At times a drop of a viscous secretion can be seen in such a Rathke's pocket. If the endoscope is rotated further medially, one can see the ostium of the tube on the *opposite* side. In this fashion, it is possible to inspect the entire nasopharynx with a 30 degree lens even when a marked septal deviation or other pathology makes it impossible to introduce the endoscope through the other side. The endoscope can now be rotated a full 360 degrees around its longitudinal axis, allowing inspection of the posterior aspect of the uvula and the nasopharyngeal surface of the palate.

Pulling the endoscope back a few millimeters and rotating it fully permits evaluation of the entire margin of the choana and the posterior end of the turbinates.

The examiner should keep in mind during this examination of the nasopharynx, that the wide-angle effect of the lens makes all curved surfaces appear much flatter in the frontal view. Thus abnormalities that are raised *above the level of the mucous membranes*, but show no alteration in color or structure, may be overlooked. For an accurate examination, the nasopharynx should be inspected in addition from the oropharynx with either a mirror or a 90 degree endoscope. The tangential view over the surface of the nasopharyngeal mucous membranes obtained with these techniques allows discrete elevations to be recognized with a greater degree of accuracy.

FIGURE 5.5　The position of the endoscope while examining the nasopharnyx. The left eustachian tube orifice is immediately distal to the tip of the endoscope.

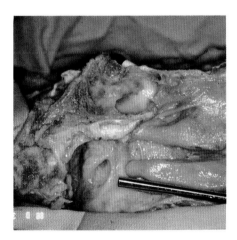

FIGURE 5.6　Endoscopic view of the left eustachian tube orifice during swallowing in a patient with AIDS. The lumen of the tube is closed. The discreet, reddish mucous membrane changes turned out to be Kaposi's sarcoma. RM = Rosenmüller's fossa.

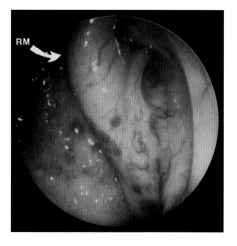

If the examiner now pulls the endoscope back, a look under the inferior turbinate can be attempted. The opening of the nasolacrimal duct, Hasner's valve, may be observed within a few millimeters from the highest point of the roof of the inferior nasal meatus or at the transition to the lateral wall. This opening of the nasolacrimal duct may be round in shape although it may have almost any form including an almost invisible slit hidden behind a fold of mucosa. Once the orifice of the nasolacrimal duct is identified, its patency can be assessed by instilling a drop of fluorescein into the conjunctival sac and observing the emergence of the dye in the inferior meatus. The easiest way to identify the opening of the nasolacrimal duct is to put light pressure on the lacrimal sac at the medial angle of the eyelid with a finger. This pressure usually expresses a few tears from the opening of the nasolacrimal duct that can be seen easily with the endoscope (Fig. 5.7).

Depending on the shape of the lower turbinate, entry into the inferior nasal meatus may be difficult, particularly if the horizontal part of the turbinate is small and the vertical part reaches down almost to the floor of the meatus or is curled up laterally. Careful elevation of the free margin of the inferior turbinate with a Freer elevator, combined, if necessary, with the use of a thinner 2.7 mm diameter endoscope usually permits a reasonable view in these cases. Nasoantral windows from previous operations can thus be evaluated for patency and even the maxillary sinus can be directly inspected.

In the second step of the diagnostic endoscopic examination, the endoscope is advanced medial to the middle turbinate in the direction of the nasopharynx to identify the posterior end of the middle turbinate. Above this the view should be directed superiorly toward the sphenoethmoidal recess. Laterally, the inferior free margin of the superior turbinate can be seen. Underneath this are the superior nasal meatus and the cells of the posterior ethmoid opening into it. Occasionally there may be a supreme (fourth) turbinate under which posterior ethmoid cells may open, too. The posterior wall of the sphenoethmoidal recess is formed by the anterior surface of the sphenoid bone. The oval or slit-like opening of the sphenoid sinus can usually be found in the medial part of the posterior wall of the sphenoethmoidal recess near the posterior insertion of the nasal septum. If the passage is very narrow or if there is evident pathology, it may be difficult to positively identify the ostium of the sphenoid sinus with the endoscope. If the sphenoid sinus is diseased, the presence of abnormal secretions of the anterior surface of the sphenoid may indicate the location of the ostium of the sphenoid sinus (Fig. 5.8 to 5.11).

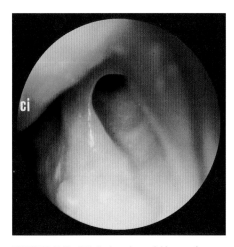

FIGURE 5.7 Well developed Hasner's valve (ostium of the nasolacrimal duct) in a left inferior meatus. ci = inferior turbinate.

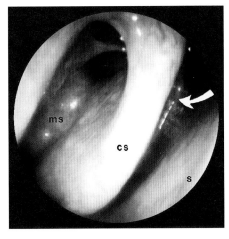

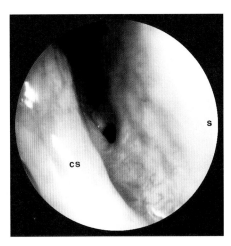

FIGURE 5.8   A view through a 30 degree lens into the right superior meatus. The opening of the posterior ethmoid cells can be seen. There are thickened secretions in the sphenoethmoidal recess medial to the superior turbinate (*arrow*). cs = superior turbinate; ms = superior meatus; and s = nasal septum.

FIGURE 5.9   View of a right sphenoethmoidal recess showing the ostium of the sphenoid sinus. cs = superior turbinate and s = nasal septum.

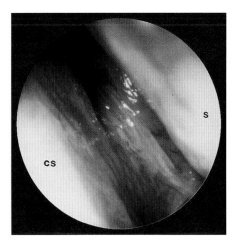

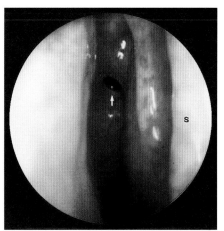

FIGURE 5.10   Tenacious secretions suggesting sphenoid sinus disease coming from the right sphenoethmoidal recess. cs = superior turbinate and s = nasal septum.

FIGURE 5.11   After the secretions were aspirated, a narrowed sphenoid sinus ostium can be seen (*arrow*). s = nasal septum.

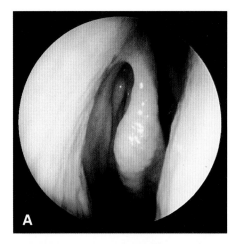

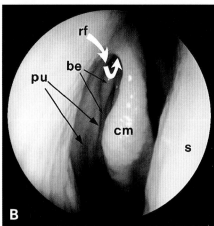

The third step of the diagnostic endoscopic examination is the exploration of the middle meatus and within it, the adjacent lateral nasal wall. This is accomplished by advancing the 30 degree endoscope to the entrance of the middle meatus and identifying the structures in this area. Viewed from the front, the examiner can usually readily identify the head of the middle turbinate, the uncinate process and, depending upon the presence of pathologic changes, parts of the ethmoidal bulla (Fig. 5.12). Occasionally it is possible to enter the middle meatus directly from the front with the endoscope and view the inferior and superior portions of the hiatus semilunaris, the sinus of the turbinate, or even the frontal recess. If the hiatus semilunaris superior is wide, it may be possible to look into the lateral sinus and see the ridge of the anterior ethmoid artery on the roof of the ethmoid (Fig. 5.13).

If it is not possible to enter the middle meatus with the 4-mm endoscope from anteriorly (Fig. 5.14), the following options are available:

It may be possible to gently displace the middle turbinate medially as far as its elasticity permits with a Freer elevator or a thin aspirator. In doing this, the examiner should take care not to fracture the middle turbinate.

FIGURE 5.12 *A* and *B*, View into a normal right middle meatus. The uncinate process and its posterior free edge, and the anterior surface of the ethmoidal bulla can be seen. The *white arrows* indicate the path into the frontal recess behind the insertion of the middle turbinate. rf = frontal recess; be = ethmoidal bulla; pu = uncinate process; cm = middle turbinate; and s = nasal septum

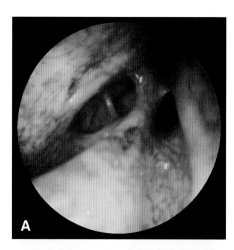

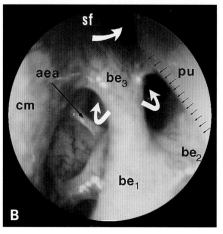

FIGURE 5.13 *A* and *B*, View into a left frontal recess through a 30 degree, wide-angle endoscope. The anterior wall of the bulla ethmoidalis passes superiorly into a bulla lamella. The bulla lamella is attached medially to the insertion of the middle turbinate and superiorly to the skull, although not along its entire length. There is a marked lateral sinus between the bulla itself and the roof of the ethmoid. The lateral sinus opens medially and laterally to the bulla lamella (*angled arrows*). The bony channel of the anterior ethmoidal artery can be seen clearly. Superiorly, the frontal recess narrows toward the ostium of the frontal sinus (*arrow*). The *thin arrows* point to the free posterior margin of the uncinate process. be₁ = anterior wall of the bulla ethmoidalis; be₂ = the insertion of the bulla ethmoidalis onto the lamina papyracea; be₃ = bulla lamella; cm = middle turbinate; aea = anterior ethmoidal artery; sf = frontal sinus; and pu = uncinate process.

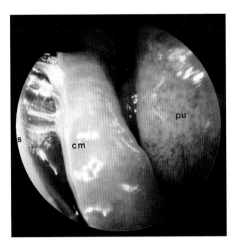

FIGURE 5.14 View from ahead and below into a left middle meatus that was too narrow to be entered from the front with a 4-mm diameter endoscope. Note the uncinate process folded over far medially. s = nasal septum; pu = uncinate process; be = ethmoidal bulla; and cm = middle turbinate.

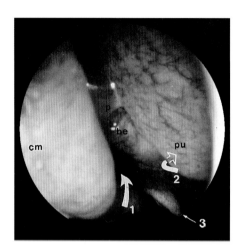

FIGURE 5.15 Inspection of the same meatus from the back and below with a 30 degree endoscope. The ethmoidal bulla can be seen clearly. A small, glassy polyp arises from its anterior surface. Between the bulla and the free posterior margin of the uncinate process is the entry into the ethmoid infundibulum, through the hiatus semilunaris (arrow 2). The middle turbinate (and its free inferior margin) is rolled far laterally and thus enfolds the structures of the lateral wall of the nose. This produces a very narrow turbinate sinus (sinus conchae, arrow 1). Deep in the meatus there is some foamy pontocaine spray (arrow 3). cm = middle turbinate; p = polyp; pu = uncinate process; and be = ethmoidal bulla.

The middle meatus can also be examined through a trocar sheath, as described by Messerklinger: The endoscope is placed into the trocar sheath which is then introduced into the nose. The flat lip of the trocar sheath can frequently be slipped under the middle turbinate and through careful rotatory movements advanced into the middle meatus. The endoscope is then advanced through the sheath and an unobstructed view of the middle meatus obtained.

The technique that we use most frequently in these cases is to inspect the middle meatus with the endoscope from the back (Fig. 5.15). The middle meatus is usually wider at the back than the front. The 30 degree endoscope is introduced past the middle turbinate posteriorly and is then laterally and superiorly rotated under the free margin of the turbinate. This usually allows the instrument to slip into the most posterior portion of the middle meatus. Careful, slow retraction of the endoscope permits inspection of the middle meatus from the rear forward. The first structure to be seen is the horizontal part of the middle turbinate (i.e., the posterior third of the basal lamella), which here forms the roof of the middle meatus and curves upward behind the ethmoidal bulla as the basal lamella to separate the anterior and posterior ethmoid sinuses. Moving forward, the bulge of the ethmoidal bulla can be seen. Between the ethmoidal bulla and the vertical part of the middle turbinate, one can look into the sinus of the Turbinate and further anteriorly into a superior hiatus semilunaris, which opens into a lateral sinus and eventually leads behind the bulla ethmoidalis. A slight rotation of the 30 degree lens laterally brings the hiatus semilunaris into view between the anterior surface of the bulla and the free posterior margin of the uncinate process. Anatomic conditions permitting, the endoscope can be directed slightly upward, the hiatus semilunaris can be followed, and the frontal recess viewed (see Fig. 5.13). The ostia and openings of the cells and spaces visible here depend on the status of the uncinate process and the lamella of the bulla (see Chapter 3).

Occasionally, a direct view into the maxillary sinus is possible provided that there is an accessory ostium in the anterior or posterior nasal fontanelle. The natural ostium of the maxillary sinus is only rarely visible from the middle meatus. It is sometimes possible to see the ostium in the depths of the ethmoidal infundibulum through a wide hiatus semilunaris from the back with a 70 degree lens.

Since the 70 degree lens does not permit forward vision and thus presents a much greater danger of injuring the nasal mucous membranes when the scope is advanced, we use the following technique:

A trocar sheath, slipped over a 0 or 30 degree lens is introduced into the nose. Under direct vision, the trocar sheath is brought to the location to be examined and fixed while the guide scope is removed and a 70 degree lens is introduced, without ever having been in contact with the mucous membranes. Examination of the area of interest may now proceed.

Because this procedure requires greater pressure on the middle turbinate or the nasal septum, it may be necessary to use nasal pledgets in addition to the spray in order to achieve more complete anesthesia. We use small cotton applicators that are dipped into a mixture of 2 percent Pontocaine and 1:1,000 epinephrine (4–5 parts Pontocaine to 1 part epinephrine). The excess anesthetic solution is squeezed out and the pledgets are placed into and around the middle meatus and left there for 5 to 10 minutes. Following this, contact with the endoscope or other instrument is usually no longer painful.

In cases in which a biopsy is contemplated, this form of anesthesia may also be indicated. When the nasopharynx is to be biopsied and the nasal cavities are narrow, we advance the endoscope on one side of the nose and the biopsy forceps on the other.

If diagnostic endoscopy is indicated in a small child, the procedure should be performed under sedation or general anesthesia, depending upon the patient's ability to cooperate. Depending on the type of general anesthesia administered, epinephrine may or may not be used for topical vasoconstriction. In these cases the proposed procedure must be discussed with the anesthesiologist.

For endoscopy of the sphenoid sinus, see Chapters 7 and 9.

Nasal Septal Deviation

A marked deviation of a portion or of the entire nasal septum may cause not only obstructed nasal breathing, but also disease within the lateral nasal wall and consecutively, within the paranasal sinuses. This is particularly true if the septal deviation forces the middle turbinate laterally and thus narrows the entrance into the middle meatus.

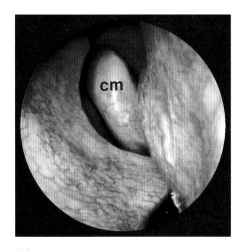

FIGURE 5.16 A large spur penetrates the lateral wall of this left nose. Such spurs usually do not require a complete septoplasty. After dissection of the mucous membrane, the spur can be chiseled off. The mucous membrane flaps are then replaced and secured with a merocel sponge. cm = middle turbinate.

Septal ridges and spurs can cause severe headaches and other functional disturbances and predispose the patient to recurrent sinusitis. This is the case particularly if these structures surround or come into intimate contact with the turbinates or other areas of the lateral wall of the nose or project far into the middle meatus.

However, clinical experience also shows that patients with massive septal deviation, ridging, or spurring may have no symptoms or only minimal complaints attributable to these changes (Figs. 5.16 to 5.19). They may instead have symptoms on the other side, i.e., on the side with the wider nasal passage (Fig. 5.18). For this reason we have become reluctant to correct septal deviation, except in extreme cases and then only if there is a clear connection between the deviation of the nasal septum and the patient's clinical symptoms. Our experience has shown that patients became free of symptoms following the correction of their ethmoid problems, *without* having the (occasionally severe) nasal septal deviation corrected at the same time. We *cannot* therefore support the dictum that *every* endonasal surgical procedure on the paranasal sinuses be preceded by correction of any pre-existing deviation of the nasal septum.

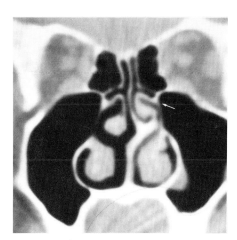

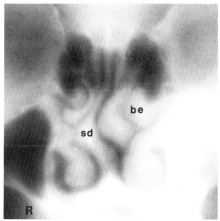

FIGURE 5.17 Radiograph of the patient shown in Figure 5.16. The septal spur can be seen plainly. It enfolds the middle turbinate from below. *Arrow* points to the insertion of the middle turbinate (the basal lamella) on the medial wall of the maxillary sinus.

FIGURE 5.18 Right nasal septal deviation. The complaints of this patient were located on the left side because of ethmoid and recurrent maxillary sinus disease. The left infundibulum is obstructed and the maxillary sinus is homogeneously opacified. sd = septal deviation and be = ethmoidal bulla.

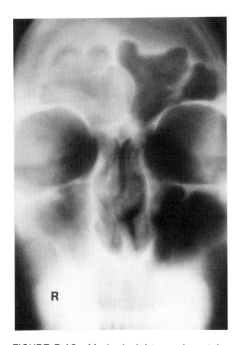

FIGURE 5.19 Marked, right nasal septal deviation. In this patient the septal deviation contributed to paranasal sinus disease. The diseased frontal recess and the consequently diseased right frontal sinus can be seen.

Our procedure in cases of unequivocally established sinus disease is therefore as follows:

If it is possible to pass a 4-mm diameter operating nasal endoscope beyond the septal deviation into the middle nasal meatus or at least visualize the anterior middle meatus and there is enough room to introduce the required surgical instruments, we first correct the ethmoid problems surgically. Only if the endoscope and the instruments *cannot* be introduced through the narrowing caused by the septal deviation, will we perform the septoplasty at the first sitting and then wait until the nose has fully recovered from this procedure before operating on the ethmoid sinuses. If the sinus complaints persist unchanged following correction of the nasal septal deviation and a repeat diagnostic endoscopy still shows the characteristic findings of ethmoid disease, then the ethmoid problems are corrected endoscopically at a second sitting. The only exception is the patient with severe polyposis and a significantly obstructing deviation of the nasal septum. In these cases we usually perform both procedures at the same time (Figs. 5.19 to 5.21). In our institution the indications for nasal septal surgery have decreased significantly since the introduction of endoscopic sinus surgery.

Smaller septal ridges and spurs that seem to be part of the disease process or which interfere with direct surgical access to the middle meatus can be resected directly without performing a complete septoplasty (Figs. 5.16 and 5.17) (see Chapter 7). Posteriorly, the septum may become pneumatized from the sphenoid sinus (Fig. 5.22).

FIGURE 5.20 The patent window (fenestra) in the inferior meatus can be seen clearly (*large arrows*). The ongoing symptoms on the left side are the consequence of involvement of the anterior ethmoid. *Thin arrows* indicate a polyp in the frontal recess. *Dotted line* shows the lateral contour of the uncinate process. sd = septal deviation; pu = uncinate process; and i = infundibulum.

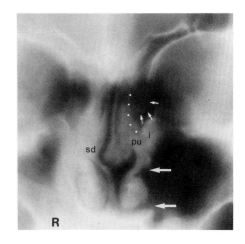

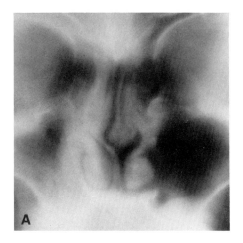
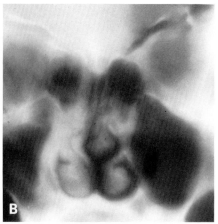
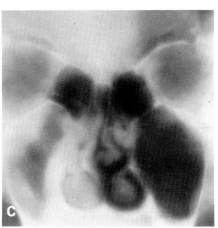

FIGURE 5.21 *A* to *C* are the same patient. The middle meatus and the right nasal cavity are significantly narrowed and the middle turbinate is compressed against the lateral nasal wall. The ethmoid infundibulum is affected, the maxillary sinus is circumferentially opacified. On the left, there is a small concha bullosa in the middle turbinate. The ethmoid infundibulum is also affected on the left side. The patient has previously had a left inferior meatal antrostomy created.

FIGURE 5.22 Pneumatization of the posterosuperior portion of the nasal septum. In most cases, this pneumatization originates from the sphenoid sinus.

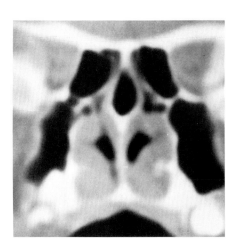

Concha Bullosa

Pneumatization (aeration) of the middle turbinate (and less commonly of the superior turbinate) can be clinically significant and is known as concha bullosa. A concha bullosa usually occurs bilaterally, however the degree of pneumatization may be variable not only from patient to patient, but also from one side to the other of a given patient. Minimal pneumatization may appear on only one section of the tomogram or CT scan. In contrast, the degree of pneumatization may be so severe that both middle turbinates, expanded like balloons, come into intimate and extensive contact with large areas of the nasal septum and the entire lateral wall of the nose (Fig. 5.23). In rare cases, a massive concha bullosa may completely obstruct the nasal vestibule.

Large differences in the degree of pneumatization between both sides are found most commonly in those patients who also have a marked deviation of the nasal septum (Fig. 5.24 and 5.25). In viewing the radiographs of such patients, it is difficult to avoid the suspicion that the concha bullosa arose "e vacuo," i.e., that the pneumatization appeared because there was an available, unfilled space that "provoked" its development. This suggests that the deviation of the nasal septum was responsible for the development of the concha bullosa.

We believe, however, that the concha bullosa and the septal deviation are only the coincidental appearance of two anatomic variants, since in many cases of marked septal deviation, the pneumatization of the turbinates is bilateral. In these cases, the concha bullosa on the side of the deviation is smaller (see Figs. 5.24 and 5.36), simply because there is more space for the turbinate to expand on the side away from the septal deviation. It seems to us unlikely that the extensive pneumatization of one middle turbinate could be the cause of the septal deviation, although this sequence of events can not be ruled out.

Clinical evidence suggests that pneumatization of the middle turbinate can continue in later life and does not necessarily cease at the end of the growth period. Many patients well past their 60th birthday present for the first time with symptoms of paranasal sinus disease as the result of a concha bullosa. In contrast, we have also seen conchae bullosae in children between 5 and 7 years of age. The pneumatization process apparently begins in middle age in some patients when there may be a renewed spurt of growth activity. This concept is unfortunately difficult to prove since there are few patients who have been followed with tomography over several decades. We do not know what stimuli initiate or control this process of pneumatization. Whether this process is similar to the hitherto unexplained formation of a pneumosinus dilatans, remains to be seen.

FIGURE 5.23 The huge conchae bullosae of both grossly enlarged middle turbinates almost fill completely the nasal cavity and come into contact with the nasal septum, the inferior turbinates, and the lateral wall of the nose. The *arrow* indicates the constricted ethmoidal infundibulum.

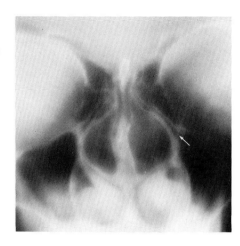

FIGURE 5.24 These conchae bullosae of both middle turbinates show pneumatization variation. The concha bullosa on the left is large, while that on the right is small. In spite of the right nasal septal deviation, the primary involvement of the ethmoid and maxillary sinus are on the left.

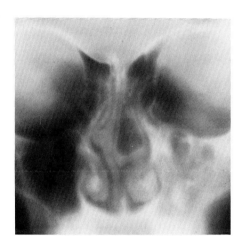

FIGURE 5.25 A concha bullosa on the left is combined with a nasal septal deviation and bilateral involvement of the anterior ethmoid.

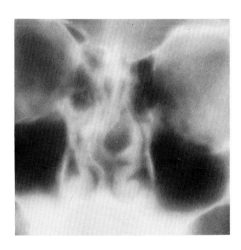

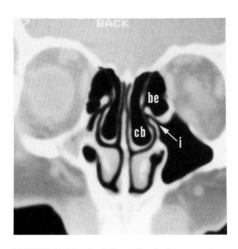

FIGURE 5.26 In this patient, the concha bullosa was pneumatized from the frontal recess and the lateral sinus. be = bulla ethmoidalis; cb = concha bullosa; and i = infundibulum.

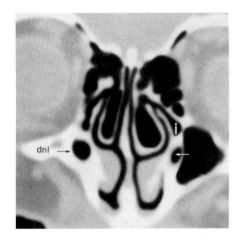

FIGURE 5.27 In this case, the concha bullosa opens into the middle meatus across from the hiatus semilunaris, i = infundibulum and dnl s = nasolac-rimal duct.

Pneumatization of the middle turbinate may originate from a variety of locations. In our experience, the most frequent site of origin is the frontal recess. Pneumatization may also originate in the agger nasi, which is itself usually pneumatized from the frontal recess, or from the lateral sinus (Figs. 5.26; 5.28; 5.30; and 5.31).

Pneumatization may also come directly from the middle meatus (Fig. 5.27), and finally, the *superior meatus* may intrude into the middle turbinate to such a degree that extensive pneumatization results. This type of concha bullosa was called an "interlaminary cell" by Grünwald. Figure 5.29 shows the early development of such an interlaminary cell.

In most cases a concha bullosa contains only a single air cell, although occasionally two and, very rarely, three air cells. These multiple air cells are usually located one behind the other. In these cases pneumatization does not necessarily originate from a single site. The anterior cell is usually pneumatized from the frontal recess and the posterior cell directly from the middle meatus. While these multiple cells may communicate, in most cases they are completely sealed off from each other.

Ventilation of the air cells within a concha bullosa comes from the area from which the pneumatization arose. Mucociliary transport is directed similarly. Thus the secretions from a concha bullosa pneumatized from the frontal recess are transported to the frontal recess where they join the regular transport pathway to the nasopharynx (see Chapter 2). This relationship indicates a reciprocal susceptibility: it is possible that a diseased frontal recess secondarily extend its disease into a connecting concha bullosa. Conversely, disease may spread from an infected concha bullosa to other areas of the ethmoid. This may explain the great variety of ways that pathologic entities can affect a concha bullosa ranging from a simple edema of the mucosal lining as part of a disease of the frontal recess; the formation of single or multiple polyps; the retention of secretions, with radiologic evidence of air fluid level (Fig. 5.34); empyemas; amorphous inspissated secretions; the formation of a mucocele or even a pyocele; and finally to fungal infections with the accumulation of mycotic concretions in the lumen of the turbinate itself (see Chapter 11).

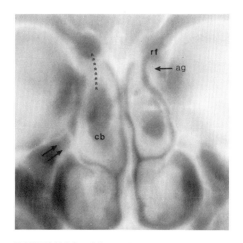

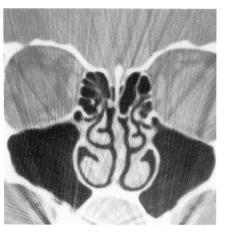

FIGURE 5.28 Bilaterally diseased concha bullosa. On the left side of the patient, an affected agger nasi cell constricts the opening of the frontal recess. On the right side, the opening of the concha bullosa into the frontal recess (*dotted line*) can be seen. *Double arrow* shows the right ethmoid infundibulum. Note: bilaterally, the reflexly swollen and enlarged inferior turbinates. After surgical management of the diseased concha bullosa, the inferior turbinates returned to normal. cb = concha bullosa; ag = agger nasi cell; and rf = frontal recess.

FIGURE 5.29 On the left side of the patient, the superior meatus enters the vertical lamella of the middle turbinate. There is a paradoxically bent middle turbinate on the right.

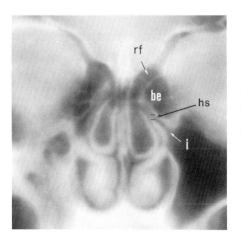

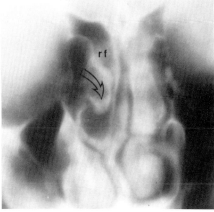

FIGURE 5.30 Pneumatization of the concha bullosa, originating in the frontal recess, can be clearly seen. rf = frontal recess; be = bulla ethmoidalis; hs = hiatus semilunaris; and i = infundibulum.

FIGURE 5.31 In this patient, a large ethmoidal bulla dips into a concha bullosa on the right side (*bent arrow*). rf = frontal recess.

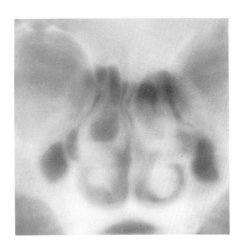

FIGURE 5.32 In this case, there is mucosal swelling inside the right concha bullosa, while polyps are present within the left concha bullosa.

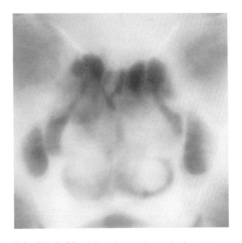

FIGURE 5.33 Massive polyposis is seen in the concha bullosa. The turbinate is almost unrecognizable on the tomogram.

In those patients who have extensive, diffuse, long-standing nasal polyposis, the recognition of a concha bullosa on a conventional tomogram may be very difficult, particularly in the older patient where the thin bony lamellae may be decalcified, thinned out by the pressure exerted by the polyps, or largely destroyed by the inflammatory process (Fig. 5.33). In such cases the definite diagnosis of a diseased concha bullosa may only be made at the time of surgery by an exploratory incision or sounding through the anterior wall of the middle turbinate with a curved blade.

The presence of a concha bullosa alone is not necessarily a pathologic finding. However, if combined with other anatomic abnormalities, such as a medially bent uncinate process or an enlarged ethmoidal bulla, even a small concha bullosa may produce a significant narrowing of the anterior and middle portion of the middle meatus. Large contact surfaces may appear that predispose to repeated and, later, persistent local complaints that may spread to involve the adjacent areas. If the pneumatization is extensive, a large concha bullosa may cause significant problems by its size alone, e.g., marked nasal obstruction (Figs. 5.16, 5.35, and 5.36). The disturbance to transportation of secretions that may result from extensive areas of mucosal contact may well be one of the major causes of the unpleasant postnasal drip of which many patients with large concha bullosa so frequently complain.

One frequently gets the impression that the bulging of the lateral lamella of the concha bullosa dents the lateral wall of the nose and displaces the uncinate process laterally. This may produce a narrowing, or even a complete blockage, of the hiatus semilunaris and the ethmoidal infundibulum. Figures 5.16, 5.19, 5.21A, and 5.35 to 5.37 show clearly that even a nondiseased concha bullosa may cause critical obstruction in the presence of otherwise unremarkable sections through the anterior ethmoid. In these cases, only a minimal amount of mucosal swelling, e.g., as the result of the mucosal cycle, a sudden change in temperature, a minor infection, or other slight irritation may partially or even completely close these narrow clefts with all the deleterious consequences on the ethmoid and on the large paranasal sinuses.

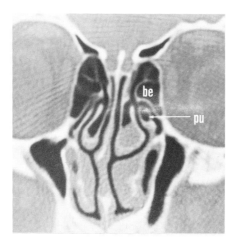

FIGURE 5.34   An air-fluid level is present in the concha bullosa on the left. A pneumatized uncinate process is an incidental finding. be = bulla ethmoidalis and pu = uncinate process.

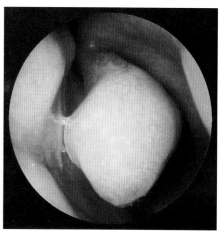

FIGURE 5.35   Endoscopic view of a large concha bullosa of the left middle turbinate.

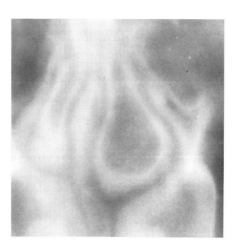

FIGURE 5.36   Tomogram of the patient in Figure 5.35. The constriction of the infundibulum can be seen clearly. At the time of tomography, the patient was essentially symptom-free.

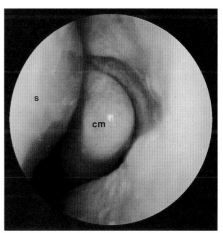

FIGURE 5.37   A concha bullosa of the left middle turbinate. The enlarged aerated turbinate "cell" bulges into the lateral wall of the nose coming into close contact with the uncinate process. cm = middle turbinate and s = septum.

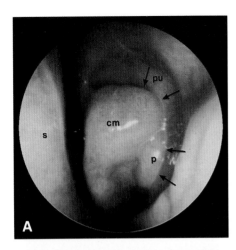

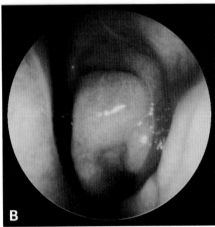

FIGURE 5.38 A concha bullosa of the left middle turbinate. The turbinate is in close contact (*arrows*) with the lateral wall of the nose in the area of the uncinate process. Polypoid mucosa spills out around the area of contact. The head of the concha bullosa shows some edematous changes. s = nasal septum; cm = middle turbinate; pu = uncinate process; and p = polyp.

The concha bullosa is a classic example of the potential of an anatomic variation to predispose the patient to sinus disease. A concha bullosa by itself does not represent a disease state per se, but it predisposes the patient (under certain conditions) to develop rhinosinusitis more readily and more frequently. Even relatively minor stimuli that in a person without a concha bullosa would only cause a temporary feeling of nasal stuffiness, somewhat increased secretions, or a minor rhinitis, may in patients with a concha bullosa cause sufficient mucosal swelling to produce a complete obstruction of the key sites in the ethmoid, thereby leading to the appearance or persistence of major symptoms.

We have frequently observed this course of events in patients with hay fever or other inhalational allergies. The slight mucosal swelling triggered by an allergic reaction is sufficient to cause major symptoms in these patients. In these cases, surgical management of the concha bullosa should be considered as an adjuvant therapy, which usually results in a marked improvement of the nasal symptoms. This facilitates the antiallergic or hyposensitization therapy and allows the use of lower doses or fewer drugs.

The concha bullosa also illustrates the significant role that mucosal contact areas play in the formation of nasal polyps. Frequently (Figs. 5.38 to 5.43) areas of mucosal contact initially show a circumscribed area of edema that may later serve as the base for extensive polyp development (Figure 5.42).

Endoscopically, a concha bullosa usually presents as an enlarged head or body of the middle turbinate that is in contact medially with the nasal septum and bulges laterally into the lateral wall of the nose, thereby making inspection of the middle meatus impossible. Typical endoscopic appearances of a concha bullosa are shown in Figures 5.35 and 5.37 to 5.39.

It should be emphasized that a concha bullosa can not always be identified with the nasal endoscope. Occasionally relatively innocuous appearing middle turbinates may contain extensive pneumatization and, conversely, not every enlarged head of a middle turbinate is pneumatized. When there is extensive pathology within the nose, endoscopic diagnosis may be extremely difficult, and the diagnosis must be made with conventional or computed tomography, although even these techniques have their limitations, as shown in Figure 5.33.

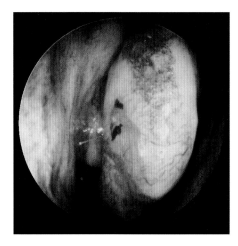

FIGURE 5.39   A right concha bullosa. For this picture, the turbinate was slightly displaced medially to demonstrate the small polyp at the site of contact between the turbinate and the uncinate process.

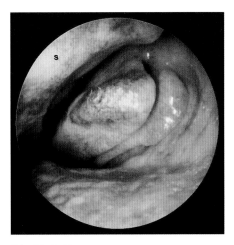

FIGURE 5.40   A concha bullosa of the left middle turbinate combined with a medially folded and anteriorly and inferiorly bent uncinate process. s = nasal septum.

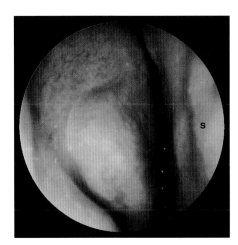

FIGURE 5.41   A concha bullosa of the right middle turbinate in close contact with the lateral wall of the nose. The concha bullosa completely obstructs the entry into the middle meatus. The ethmoidal infundibulum and the concha bullosa are both diseased. s = nasal septum.

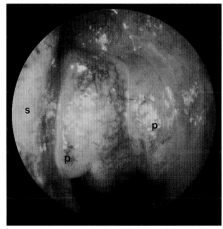

FIGURE 5.42   A concha bullosa of the left middle turbinate. Obvious polypoid mucous membrane changes are seen in the area of contact between the turbinate and lateral wall of the nose (in the uncinate process) and also with the nasal septum. s = nasal septum and p = polypoid mucous membrane changes.

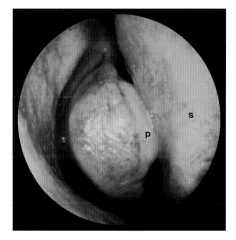

FIGURE 5.43   A huge concha bullosa of the right middle turbinate. Entry into the middle meatus is severely constricted. There are some secretions in the infundibulum. There is a polypoid and edematous change of the mucosa at the site of contact between the concha bullosa and the septum. s = nasal septum and p = polypoid and edematous membrane changes.

Pneumatization of the superior turbinate, i.e., a supreme concha is extremely rare and only a few cases have been reported where the symptoms of a superior turbinate concha bullosa were sufficiently severe to require surgical correction (Fig. 5.44). In these rare cases, the pneumatization of the superior turbinates was bilateral and forced the turbinate so far anteriorly between the nasal septum and the middle turbinate that headaches and a loss of olfactory sense resulted.

We have never encountered a case of pneumatization of the inferior turbinate. In rare cases, a tomogram may show a deeply depressed floor of the ethmoidal infundibulum, which has sunk to the level of the attachment of the inferior turbinate. This should not be mistaken, however, for a true pneumatization of the body of the turbinate. Infundibula that penetrate deeply into the inferior turbinate may cause, in cases of disease, a significant secondary hyperemia and swelling of the inferior turbinate, which may appear clinically as hyperplasia or hypertrophy. In these cases, mucosal hyperplasia of the inferior turbinate regresses as soon as the disease in the ethmoidal infundibulum is cured.

In a single instance, we have observed a presumptive, extensive turbinate cell in a right inferior turbinate that opened caudally into the common nasal passage. Purulent secretions were seen to come from the opening of the alleged cell and this was interpreted by the patient as a postnasal drip and as foul tasting secretions. Tomography (Fig. 5.45) clearly showed that this was not a true turbinate air cell, but rather an unusual slit formation with a saccular enlargement in the inferior turbinate.

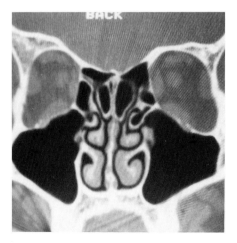

FIGURE 5.44 Bilateral concha bullosa of the superior turbinates.

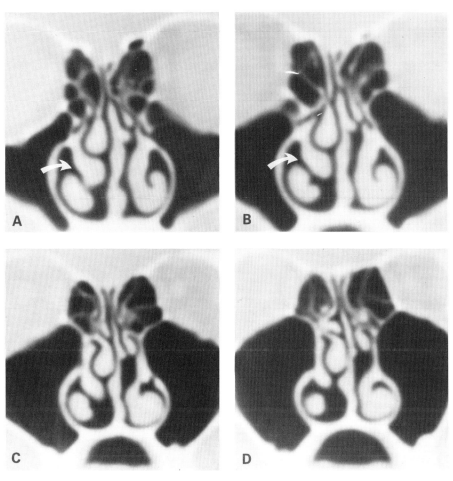

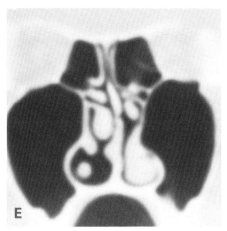

FIGURE 5.45   This is a CT sequence of an unusual groove and fossa formation of the right inferior turbinate (*arrows*). For details, see text.

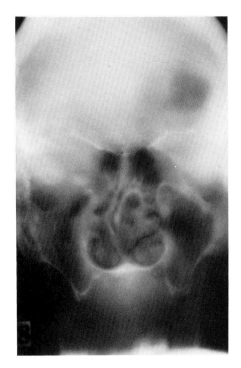

FIGURE 5.46   A combination of anatomic variants. Right septal deviation, marked and obvious involvement of a left concha bullosa, and bilateral ethmoid and maxillary sinus disease.

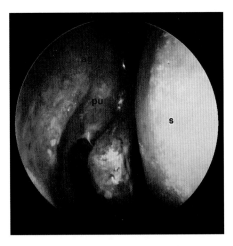

FIGURE 5.47   A paradoxically bent right middle turbinate and a diseased ethmoid infundibulum and agger nasi. The bulging of the agger nasi and of the upper part of the uncinate process is clearly visible. s = nasal septum; ag = agger nasi; and pu = uncinate process.

Variations of the Middle Turbinate

In addition to a concha bullosa, the middle turbinate can show other anatomic variations that can narrow the middle meatus and lead to mucosal contact sites. In so-called "paradoxically bent middle turbinates" the concavity of the turbinate points towards the septum and its convexity towards the lateral nasal wall. This anatomic variation usually occurs bilaterally. A paradoxically bent middle turbinate is also not a pathologic finding per se, although the paradoxic curvature can become quite pronounced and thereby cause a significant narrowing of the entrance to the middle meatus. In this instance, the paradoxically bent turbinate is usually combined with other anatomic abnormalities that together produce a significant narrowing of the entrance to the middle meatus and extensive mucosal contact areas (Fig. 5.47). Here, the most important additional anatomic abnormality is the medially bent uncinate process. Figure 5.48 shows such a case: this patient had recurrent maxillary sinus empyema that responded well to conservative management (irrigation, antibiotics, decongestants), however, after discontinuation of the therapy the symptoms recurred promptly. On endoscopy, only a paradoxically curved middle turbinate was found that narrowed the entrance to the middle meatus. There was also a medially curved uncinate process that was in contact with the lateral surface of the middle turbinate (not visible on the illustration). As shown in Figure 5.48A, the middle meatus is narrow but otherwise unremarkable during the symptom-free period. Figure 5.48B shows the same patient during an acute phase (primary finding: maxillary sinus empyema). The medial infundibular wall bulges forward massively, and is adjacent to the equally congested mucosa of the paradoxically curved middle turbinate. No free passage can be found in the middle meatus. Through a small perforation in the uncinate process, pus empties from the infundibulum, as evidence of a serious problem in the area. The radiograph taken during the symptom-free period (Fig. 5.49) shows the paradoxical curve of the middle turbinate. A narrowing of the hiatus semilunaris and the ethmoid hiatus are clearly shown. The uncinate process appears jammed up against the lateral wall and it is obvious that it requires minimal mucosal swelling in this area to close this narrow passage completely. Marked paradoxically curved middle turbinates can occasionally make endoscopic surgical manipulations in the ethmoid sinuses extremely difficult (Figs. 5.50 and 5.51).

FIGURE 5.48 *A*, A minimally bent paradoxical left middle turbinate. The patient is in a symptom-free interval. s = nasal septum. *B*, The patient is seen at the time of acute symptoms. For explanation, see text. Notice the pus coming from a perforation in the uncinate process (*arrow*). s = nasal septum.

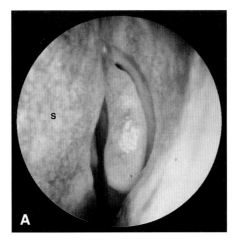

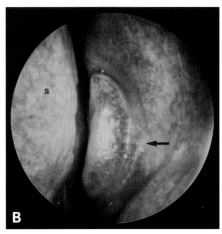

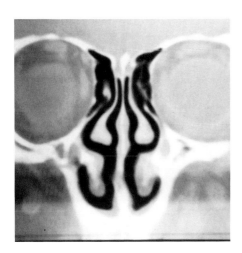

FIGURE 5.49 The CT of the same patient seen in Figure 5.48 during a relatively symptom-free period.

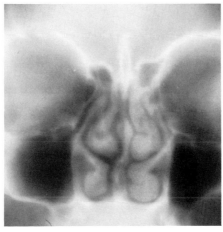

FIGURE 5.50 Marked, bilateral, paradoxically bent middle turbinates. The relative constriction of the middle meatus and particularly of the ethmoidal infundibulum is clearly visible.

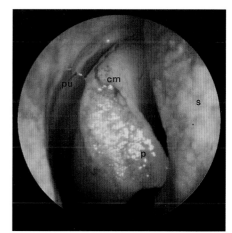

FIGURE 5.51 A paradoxically bent, right middle turbinate. At the site of contact between the free margin of the head of the turbinate and the uncinate process, polypoid mucous membrane hyperplasia has developed.

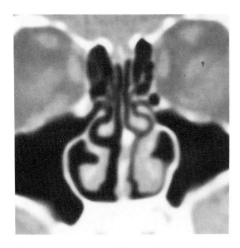

FIGURE 5.52 A middle turbinate with a marked horizontal lamella, particularly on the left where the horizontal lamella encircles practically the lateral wall of the nose from below. On the left side of the patient, the overlap between uncinate process and the horizontal lamella of the turbinate can be seen.

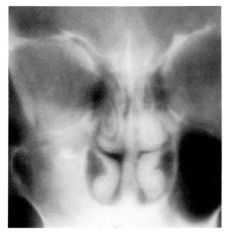

FIGURE 5.53 A middle turbinate surrounds the ethmoidal bulla on the right. On the left side of the turbinate and bulla complex are uniform opacities. There was significant mycotic disease in the opacified right maxillary sinus.

A normally convex middle turbinate may occasionally be so tightly rolled up laterally that it may simulate a concha bullosa in the X-ray image. The free margin of such a middle turbinate may be curved so far laterally that it envelops the middle meatus and makes the introduction of an endoscope almost impossible (Fig. 5.52). The space under the concavity of such a middle turbinate, frequently filled by a large bulla ethmoidalis, has been called a "sinus conchae" or turbinate sinus (Fig. 5.53). A distended head of the middle turbinate is not always due to abnormalities of the mucous membrane.

The vertical bony lamella of the middle turbinate can assume a variety of curvatures. The head of the middle turbinate may be normally medially convex, but in the posterior two-thirds it may occasionally show a considerable paradoxical curvature. This is most frequently seen when the anterior third of the turbinate contains a concha bullosa (Fig. 5.54).

The sagittal groove formation of the middle turbinate that is occasionally seen has pathologic significance only in the rarest of cases. These grooves should not be mistaken for the depressions in the superior meatus caused by a relatively far forward-reaching attachment of the superior turbinate. An L- or T-shape of the underlying bony lamellae of the turbinate is the usual cause of the "triangular" middle turbinate.

It is important to remember during surgery that the shape and contour of the head of the middle turbinate is not a reliable topographic landmark.

Normally the head of the middle turbinate extends anterior to its attachment by only a few millimeters and follows in its contours the projection of the attachment of the uncinate process along the lateral nasal wall. There are, however, frequent variations in which the head of the middle turbinate extends anteriorly beyond its attachment by more than 1 centimeter and thus overlaps the uncinate process by a considerable margin and may even overlie a portion of the agger nasi.

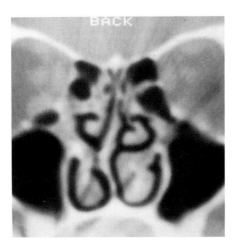

FIGURE 5.54 Paradoxical bending of the posterior segment of the left middle turbinate. There is obvious bilateral ethmoid disease.

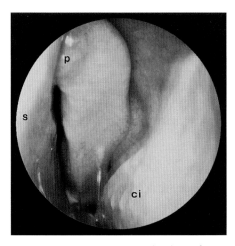

FIGURE 5.55 An endoscopic view of a laterally bent, left middle turbinate. The structures of the lateral wall of the nose could not be identified. s = septum; p = small polyp at the contact site between the head of the turbinate and the septum; and ci = inferior turbinate.

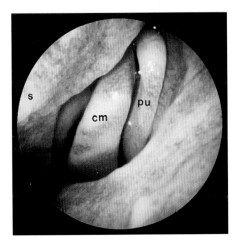

FIGURE 5.56 A "doubled" middle turbinate. The uncinate process on the left side is bent medially anteriorly and inferiorly so that it protrudes from the middle meatus, parallel to the middle turbinate. It thus appeared as though there was a second middle turbinate. s = septum; cm = middle turbinate; and pu = uncinate process.

These variations of the head of the turbinate must be considered when opening the infundibulum and when the attachment of the uncinate process must be identified (see Chapter 7).

Uncinate Process

The uncinate process may show a large number of anatomic variations. Normally the uncinate process extends from its sickle-shaped attachment on the lateral wall of the nose and the inferior turbinate posteriorly and medially to its posterior free margin, so that only a 1- to 3-millimeter wide fissure, the hiatus semilunaris, remains between the uncinate process and the anterior surface of the ethmoidal bulla. The distance between its free posterior edge and the lamina papyracea varies between 1.5 and 5 millimeters. The most frequent, pathologically significant variation of the uncinate process is a marked medial curvature or bend. This medial bending may involve the entire uncinate process or only certain portions of it so that, at times, the uncinate process may appear like a twisted band. This medial curvature can be so marked that contact is established between its free edge and even its entire medial surface and the lateral surface of the middle turbinate.

The uncinate process can be bent medially and folded anteriorly so far that it protrudes anteriorly and inferiorly out of the middle meatus like the curled brim of a hat. This may give the impression that two middle turbinates are present (Figs. 5.56, 5.57, and 5.58). In fact, this finding was labelled by Kaufmann as a "doubled middle turbinate." By increased posterior extension, the uncinate process may impinge its free, posterior margin on the ethmoidal bulla and thereby significantly narrow the hiatus semilunaris. The same result is achieved if the uncinate process overlaps the bulla medially and posteriorly. In combination with anatomic variations such as a paradoxically curved

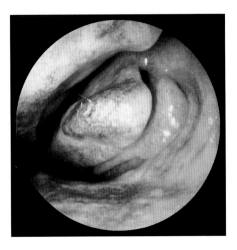

FIGURE 5.57 A similar case, but here the anteriorly bent uncinate process is combined with a concha bullosa of the middle turbinate.

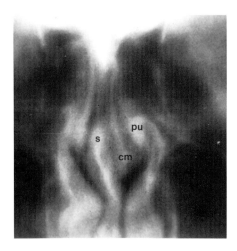

FIGURE 5.58 Conventional tomogram of a folded left uncinate process. s = septum; cm = middle turbinate; and pu = uncinate process.

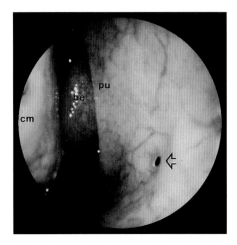

FIGURE 5.59 This is an endoscopic view into a left middle meatus. The small perforation seen just anterior to the inferior insertion of the medially bent uncinate process is an accessory maxillary sinus ostium located in the anterior nasal fontanelle (*arrow*). be = ethmoidal bulla; cm = middle turbinate; pu = uncinate process.

middle turbinate, a concha bullosa, or an extensively pneumatized ethmoidal bulla, a medially bent uncinate process may produce significant functional blockage of the narrow spaces of the anterior ethmoid and the related frontal and maxillary sinuses.

A markedly medially bent or folded uncinate process with a corresponding area of extensive contact with the middle turbinate is one of the most frequent pathologic findings in our population of patients with sinusitis.

Septal ridges or spurs may project into the uncinate process or into the hiatus semilunaris and thereby cause additional problems. In its projection superiorly, the uncinate process may bend laterally and insert into the lamina papyracea (see the Chapter on Anatomy) thereby closing off blindly the ethmoidal infundibulum superiorly and forming a recessus terminalis. In this event the secretions from the frontal recess are carried past the ethmoidal infundibulum medially and arrive inferiorly in the hiatus semilunaris. Through accessory ostia in the fontanelles, secretions may even be transported *into* the maxillary sinus (Figs. 5.59 and 5.60).

The uncinate process may alternatively extend gradually upwards and reach the base of the skull. When this happens, the frontal recess opens inferiorly directly into the ethmoidal infundibulum. The superior portion of the uncinate process may also be twisted medially and undergo a bony fusion with the attachment of the middle turbinate, or even with a portion of the head of the turbinate (Figs. 5.61, 5.62, 5.63, and 5.64). In extreme cases, this may produce an almost frontally oriented bony plate that can narrow the entrance to the middle meatus and the frontal recess anteriorly very much like a postoperative adhesion.

The uncinate process may also be bent laterally, either along its entire length or in only one portion. This lateral bend may also narrow the ethmoidal infundibulum, especially when the insertion of the uncinate process is far laterally on the inferior turbinate (for a discussion of traumatic lateral displacement of the uncinate process, see Chapter 11).

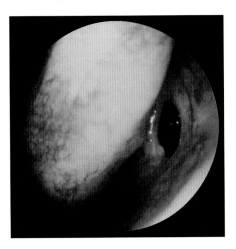

FIGURE 5.60 This patient has a larger accessory maxillary sinus ostium.

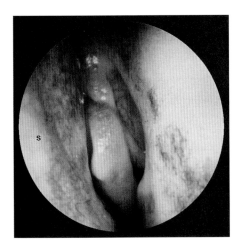

FIGURE 5.61 There is a medially bent left uncinate process that blocked the upper part of the opening into the middle meatus. Note the extensive area of contact with the middle turbinate. s = nasal septum.

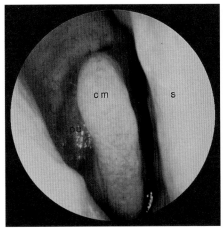

FIGURE 5.62 A very thin and translucent uncinate process is bent so far medially that on the right side, it has come into contact with the middle turbinate almost along its entire length. As a result, entry into the middle meatus is almost completely obstructed. pu = uncinate process; cm = middle turbinate; and s = nasal septum.

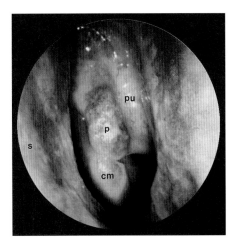

FIGURE 5.63 In this patient, the uncinate process has folded medially along a wide area and fused with the upper third of the middle turbinate. The uncinate process forms an almost completely vertical bony plate at the entrance to the middle meatus. s = nasal septum; p = polypoid mucous membrane at the anterior end of the uncinate process; cm = middle turbinate; and pu = uncinate process.

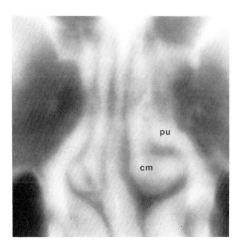

FIGURE 5.64 Conventional tomogram of a medially folded uncinate process. cm = middle turbinate and pu = uncinate process.

In the radiologic assessment of the uncinate process, in coronal sections, its anatomic course must always be kept in mind. The arc-shaped course of the process from anterosuperior to posteroinferior means that in coronal views the most anterior sections show the process at its longest. If the infundibulum ethmoidale is very "deep," the uncinate process may directly insert at the posteromedial wall of the nasofrontal duct in the middle third of its course (Fig. 5.65). In the more posterior sections, the uncinate process appears increasingly smaller (see Chapter 4).

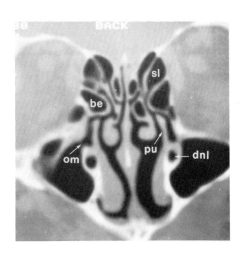

FIGURE 5.65 This CT picture clearly shows the relationship of the uncinate process to the nasolacrimal duct. om = maxillary ostium; pu = uncinate process; dnl = nasolacrimal duct; be = bulla ethmoidalis; and sl = sinus lateralis.

The strength of this small bony plate varies enormously. In cases of chronic nasal polyposis or other inflammatory diseases, the bony base may be so demineralized that it may become invisible on X-ray and even defy identification at the time of surgery.

Since the uncinate process forms the bony base of the medial wall of the ethmoidal infundibulum, any changes in the uncinate process or in its medial mucous membrane surface are important indicators of an inflammatory process in the infundibulum itself. Changes in the mucous membrane covering the medial surface of the uncinate process suggest changes in the infundibulum, the recessus frontalis and the adjacent areas of the ethmoid. Frequently these changes appear as discrete, circumscribed mucosal swellings at the site of contact. In some patients, these changes may appear as more or less pronounced polypoid changes. These polyps, which originate on the free margin of the uncinate process or in the infundibulum proper, may protrude around the free edge of the uncinate process and into the nasal cavity (Figs. 5.66 to 5.68). Frequently the entire medial wall of the infundibulum bulges medially, indicating the presence of a significant pathologic process in the anterior ethmoid (Figs. 5.69 and 5.70). The changes consist of chronic edema and may in acute exacerbations develop perforations from which pus or other pathologic secretions may pour forth (see Figs. 5.48B and 5.72) (see also Disease of the Ethmoidal Infundibulum).

This extensive contact between the uncinate process, the middle turbinate, and also the bulla ethmoidalis can be diagnosed in many patients by carefully displacing the middle turbinate with a Freer elevator (see Fig. 5.66).

FIGURE 5.66 *A*, A medially folded, right uncinate process. A mucosal polyp is seen to arise from the contact site between the middle turbinate and the free margin of the uncinate process. pu = uncinate process; p = mucosal polyp; cm = middle turbinate; and s = septum. *B*, This small polyp is more easily seen after gentle retraction of the middle turbinate. p = mucosal polyp; be = bulla ethmoidalis; and f = Freer elevator.

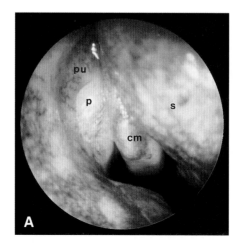

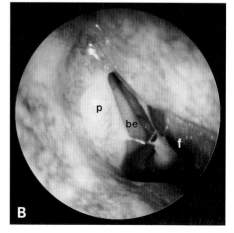

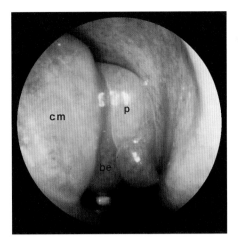

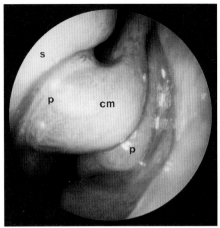

FIGURE 5.67   Massive polyp development at the site of contact between the uncinate process and the bulla ethmoidalis on the left. p = polyps and cm = hyperplastic head of the middle turbinate.

FIGURE 5.68   A paradoxically bent right middle turbinate and a medially bent uncinate process. There are marked polypoid changes at the extensive area of contact between the turbinate and the uncinate process and between the turbinate and the septum. s = septum; cm = middle turbinate; and p = polyps.

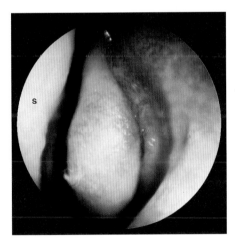

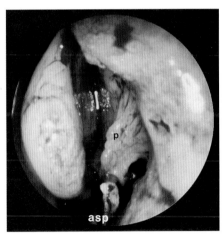

FIGURE 5.69   The left middle meatus of this patient appears relatively "healthy." Note how the uncinate process is bent medially and comes into close contact with the middle turbinate. s = septum.

FIGURE 5.70   The same patient shown in Figure 5.69 after resection of the uncinate process. Note the marked polypoid mucous membrane changes in the ethmoidal infundibulum. p = polyps and asp = suction tip.

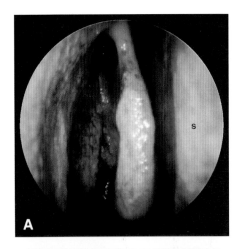

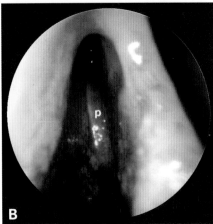

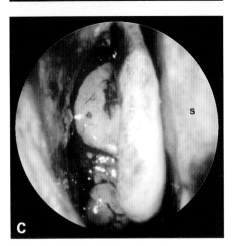

FIGURE 5.71 Diseased ethmoidal infundibulum. *A*, A medially bent uncinate process. A small polyp is seen emerging from the middle meatus between the uncinate process and the middle turbinate. s = septum. *B*, This very small polyp is more obvious in the close-up view. p = polyp. *C*, The same area immediately after resection of the uncinate process. Note the massive protrusion of polypoid mucous membrane that was obviously under considerable pressure in the anterior ethmoid. s = septum.

The mucosa on the posterior margin and lateral surface of the uncinate process (in the ethmoidal infundibulum) appears to be particularly sensitive to inflammatory stimuli and responds readily with engorgement and polyp formation (Fig. 5.71). We have frequently observed, even in cases of extensive nasal polyps, that resection of the uncinate process usually removes the most anterior large polyps, thus indicating that these polyps arose from the uncinate process and the ethmoidal infundibulum. This clinical observation is the reason that in severe polyposis we always try to identify and resect the uncinate process first and *not* just remove the polyps that seem to be obstructing the passage towards it. This technique is much less bloody, provides improved exposure, and permits a tissue sparing, goal-oriented operation.

In more than a quarter of all patients, "holes" can be found in the lateral nasal wall that open into the maxillary sinus. These are located both anteriorly and posteriorly to the posterior third of the uncinate process. These "holes" are not the natural ostium of the maxillary sinus, but they are accessory maxillary ostia located in the anterior and posterior nasal fontanelles (see Figs. 5.59 and 5.60) or they are perforations in the uncinate process (Figs. 5.72 and 5.73). The primary ostium of the maxillary sinus can almost never be seen directly from the middle meatus, since it is hidden in the depths of the posterior third of the ethmoid infundibulum, lateral to the uncinate process (see Chapter 3). It is not unusual to find secretions moving through the accessory ostia *into the maxillary sinus*, only to then leave the maxillary sinus through the primary ostium. The secretions now appearing in the ethmoidal infundibulum may mingle with the secretions carried into the maxillary sinus through the accessory ostium and thus recycle through the sinus. This mechanism is one of the possible routes by which pathogens may enter the maxillary sinus when the natural ostium of the sinus is occluded (see Chapter 2).

Pneumatization of the uncinate process must be mentioned even though it is a very rare occurrence (see Fig. 5.34). When the uncinate process is pneumatized, the additional space occupied by this widened structure causes further narrowing of the already narrow spaces of the ethmoidal infundibulum and creates new areas of mucosal contact.

The uncinate process may be entirely absent or markedly thinned. This may occur in chronic inflammatory diseases, polyposis, and mycotic infections. When this occurs, it is essential to exclude granulomatous or neoplastic diseases by consideration of the differential diagnosis (Figs. 5.74 and 5.75). If doubt exists, an endoscopic examination and biopsy should be performed before surgically approaching what may turn out to be an unexpected disease.

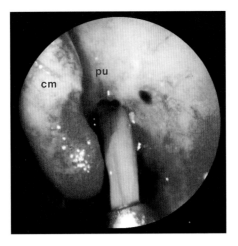

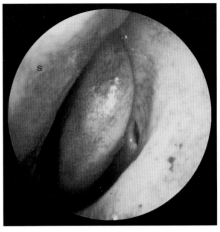

FIGURE 5.72   Acute sinusitis. A large amount of purulent viscous secretions is aspirated through a small perforation in the uncinate process on the left side. cm = middle turbinate and pu = uncinate process.

FIGURE 5.73   The same patient as in Figure 5.72. After medical management of the acute symptoms, the perforation can be seen. As the mucosal edema is less, the perforation appears larger than during the acute phase of inflammation.

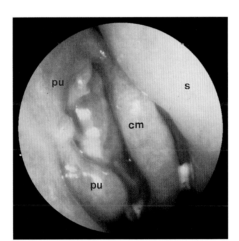

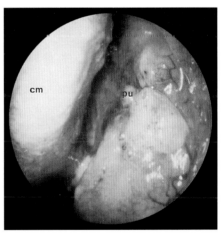

FIGURE 5.74   A right uncinate process, which has been largely destroyed following recurrent episodes of infection. Polypoid mucous membrane can be seen spilling out from the anterior surface of the ethmoidal bulla, while pus emerges from the frontal recess. pu = remnants of the uncinate process; cm = middle turbinate; and s = septum.

FIGURE 5.75   Polypoid granulomatous tissue on the medial wall of the left uncinate process. Biopsy revealed a squamous cell carcinoma. pu = uncinate process and cm = middle turbinate. Note the strikingly similar appearance to the nonspecific disease in Figure 5.74.

Ethmoidal Bulla

The ethmoidal bulla (bulla ethmoidalis) is usually the largest, most constant and most easily demonstrable air cell of the anterior ethmoid. It rests laterally on the lamina papyracea, but its other relationships are highly variable. The bulla can extend superiorly to the roof of the ethmoid and posteriorly to the basal lamella of the middle turbinate. Depending on the development of a lateral sinus or other anterior ethmoid cells, the bulla may lose contact with the roof of the ethmoid and also with the basal lamella (see Chapter 3). The ethmoidal bulla can develop independent pathology, but clinical experience shows that most diseases of the bulla originate more frequently at contact sites with other structures than from the interior of the cell.

The extent of pneumatization of the ethmoidal bulla is quite variable, ranging from no pneumatization at all to extreme pneumatization where the bulla extends far anteriorly under the middle turbinate (Fig. 5.76). This excessive pneumatization may be directed anteriorly and establish intimate contact with the posterior free margin of the uncinate process, thereby narrowing or partially blocking the hiatus semilunaris. The bulla may also extend medially beyond the hiatus semilunaris and block it in this fashion (Fig. 5.80). Finally, the pneumatization may extend so far anteriorly that the bulla forces its way between the uncinate process and the head of the middle turbinate (Fig. 5.81). When examined from anteriorly, the bulla may completely obscure the middle turbinate and make the initial endoscopic diagnosis very difficult.

More commonly, there is a general enlargement of the ethmoidal bulla that completely fills the space under a somewhat laterally curled middle turbinate (the "turbinate sinus"). In severe cases, this general enlargement produces an extensive area of surface contact between the medial surface of the ethmoidal bulla and the mucosa of the lateral surface of the middle turbinate (Figs. 5.77 to 5.79). In our experience, this is one of the most common sites from which polyps originate. Thus even a nondiseased but enlarged bulla may fill the entire middle meatus tightly like a balloon and give rise to considerable symptoms. The most frequent symptoms are a strong, unpleasant pressure above or behind the eyes, headaches (particularly frontal headaches), impeded or blocked nasal breathing, the feeling that something is "stuck" in the nose causing a continuous sneezing or blowing urge without being able to "blow anything out." A large or diseased bulla ethmoidalis, by virtue of its contact surfaces, may also be responsible for a postnasal discharge.

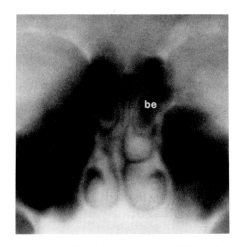

FIGURE 5.76 This scan shows bilateral large ethmoidal bullae. Even though the bullar air cells are healthy in this case, such extensive pneumatization can be the cause of numerous symptoms.
be = bulla ethmoidalis.

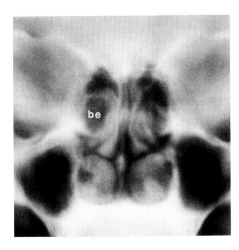

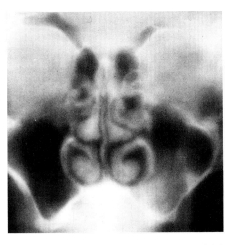

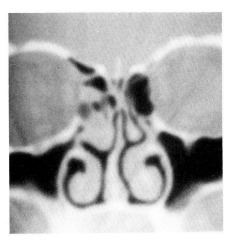

FIGURE 5.77 Note the large right ethmoidal bulla that almost completely fills the middle meatus and comes into extensive contact with the middle turbinate. There is swelling of the mucosa within the bulla. This patient complained of headaches, obstructed nasal breathing, and postnasal drip.

FIGURE 5.78 There is bilateral ethmoidal bulla disease. The mucosal swelling has extended to the ethmoidal infundibulum on both sides. The left maxillary sinus is partially opacified.

FIGURE 5.79 Note the ethmoidal bulla disease on the right side. The space between the middle turbinate and the bulla (the "turbinate sinus") is also diseased.

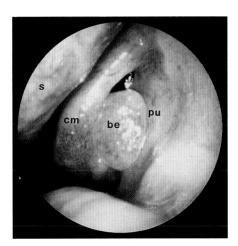

FIGURE 5.80 Note the large bulla herniating from the middle meatus. Extensive pneumatization has caused the bulla to extend anteriorly. The mucous membrane shows polypoid changes. s = septum; cm = middle turbinate; be = ethmoidal bulla; and pu = uncinate process.

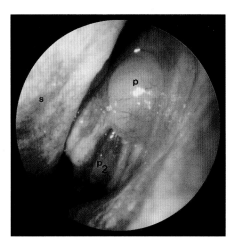

FIGURE 5.81 In addition to the edematous polyp arising from the upper part of the uncinate process, there are two polyps deep in the middle meatus. These polyps originated from the anterior surface of the ethmoidal bulla and from the turbinate sinus. s = septum; p = edematous polyp; and P_2 = polyps in the middle meatus.

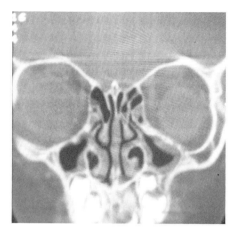

FIGURE 5.82 This is the CT of a 7-year-old patient with chronic, recurring sinusitis that was resistant to all forms of medical therapy. This patient's adenoids had been removed and there were no known allergies. Note the obvious bilateral ethmoidal bullar disease, with involvement of the infundibulum and resulting edema of the maxillary sinus mucosa.

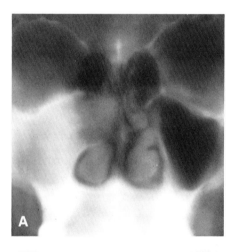

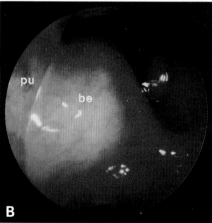

FIGURE 5.83 For explanation see text. be = ethmoidal bulla and pu = uncinate process.

Because of its central location and its multiple intimate anatomic relationships to the other key areas of the ethmoid sinus, the ethmoidal bulla is frequently involved in those disease processes that affect the anterior ethmoid sinus. Even minor mucosal swellings may affect the hiatus semilunaris and the ethmoidal infundibulum. The frontal recess, the agger nasi, and the lateral sinus may also be involved.

When reviewing the tomograms, it must be kept in mind that there need not be a marked opacification of the bulla or its immediate surroundings in order to identify the bulla as an etiologic factor in the disease process. As shown in Figure 5.76, a normally aerated albeit enlarged bulla may be the principal cause of the patient's complaints. In Figure 5.77, there are marked contact areas between the bulla and the middle turbinate. Through its extensive downward growth, the ethmoidal bulla has significantly blocked the ethmoidal infundibulum and the ostium of the maxillary sinus. The radiographic interpretation of a "normally aerated ethmoid" is correct, but insufficient, since it may lead to the conclusion that there is no pathologic process. This is an example where good communication between the surgeon and the radiologist is particularly important.

Figures 5.83 A and B are of a patient who had recurrent maxillary sinus empyemas for several years. With conservative management (irrigation, antibiotics, etc.) the symptoms always improved, but the sinus infections recurred regularly and rapidly. Tomography showed diffuse shadows in the right maxillary sinus and filling the middle meatus, with the suggestion of destruction of a portion of the lateral nasal wall since its individual features could no longer be identified. Nasal endoscopy, performed after conservative therapy and during a quiescent period, showed a very large bulla ethmoidalis that extended over the hiatus semilunaris anteriorly, covering the hiatus semilunaris completely, and totally blocking the ethmoidal infundibulum and the ostium of the maxillary sinus. When infection recurred, the patient developed an acute maxillary sinusitis with the symptoms of this sinusitis dominating the clinical picture. The reasons for the recurrent maxillary sinusitis were not in the maxillary sinus itself, but in the anatomic changes and relationships of the ethmoidal bulla. The endoscopic solution to this problem consisted of a resection of the bulla ethmoidalis combined with excision of the uncinate process and enlargement of the natural ostium of the maxillary sinus. The maxillary sinus was not touched.

Figures 5.84 to 5.87 show further examples of bulla-associated problems.

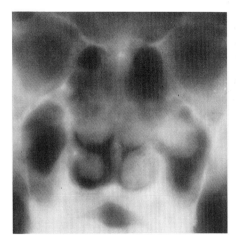

FIGURE 5.84 This patient has very large ethmoidal bullae, bilaterally. They are not diseased, but they are in extensive contact with the middle turbinate. The turbinate sinus is opaque on both sides. Note the polypoid mucosal edema in the area of the posterior fontanelle of the left maxillary sinus.

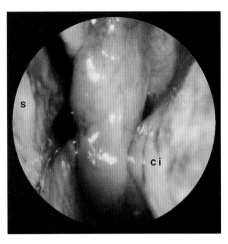

FIGURE 5.85 There is a choanal polyp, originating from the anterior surface of this left ethmoidal bulla and the turbinate sinus. It reaches the choana along the floor of the nose. s = septum and ci = inferior turbinate.

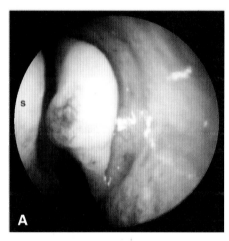

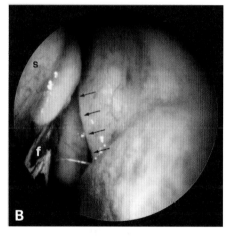

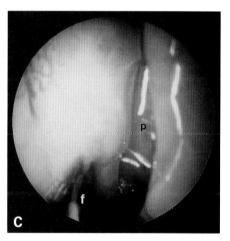

FIGURE 5.86 This patient had marked disease in the left anterior ethmoid. *A*, Note the tight contact between the slightly paradoxically bent middle turbinate and the uncinate process. The mucosa of uncinate process is edematous at the site of contact. s = septum. *B*, After retraction of the middle turbinate, the free posterior margin of the uncinate process becomes visible (*arrows*). s = septum. *C*, Behind the uncinate process, a polypoid edematous mucosa bulges forward from the anterior surface of the bulla ethmoidalis (*arrows*). p = polypoid edematous mucosa and f = Freer elevator.

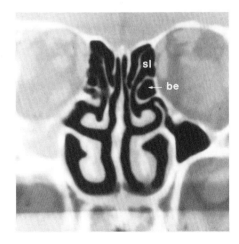

FIGURE 5.87 Note the position of the lateral sinus just above the bulla ethmoidalis in this coronal CT section. sl = lateral sinus and be = bulla ethmoidalis.

Lateral Sinus

The lateral sinus (sinus lateralis) is a highly variable space located between the ethmoidal bulla, the roof of the ethmoid, the basal lamella of the middle turbinate, and the lamina papyracea (Fig. 5.87). Localized disease may develop within the lateral sinus without involving the ethmoidal bulla (Figs. 5.88 and 5.89). Disease in the lateral sinus can be very difficult to diagnose endoscopically, and occasionally the only indication of pathology in this area is the observation of a small amount of abnormal discharge coming from the superior hiatus semilunaris. Small polyps or mucosal swellings that appear medial to the ethmoidal bulla and exert pressure inferiorly may also indicate disease in the lateral sinus (Figs. 5.90 and 5.91). If the lateral sinus is well developed and extends far posteriorly, the ethmoidal bulla may open into the lateral sinus, thereby creating a pathway through which disease can spread from the bulla to the lateral sinus and vice versa.

In our experience, the lateral sinus is *the* ethmoidal fissure from which pathology most frequently spreads across the basal lamella into the posterior ethmoid. This spread of infection occurs either through bony dehiscences of the basal lamella or through circumscribed areas of destruction secondary to inflammation (see Chapter 3).

Depending upon its anatomic shape and relations, disease within the sinus lateralis may spread to the frontal recess and to the agger nasi and vice versa. The so-called "supraorbital ethmoid cells" are usually only extensions of the lateral sinus that extend deeply into the roof of the orbits.

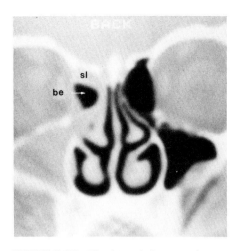

FIGURE 5.88 The lateral sinus on the right is diseased. The turbinate sinus and the infundibulum are also involved, and disease has spread to the maxillary sinus. The ethmoid bulla is only slightly involved. sl = sinus lateralis and be = ethmoidal bulla.

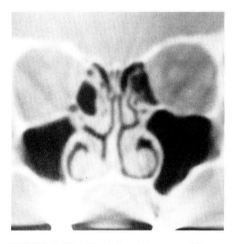

FIGURE 5.89 The lateral sinus and the turbinate sinus on the right side are diseased, but in this patient the maxillary sinus is not involved.

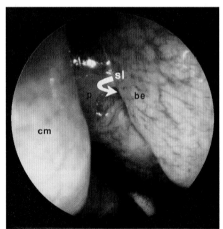

FIGURE 5.90 This edematous polyp originated from the left lateral sinus. The entrance to the lateral sinus is indicated by the curved white arrow. sl = lateral sinus; cm = middle turbinate; be = bulla ethmoidalis; and p = polyp.

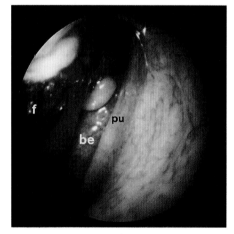

FIGURE 5.91 In this patient, the polyps originated from the superior hiatus semilunaris. They were a manifestation of involvement of the left lateral sinus. The slight pressure of the Freer elevator displacing the middle meatus medially has caused a small hemorrhage. pu = uncinate process; be = bulla ethmoidalis; p = polyp; and f = Freer elevator.

Disease of the Ethmoidal Infundibulum

The ethmoidal infundibulum (infundibulum ethmoidale) is *the* key area in inflammatory diseases of the paranasal sinuses. The majority of the drainage pathways from the anterior ethmoid join in the infundibulum and in its immediate vicinity with those from the frontal and maxillary sinuses. Ventilation and drainage of the maxillary sinus and, depending upon the anatomic configuration, of a portion of the frontal recess takes place through the infundibulum. Because of its anatomic shape, i.e., a long, narrow fissure, the patency of the infundibulum is affected early and quickly by even minor and localized changes in the adjacent structures. Conversely, primary disease in the infundibulum quickly spreads to involve the adjacent structures and especially to the large sinuses.

Since even normally the view through a diagnostic endoscope is limited to the hiatus semilunaris and includes the infundibulum only in the rarest of instances, endoscopic diagnosis is limited to the recognition and evaluation of those physical signs that point directly or indirectly to infundibular pathology.

A routine plain survey X-ray film of the sinuses for all practical purposes fails to show the area of the infundibulum and thus the information provided by plain radiographs does not allow any conclusions to be drawn about the presence or absence of diseases in the infundibulum. This is the major reason we must combine diagnostic endoscopy with conventional or computed tomography to properly investigate patients with sinus disease.

The diagnostic endoscopic examination provides the indications for tomography by observing direct or indirect evidence of disease, while the tomograms reveal the hidden disease processes that are not endoscopically visible. The tomograms also enable us to decide if a more invasive diagnostic procedure or an endoscopic surgical operation is indicated.

There are four prime endoscopic clues that suggest the presence of disease within the infundibulum:

1. Obvious pathologic changes in the infundibulum or the hiatus semilunaris.
2. The observation of pathologic discharge coming from the infundibulum via the hiatus semilunaris.
3. The identification of anatomic variants that are capable of constricting the infundibulum.
4. The observation of mucosal changes on the medial surface of the uncinate process that suggest infundibular pathology.

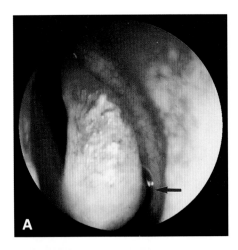

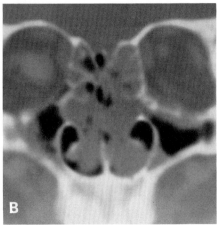

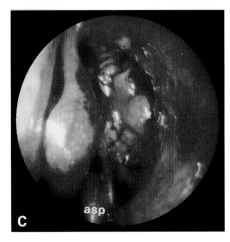

FIGURE 5.92 The infundibulum is diseased and the uncinate process is medially bent. The *arrow* shows pathologic secretions coming from the infundibulum. *B*, This is the CT scan of the patient. Note the opacification of the infundibulum, the remainder of the anterior ethmoid. The maxillary sinuses are diseased bilaterally. *C*, After resection of the uncinate process, the massive disease of the infundibulum becomes evident. asp = suction tip.

The endoscopic or radiologic findings may uncover hidden disease in the infundibulum that causes the patient to have severe problems. In the patient shown in Fig. 5.92A, the diagnostic nasal endoscopic examination revealed some abnormal secretions coming from the infundibulum. The middle turbinate was paradoxically curved and the uncinate process appeared to be bent medially. On the basis of the patient's history of symptoms, which had been present for several years and which were associated with recurrent empyemas of the maxillary sinus, headaches, and obstructed nasal breathing that had not responded to repeated conservative management, computerized tomography was performed. CT showed a definite shadow in the infundibulum and in the more anterior portions of the ethmoid (Fig. 5.92B). Subsequent opening of the infundibulum at the time of endoscopic surgery (Fig. 5.92C) showed obvious pathology that was hidden behind the uncinate process. The entire infundibulum was blocked by a polypoid mass that was responsible for the recurrent episodes of acute maxillary sinusitis.

Conversely, an impressive endoscopic finding need not necessarily be responsible for significant symptoms, as is frequently seen in those patients who have a moderate number of nasal polyps (Figs. 5.93 and 5.94). While these patients may in some cases complain of partially obstructed nasal breathing, a limitation in the sense of smell, or blockage of the eustachian tube, they frequently have no other serious complaints.

All of these factors must be taken into account when a surgical procedure is being considered. Such a procedure should not be undertaken on the basis of radiologic findings alone, but should always be the result of an assessment of the radiologic and endoscopic findings, in combination with the patient's clinical symptoms.

The endoscopic picture of infundibular disease is extremely variable, as there is a continuous spectrum from minor, isolated and circumscribed pathology to a massive involvement of the entire ethmoid and related paranasal sinuses.

In relatively circumscribed disease, the typical mucosal changes are best seen in the area of the hiatus semilunaris, where abnormal or adherent discharge provides evidence of disease within the infundibulum. If the disease spreads further within the infundibulum, one usually sees edematous, inflammatory changes in the mucosa of the free posterior margin of the uncinate process and on the anterior surface of the ethmoidal bulla. There may also be polypoid changes in both of these areas. Individual polyps or irregular mucosal folds may obstruct the infundibulum and the hiatus semilunaris and extend into the middle meatus prolapsing anteriorly or inferiorly. Depending upon the nature of the disease process, the medial wall of the infundibulum (whose bony base is the uncinate process) may curve markedly medially or anteriorly. This is seen clearly in cases of acute sinus infection. The mucous membrane covering the uncinate process medially need not show any changes. At times, increased vascular markings are the only indication of an inflammatory process deep in the infundibulum. Finally, an inflammatory edematous engorgement of the mucous membrane may be seen on an anterior bulging uncinate process. This is most commonly seen in chronic cases, and this edematous swollen mucosa frequently blocks the entrance to the middle meatus either partially or completely.

Granulomatous changes and polyps may also be seen, not only at the sites of contact between the wall of the uncinate process and the middle turbinate, but also projecting anteriorly and inferiorly from the anterior surface of the ethmoidal bulla and from the more superior ethmoid fissures. The bony base of the uncinate process may be partially destroyed and perforations may appear through the uncinate process into the middle meatus. Granulation tissue, polyps, or abnormal secretions may be seen emerging from these perforations.

If the endoscopic findings are this severe and especially if there is an additional inflammatory component, it is advisable to use a more substantial anesthetic by applying Pontocaine and epinephrine soaked cotton pledgets as described in Chapter 8, even for the first examination, since satisfactory anesthesia may not be obtained with only the application of a topical anesthetic and vasoconstrictor spray. Following decongestion and anesthesia, it is at times possible to lift the middle turbinate medially with a Freer elevator and look directly into the middle meatus in spite of the pathologic process.

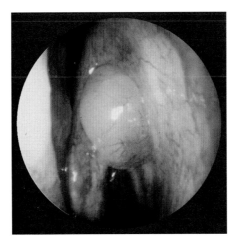

FIGURE 5.93 Note the edematous polyp originating from the upper part of the infundibulum.

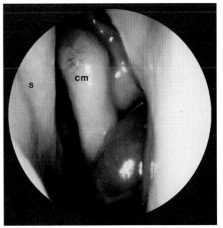

FIGURE 5.94 Note the large polyps from the left middle meatus in this patient with infundibular disease. s = septum and cm = middle turbinate.

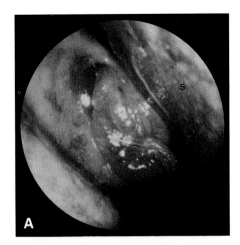

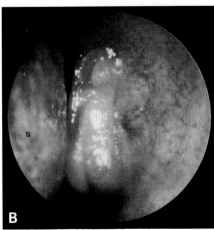

FIGURE 5.95 *A*, This patient shows the typical endoscopic appearance of chronic infundibular disease (right). Glassy-polypoid mucous membrane masses protrude from the middle meatus. The middle turbinate is pushed medially against the septum and the uncinate process is also medially bent. s = septum. *B*, Note the identical appearance of the opposite side of the patient. c = coptum.

The topical decongestion of the nose may in some cases make the abnormal secretions drain spontaneously. This gives a good indication of the location of the problem and of its suitability for medical or surgical approach. If decongestion alone permits the drainage of secretions from an empyema of the frontal or maxillary sinus through the middle meatus, this strongly suggests that treatment of the obstruction in the lateral wall of the nose will permit drainage, ventilation, and the subsequent normalization of the conditions in these larger paranasal sinuses without the sinuses themselves being subjected to any direct surgical manipulation.

In the initial episode of acute maxillary or frontal sinusitis with an air-fluid level on X-ray study, a cure can frequently be achieved by introducing a vasoconstrictor-soaked cotton pledget (with anesthetic, if indicated) under direct endoscopic vision directly to the afflicted site in the middle meatus. With this technique, puncture, fenestration, or other surgical procedures may be avoided.

Tomography is indicated in acute sinusitis only if complications are suspected. In chronic sinusitis, the tomography should be performed when the patient's infection is quiescent. The purpose of the radiologic examination is to demonstrate the underlying predisposing changes in the area of the ethmoid. During the acute phase, the diffuse opacities that result from the acute inflammation do not allow this to be done with any degree of accuracy.

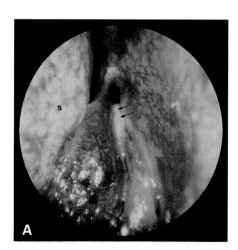

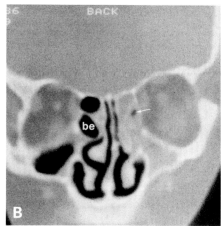

FIGURE 5.96 *A*, In this patient, inflamed polyps are seen protuding from the entrance to the middle meatus. Note the pathologic secretions coming from the infundibulum above the polyps (*arrows*). s = septum. *B*, This is the CT scan of the patient. On the patient's right side there is a relatively circumscribed area of disease in the turbinate sinus and in the infundibulum. There is a mucosal swelling in the maxillary sinus as well. The ethmoidal bulla is not affected. On the patient's left, the entire infundibulum is opacified, as is the remainder of the anterior ethmoid. A small air-containing space can be seen in the ethmoidal bulla (*arrow*). The left maxillary sinus is also completely opacified. be = ethmoidal bulla.

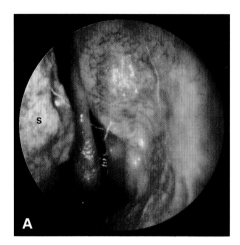

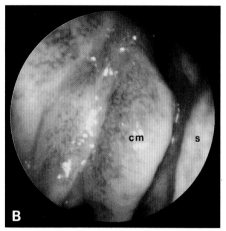

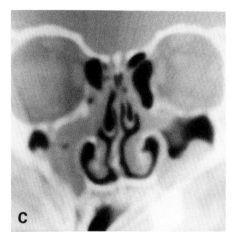

FIGURE 5.97 *A*, This patient had a long history of recurrent maxillary sinus empyemas. Note on the left side, the typical appearance of a diseased infundibulum with a massively bulging mucosa over the medial wall of the infundibulum. There is also contact between the uncinate process and the middle turbinate. s = septum. *B*, On the right side of the patient, there is a large concha bullosa of the middle turbinate. At the area of contact between the uncinate process and widened middle turbinate, polypoid mucosa protrudes. cm = middle turbinate and s = nasal septum. *C*, In this CT scan of the patient, the infundibular involvement and the consequent maxillary sinus disease can be seen clearly. The ethmoidal bulla itself is not significantly involved, but there is a disease in the space between the bulla and the concha bullosa (the so-called "turbinate sinus").

Figures 5.93 to 5.105 show the typical endoscopic and radiologic findings in patients with anterior ethmoidal disease in which the infundibulum is clearly involved.

If the large paranasal sinuses become secondarily affected by the disease in the infundibulum, the clinical picture is dominated by the symptoms of the secondary infection in these larger sinuses. The symptoms of isolated infundibular disease are usually mild and nonspecific. Headaches, often only a mild, dull pressure between the eyes or in the area of the inner canthus, a feeling of fullness in the nose, or impeded nasal breathing in spite of an open nasal passage are suggestive of infundibular diseases.

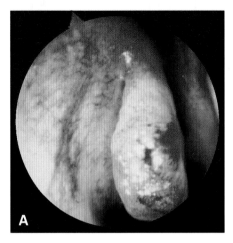

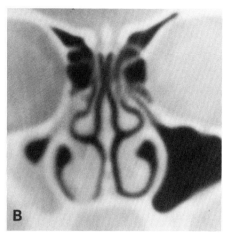

FIGURE 5.98   *A*, Note the endoscopically, relatively nondiseased appearance of this right middle meatus. The uncinate process is slightly bent medially. At the time of the examination, no pathologic secretions were present. *B*, In view of the patient's history (recurrent maxillary sinus empyema), a CT scan was performed. This showed a very narrow diseased infundibulum and the ensuing opacifications in the maxillary sinus on the right side.

FIGURE 5.99   *A*, Chronic maxillary sinusitis can be caused not only by massive ethmoidal disease, but also by discrete, localized disease. The medially folded uncinate process is in contact with the middle turbinate, which has been pushed laterally by a septal deviation. *B*, The CT scan shows obstruction of the infundibulum and the ensuing retention of secretions in the left maxillary sinus.

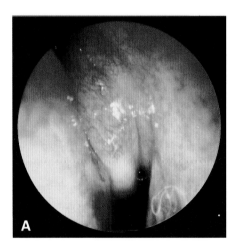

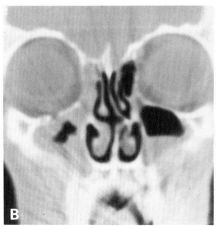

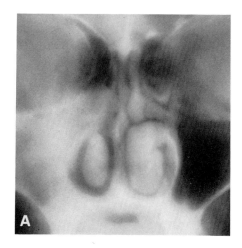

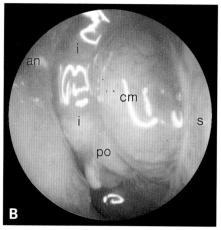

FIGURE 5.100 *A*, This is the conventional tomogram of a severely diseased infundibulum. The patient's principal clinical symptom was recurrent episodes of acute maxillary sinusitis. *B*, The endoscopic findings show that the medial wall of the infundibulum bulges massively in a medial direction, in the area of the agger nasi between the middle turbinate and the lateral wall of the nose. The mucosa of the middle turbinate shows edematous changes. The entire mucosa also shows edematous-polypoid changes. Individual polyps protrude from the middle meatus. There are pathologic secretions coming from the infundibulum. an = agger nasi; i = bulging medial wall of infundibulum ethmoidale; po = polyps; cm = middle turbinate; and s = septum.

FIGURE 5.101 *A*, This is a typical CT of infundibular disease. (Clinically the chief complaint was recurrent maxillary sinusitis.) The infundibulum is blocked by edematous mucous membrane between the uncinate process, the bulla, and the lamina papyracea. Note the ensuing mucosal edema in the right maxillary sinus. *B*, At endoscopy, the swollen head of the middle turbinate obstructs the view into the middle meatus. *C*, After the turbinate has been carefully retracted medially, polypoid mucosa appears on the medial wall of the infundibulum, where it and the turbinate were in contact (*arrows*). *D*, The posterior edge of the uncinate process is in close contact with the bulla ethmoidalis and thus completely closes the hiatus semilunaris (*arrows*). f = Freer elevator.

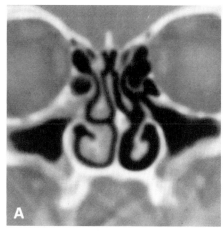

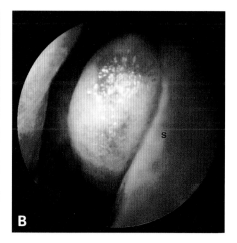

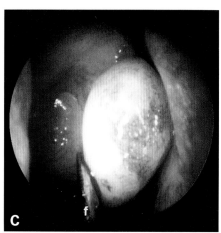

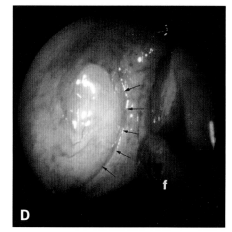

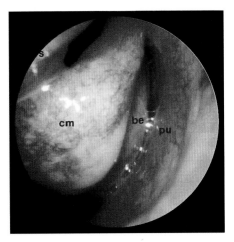

FIGURE 5.102 The acute phase of chronic, recurrent maxillary sinusitis. Note the hyperemia of the mucosa of the uncinate process. The uncinate process is overlapped by an anteriorly extended bulla ethmoidalis, which closes off the hiatus semilunaris and the ethmoidal infundibulum. pu = uncinate process; be = ethmoidal bulla; cm = middle turbinate; and s = septum.

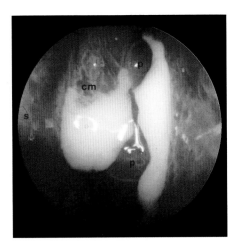

FIGURE 5.103 Acute, purulent sinusitis. Note the typical endoscopic appearance of the left middle meatus. There is a massive and occlusive protrusion of inflammatory, hyperemic mucosa from the middle meatus, and copious purulent secretions. cm = middle turbinate; p = polyps; and s = nasal septum.

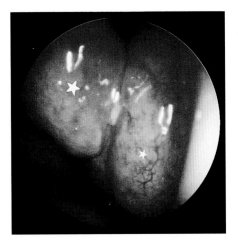

FIGURE 5.104 Purulent left maxillary sinusitis. The infundibular wall is massively arched medially. It is in close contact with the middle turbinate and represents an acute infundibular disease. Large star = middle turbinate and small star = medial wall of the infundibulum.

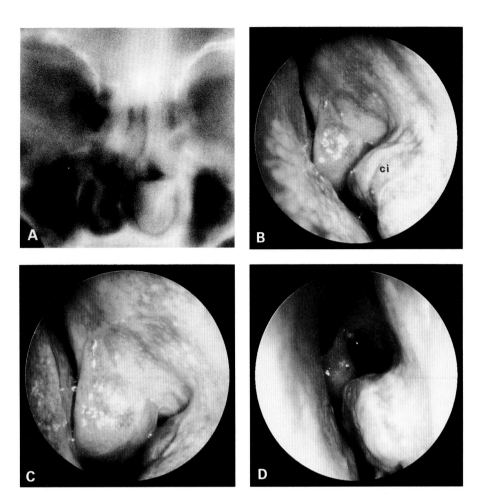

FIGURE 5.105 Hypertrophy of the turbinates, requiring surgical correction is rare in our practice. In most cases, the swelling of the turbinate is secondary to disease in the ethmoid. *A*, A markedly enlarged left inferior turbinate, but also note the evident anterior ethmoid disease. The ethmoid on the right is also involved, but not as severely as on the left. On the left side, the infundibulum extends far inferiorly, almost to the insertion of the inferior turbinate. *B*, A view along the hypertrophied inferior turbinate into the middle meatus, following the insertion of vasoconstrictor pledgets. ci = inferior turbinates. *C*, A close-up view of the same area. The medially folded uncinate process can be seen clearly, blocking the entrance to the middle meatus. At the time of surgery (see Chapter 11) massive ethmoidal disease was encountered. *D*, When this was cured, the inferior turbinate "shrunk back" to its normal size approximately 4 weeks postoperatively.

Disease of the Frontal Recess

The frontal recess is most commonly affected by disease that originates in the adjacent areas of the ostiomeatal complex, e.g., in the ethmoidal infundibulum, the hiatus semilunaris, the sinus of the turbinate, or the lateral sinus. Disease, however, can develop in the frontal recess as an isolated lesion. The involvement of the various compartments of the ethmoid by the internal spread of disease in the ethmoid depends not only upon the type and virulence of the inflammatory process but also, more importantly, upon the anatomic configuration of the individual components of the ethmoid (see Chapter 3).

Since the frontal recess is the ethmoidal antechamber of the frontal sinus, many of the changes that ultimately lead to actual disease of the frontal sinus are found in the frontal recess. Just as in the maxillary sinus, the frontal sinus is usually involved only secondarily, with infections reaching it through the nose by way of the frontal recess. Even when the symptoms of a frontal sinusitis dominate the clinical picture, the source of the complaints can usually be found not in the frontal sinus itself, but in the adjacent ethmoid. It should be emphasized that when plain survey radiographs of the paranasal sinuses show opacities or a fluid level in the frontal sinus, these changes are usually the result of a disease process in the frontal recess. Even in the presence of massive frontal sinus involvement, the changes in the frontal recess may appear very slight and can be identified only with conventional or computed tomography.

The endoscopic findings may also be minimal in disease of the frontal sinus. Abnormal secretions arising from the middle meatus may be the only endoscopic indication of frontal recess disease. Depending upon the shape of the uncinate process, these secretions may go directly into the infundibulum and appear only at the posterior portion of the hiatus semilunaris. From there they drain medially across the uncinate process. Frequently, circumscribed inflammatory mucous membrane changes in the frontal recess can only be detected if a 30 or 70 degree nasal endoscope can be introduced into the middle meatus. Occasionally, small polyps may be seen pressing forward and downward, just below the attachment of the middle turbinate. Larger polyps may bulge out of the middle meatus and block any view of the meatus or the attachment of the middle turbinate. An inflammatory bulging of the uppermost portion of the uncinate process, spreading eventually to the mucosa of the attachment of the middle turbinate, may also be an indication of a disease process in the frontal recess. If the drainage of secretions from the frontal recess (and thus from the frontal sinus) is completely blocked, a mucocele or a pyocele may develop from the retained secretions, which may result in a frontal sinus empyema.

In such cases, the medial wall of the frontal recess, i.e., that part of the middle turbinate immediately above the most anterior part of its attachment, may be bulging medially and may even come into contact with the nasal septum. The mucous membrane in this area may be only minimally affected, although frequently increased vascular markings can be observed over the protruding area. Inflammatory changes and polyp formation at the point of contact with the septum are not rare. Mucosal engorgement and polyp formation in this area are a frequent cause of blockage of the olfactory fissure.

Disease of the frontal recess does not necessarily produce all the symptomatology of a sinusitis. The chief complaints may be limited to an unpleasant sensation of pressure in the inner canthus or at the inferomedial aspect of the frontal sinus and, most commonly, headaches. In such patients, when there is adequate clinical suspicion, it is important to perform a careful endoscopic examination of the frontal recess. This is particularly important if the plain films of the sinuses reveal no appreciable changes. Since it may be impossible to inspect the sinus, even with a slender 2.7-mm diameter endoscope, the examiner must try to get a view of the recess by medially displacing the middle turbinate with a Freer elevator, or by using the Messerklinger technique of introducing the endoscope through a small trocar sheath.

Almost all anatomic variations of the structures of the anterior ethmoid can produce stenosis in the area of the frontal recess. Prominent among these variations are those of the uncinate process, the ethmoidal bulla, the formation of a concha bullosa of the middle turbinate, or a marked pneumatization of the agger nasi cells. Figures 5.106 to 5.113 demonstrate a variety of endoscopic and radiographic findings in diseases of the frontal recess.

Endoscopic diagnosis has proven to be of value in the conservative medical therapy of primary, acute frontal sinusitis. It is usually possible to pinpoint the etiologic focus in the frontal recess. Even in an empyema or in cases with a fluid level in the frontal sinus, it is frequently possible to introduce a decongestant, perhaps with the addition of a topical anesthetic, directly into the frontal recess, under direct endoscopic control. This almost always results in an improvement of the symptoms by promoting the drainage of secretions. With simultaneous antibiotic therapy, most cases of acute frontal sinusitis can be managed conservatively, if the pledgets are placed 2 or 3 times each day. If these maneuvers do not produce a definite improvement in the symptoms, or if the symptoms recur promptly after a period of improvement, we perform tomography and, if indicated, a surgical exploration of the frontal recess. Only in very exceptional cases (e.g., a threat of complications such as incipient osteomyelitis or intracranial complications and a very fulminant course) do we resort to an external surgical approach. With the endoscopic-conservative management of frontal sinusitis, we have not needed to perform trephination of the frontal sinus during the past decade.

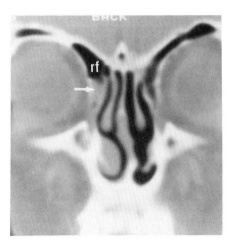

FIGURE 5.106 This coronal CT scan shows the relationship of the ethmoidal infundibulum (*arrow*) to the frontal recess in a patient in whom the uncinate process entends up to the skull base. rf = frontal recess.

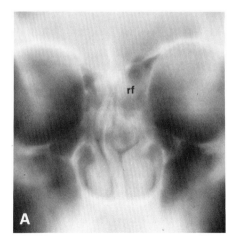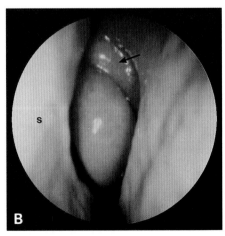

FIGURE 5.107 *A*, This CT scan shows an obviously bilaterally diseased left frontal recess. There is a concha bullosa on the left and septal deviation on the right.

rf = frontal recess. *B*, The endoscopic finding. Note the bulging of the uppermost segment of the medial wall of the infundibulum (*arrow*). s = septum.

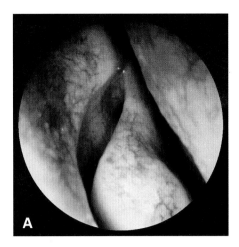

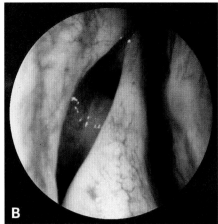

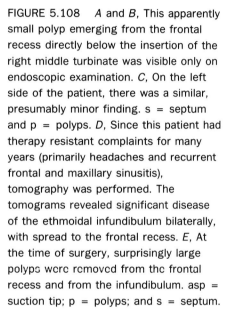

FIGURE 5.108   *A* and *B*, This apparently small polyp emerging from the frontal recess directly below the insertion of the right middle turbinate was visible only on endoscopic examination. *C*, On the left side of the patient, there was a similar, presumably minor finding. s = septum and p = polyps. *D*, Since this patient had therapy resistant complaints for many years (primarily headaches and recurrent frontal and maxillary sinusitis), tomography was performed. The tomograms revealed significant disease of the ethmoidal infundibulum bilaterally, with spread to the frontal recess. *E*, At the time of surgery, surprisingly large polyps were removed from the frontal recess and from the infundibulum. asp = suction tip; p = polyps; and s = septum.

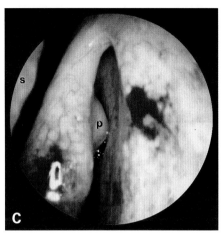

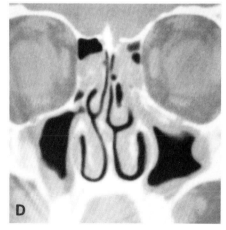

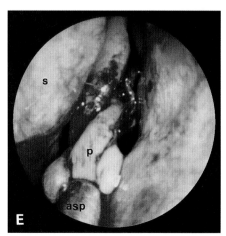

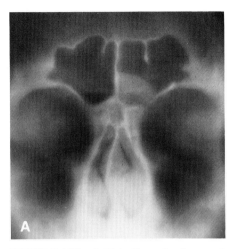

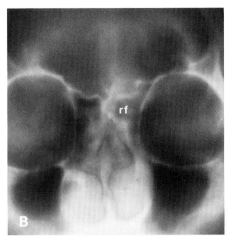

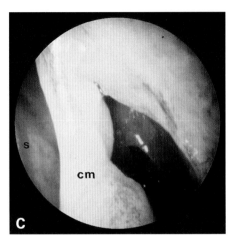

FIGURE 5.109 *A*, Note the retention cyst at the floor of the left frontal sinus. *B*, There was also disease in the frontal recess. During the endoscopic surgical management of the frontal recess, this cyst was grasped and removed in toto without having to enter the frontal sinus. *C*, The endoscopic findings. Note the edematous mucous membrane in the frontal recess. cm = middle turbinate and s = septum.

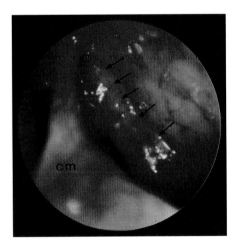

FIGURE 5.110 The endoscopic appearance of a patient with recurrent frontal sinusitis (acute phase). The mucosa of the free margin of the uncinate process is inflamed and acutely swollen and blocks entry into the frontal recess (*arrows*). cm = middle turbinate.

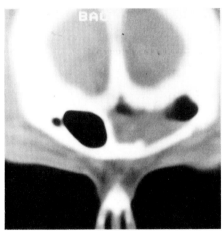

FIGURE 5.111 This tomogram shows an air-fluid level in the left frontal sinus.

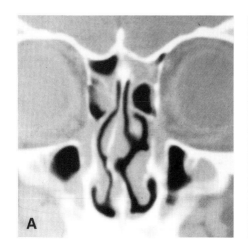

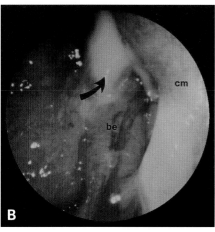

FIGURE 5.112 *A*, This is the CT of a patient with recurrent bilateral frontal sinus empyemas. Note the disease in both frontal recesses (and also of the rest of the ethmoid). *B*, The endoscopic findings after decongestant pledgets had been placed into the right frontal recess. Purulent secretions can be seen pouring out of the frontal sinus (*arrow*). (70 degree lens.) cm = the lateral side of the middle turbinate and be = anterior aspect of the bulla ethmoidalis.

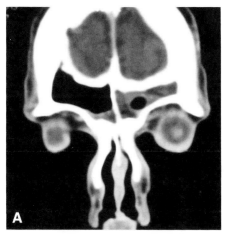

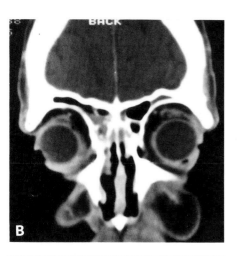

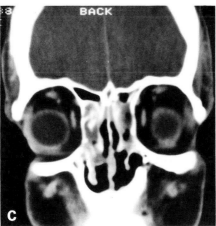

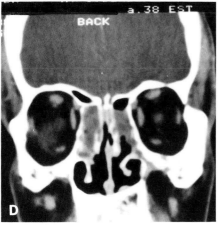

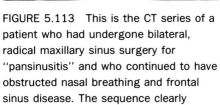

FIGURE 5.113 This is the CT series of a patient who had undergone bilateral, radical maxillary sinus surgery for "pansinusitis" and who continued to have obstructed nasal breathing and frontal sinus disease. The sequence clearly shows that the reason for the persistent complaints is disease in both frontal recesses and involving the entire anterior ethmoid as well. After these problems were treated, the frontal sinus recovered without ever having been touched.

Agger Nasi

The pneumatized agger nasi is an anatomic variant that appears as an elevation of the lateral wall of the nose just anterior to the attachment of the middle turbinate. Endoscopically, the agger nasi can appear as a small eminence just anterior to the insertion of the middle turbinate. In some individuals, the agger does not rise above the surrounding structures. The area of the agger nasi may become pneumatized, usually from the frontal recess to form the "agger nasi cells." When there is extensive pneumatization, an enlarged agger nasi air cell may displace the attachment of the middle turbinate medially and superiorly. When this occurs, the agger may appear as a distinct bulge on endoscopy. When an agger nasi cell is very large, or if it extends posteriorly, it may mechanically constrict the frontal recess. From the clinical diagnostic perspective it is important to remember that the agger nasi cells abut laterally onto the paper-thin lacrimal bone, which can have dehiscences per se. Any disease process affecting the lateral wall of the agger nasi can therefore spread to the adjacent lacrimal sac and produce epiphora and other inflammatory conditions of the lacrimal system. When the ophthalmologist is unable to find local causes for such problems, then an intranasal endoscopic examination and, if indicated, tomography, may reveal the underlying intranasal cause. Complaints arising from isolated agger nasi cell disease may be very atypical, and usually there is only a sensation of pressure between the eyes, with tenderness or pain over the medial palpebral ligament.

The involvement of the agger nasi cells in disease processes of the frontal recess and the ethmoidal infundibulum occurs much more commonly than a true isolated agger nasi pathology. Depending upon the anatomic configuration of the sinuses, there may be a connection between the agger nasi and the lateral sinus and consequently, disease may spread between these two areas. Large agger nasi cells may, by themselves, be a frequent cause of disease in the frontal recess. We have repeatedly found enlarged agger nasi cells as the sole etiologic factor in divers and aviators who have experienced difficulty in equalizing pressure changes (Figs. 5.114 to 5.119).

Endoscopically, a marked bulging anterior and sometimes superior to the attachment of the middle turbinate may indicate disease in this agger nasi. These endoscopic findings are significant only if the changes are pronounced. A definitive diagnosis of the presence of disease in the agger nasi can only be made by tomography. It is important that the tomograms be taken in a coronal plane when looking for disease in the agger nasi. Coronal views clearly demonstrate the anatomic relationship of the agger nasi to the lacrimal fossa. In coronal sections, those cells seen below the level of the

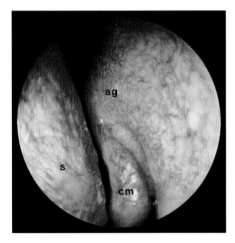

FIGURE 5.114 An agger nasi cell can be seen arching the lateral nasal wall above and anterior to the insertion of the middle turbinate. The uncinate process is slightly bent medially. s = septum; cm = middle turbinate; and ag = agger nasi area.

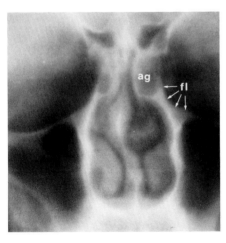

FIGURE 5.115 This is a conventional tomogram through bilateral agger nasi cells. The anatomic relationship of the agger nasi to the lacrimal sac is clearly seen. The medial bony wall of the lacrimal fossa (arrows) is also the lateral bony wall of the agger nasi cell. ag = agger nasi cell and fl = lacrimal fossa.

frontal sinus and frontal recess and that are located anterior to the attachment of the middle turbinate, are always agger nasi cells.

If the agger nasi is opacified, delineation of the posterior border of the agger may be difficult, since in some patients the agger nasi may have wide communication with the frontal recess and even with the lateral sinus. If the distance between sections is greater than 4 mm, the next section may cut through the ethmoidal bulla beyond the agger, thus making a delineation between these two structures difficult.

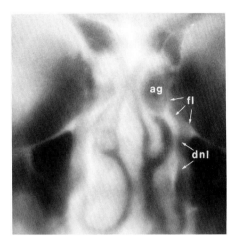

FIGURE 5.116 A conventional tomogram through the agger nasi cells bilaterally. The right agger nasi cell is diseased. This tomogram shows not only the lacrimal fossa, but most of the nasolacrimal ducts on both sides. ag = agger nasi cell; fl = lacrimal fossa; and dnl = nasolacrimal duct.

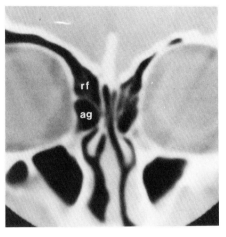

FIGURE 5.117 In this tomogram, bilateral large agger nasi cells are seen constricting (by their size) the frontal recess from inferiorly. rf = frontal recess and ag = agger nasi.

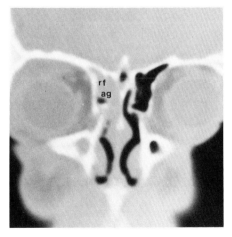

FIGURE 5.118 In this CT scan, disease in the frontal recess has spread to involve an agger nasi cell. rf = frontal recess and ag = agger nasi.

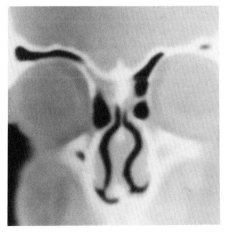

FIGURE 5.119 This CT scan shows a "healthy" agger nasi air cell and a diseased right frontal recess.

Haller's Cells

Haller's cells are yet another anatomic variant that may play an important role in the development of maxillary sinusitis. Haller's cells are ethmoidal cells that develop into the floor of the orbit (i.e., the roof of the maxillary sinus) adjacent to and above the maxillary sinus ostium, and which if enlarged can significantly constrict the posterior aspect of the ethmoidal infundibulum and the ostium of the maxillary sinus from above. If a Haller's cell becomes diseased, the natural ostium of the maxillary sinus may rapidly become obstructed with a secondary maxillary sinusitis developing.

Because Haller's cells are located lateral to the infundibulum, diagnostic endoscopy does not show any specific changes when Haller's cells are present. Changes secondary to infundibular disease such as a slight bulging in the lateral wall of the nose below the bulla ethmoidalis and a narrowing of the most posterior part of the hiatus semilunaris may suggest the presence of a Haller's cell. During an endoscopic examination of the maxillary sinus, on the other hand, the presence of an enlarged or diseased Haller's cell becomes obvious (Fig. 5.120).

The diagnosis of Haller's cell is thus primarily made by radiography. Figures 5.121 to 5.123 clearly show enlarged pneumatized Haller's cells and how this enlargement can produce a constriction of the ostium of the maxillary sinus. These illustrations show clearly how even a minor swelling of the mucous membranes (from any cause) can block the ostium of the maxillary sinus completely. Some horizontal septations or a complete division of the maxillary sinus, as seen in Fig. 5.193, may be due to an invasion of the maxillary sinus by a large Haller's cell. The resulting situation can only be visualized by tomography. Both sinuses had their own ostium and did not communicate with each other. The posterior, superior sinus opened into the middle meatus posterolaterally from the bulla ethmoidalis.

The site of origin of Haller's cells has not yet been established, and indeed discussion continues whether these cells belong to the anterior or the posterior ethmoidal cells. In our patients, we have gained the impression that their Haller's cells consistently opened into the middle meatus, i.e., before the basal lamella of the middle turbinate. This would suggest an anterior ethmoid origin. Unfortunately, it is not always possible to identify the exact location of the opening of such cells with any degree of certainty at operation.

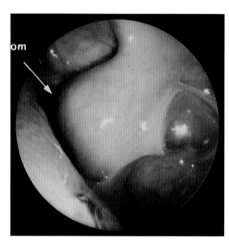

FIGURE 5.120 This is the endoscopic finding inside a left maxillary sinus. The bulging of the Haller's cell from the roof of the orbit can be clearly seen. The ostium of the maxillary sinus is severely constricted by this large cell (*arrow*). After removing the empyema by suction, residual foamy secretions can still be seen along the Haller's cell. om = maxillary sinus ostium.

FIGURE 5.121 This tomogram shows bilateral Haller's cells with obvious narrowing of the ethmoidal infundibulum on the right side (*arrow*). i = infundibulum and h = Haller's cell.

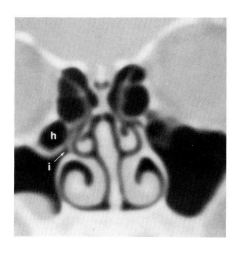

FIGURE 5.122 In this scan, Haller's cells can be seen invading the floor of the orbits. Note the narrow infundibulum on the right (arrow). i = infundibulum and h = Haller's cell.

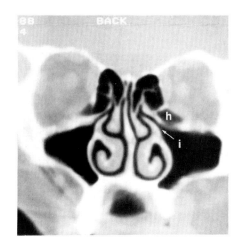

FIGURE 5.123 The scan was taken during a symptom-free interval in a patient with recurrent maxillary sinus empyema. Note the bilateral large Haller's cells compromising both infundibula. i = infundibulum.

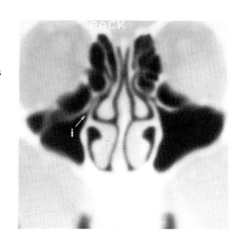

Disease of the Posterior Ethmoid

The posterior ethmoidal sinus is located, by definition, between the basal lamella of the middle turbinate anteroinferiorly, the lamina papyracea of the orbit laterally, and the superior and/or supreme turbinate medially. Posteriorly, the posterior ethmoidal sinus may extend up to the anterior wall of the sphenoidal sinus, and in some cases the cells of the posterior ethmoid may project laterally well beyond the sphenoidal sinus.

Isolated inflammatory diseases of the posterior ethmoid are extremely rare. In our patients, disease in the posterior ethmoids is usually combined with disease in the anterior ethmoid and, less commonly, with diseases in the sphenoidal sinus. Even those mucoceles that we encountered in this area have always involved either the anterior and posterior ethmoid or the sphenoid and the posterior ethmoid.

The posterior ethmoid is most frequently involved in diffuse polypoid sinusitis. Otherwise, the posterior ethmoid is involved in only about one-third of the cases of chronic sinusitis of inflammatory origin (Table 5.2).

Endoscopically, a drainage of secretions from the superior or supreme meatus or from the sphenoethmoidal recess may be the only indication of posterior ethmoidal sinus disease (Fig. 5.124). Inflamed mucosa may protrude from the superior or the supreme meatus and smaller or larger polyps may be present (Fig. 5.125). In our experience, larger polyps found between the middle turbinate and the septum may have three sites of origin. They may come from the mucosa of the olfactory fissure in cases of diffuse polyposis. They may originate at the site of mucosal contact between the septum and the middle turbinate or, less commonly, the superior turbinate, arising either from the septum or from the turbinate. Lastly, the polyps may originate from the posterior ethmoid, extend anteriorly and medially through the superior meatus, and appear in the nasal cavity medial to the middle turbinate. In severe polyposis, polyps originating from the posterior ethmoid and the margin of the superior turbinate are frequently found in the sphenoethmoidal recess.

If the posterior ethmoidal sinus is extensively pneumatized, and particularly if the pneumatization extends laterally along the sphenoid, the posterolateral portions of the posterior ethmoid may come into intimate contact with the optic nerve. We have encountered cases where the optic nerve, covered only by a very thin bony layer, passed almost freely through the posterior ethmoid, i.e., the nerve was surrounded by pneumatic spaces laterally as well as medially. This possibility must always be kept in mind during surgery for the correction of diffuse polyposis. Such Onodi cells can not always be

TABLE 5.2 Origination of Polyps in 200 Consecutive Patients*

80%	Uncinate—Turbinate—Infundibulum
65%	Face of Bulla—Hiatus—Infundibulum
48%	Frontal Recess
42%	"Turbinate Sinus"
30%	Inside Bulla
28%	"Lateral Sinus"
27%	Posterior Ethmoid (Superior Meatus)
15%	Middle Turbinate

Secondary Sinuses Affected

65%	Maxillary Sinus (Mucosal Swelling)
23%	Frontal Sinus (Mucosal Swelling)
8%	Sphenoid Sinus

* Not including diffuse polypoid rhinosinopathy.

identified accurately by endoscopy and only tomography can identify these cells and their relationship to the optic nerve with certainty. By changing the plane of the tomographic examination, the ocular muscles, the course of the optic nerve and its relationship to the posterior ethmoid can be clearly shown, particularly on axial CT.

In extensive pneumatization, both the sphenoid sinus and the posterior ethmoid may be in close contact with the foramen rotundum. In rare cases, the foramen rotundum may even be surrounded by pneumatic spaces laterally. The second division of the trigeminal nerve can thus become involved when the posterior aspects of the posterior ethmoid become diseased.

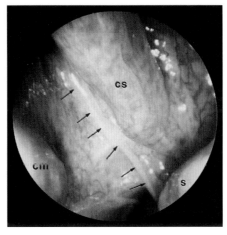

FIGURE 5.124 The tenacious secretions in the right superior meatus (*arrows*) suggest posterior ethmoidal sinus disease. cm = posterior end of the middle turbinate; cs = superior turbinate; and s = posterior end of the septum.

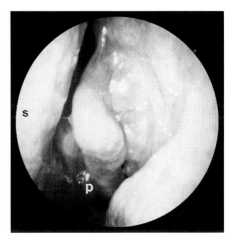

FIGURE 5.125 In this patient, polyps from the posterior ethmoid can be seen emerging between the middle turbinate and the septum in the posterior portion of the nasal cavity. s = septum and p = polyp.

Since even the root of the pterygoid process may be reached by extensive pneumatization, this area and the critical structures it contains may also become involved in inflammatory diseases of the posterior ethmoid. The same is also true for the nerve of the pterygoid canal (Vidian nerve) (see Disease of the Sphenoidal Sinus). In cases of midface neuralgias, the possibility of an irritation of the second division of the trigeminal nerve originating from the posterior ethmoid should be considered. Figures 5.126 to 5.129 show the typical radiographic findings in diseases of the posterior ethmoid.

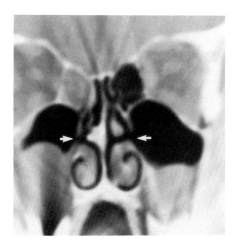

FIGURE 5.126 In this tomogram, the disease seen in the right posterior ethmoid is only part of the overall polypoid involvement of the entire ethmoid. The opacities in both maxillary sinuses are not cysts, but retained secretions that are unable to leave the maxillary sinus, because the infundibula are also involved (this, in spite of the presence of patent accessory ostia in the posterior fontanelles bilaterally, *arrows*).

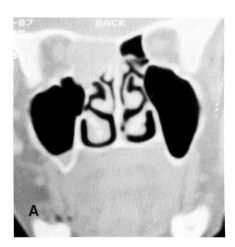
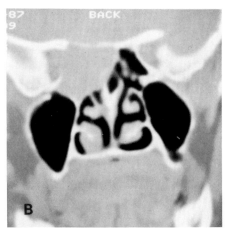

FIGURE 5.127 *A* and *B*, In this CT scan, the homogeneous opacification of the right posterior ethmoid is a large mucocele that includes the posterior ethmoid and the maxillary sinus. The medial wall of the orbital apex has been destroyed. The mucocele caused blindness and ophthalmoplegia in this patient. The ophthalmoplegia disappeared postoperatively, but unfortunately, the vision could not be restored.

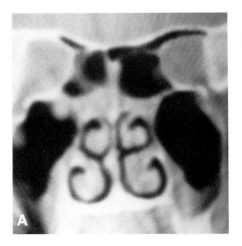

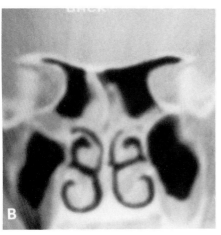

FIGURE 5.128 *A* and *B*, In these tomograms, there is extensive pneumatization of the posterior ethmoid, which extends into the roof of the orbits and the lesser wing of the sphenoid.

Under these anatomic conditions, particular care must be taken at the time of surgical management of the posterior ethmoid, not to injure the apex of the orbits.

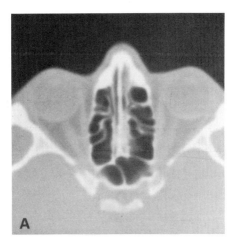

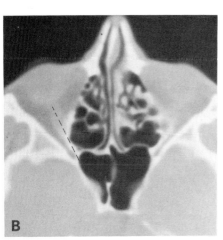

FIGURE 5.129 *A* and *B*, These CT scans show the relationship of the optic nerve to the posterior ethmoids. The most posterolateral portion of the posterior ethmoid can lie very close to the optic nerve. The posterior ethmoidal cells may even be closer to the nerve than the walls of the sphenoid sinus. The section in *B* is 4 mm higher than the section in *A*. It shows how the most posterior cells of the ethmoid may extend far laterally, even beyond the sphenoidal sinus. They thus may envelop the optic nerve (*line of dashes*) from above and cause the optic nerve to produce a marked bulge in the lateral wall of these posterior ethmoidal cells. These posterior ethmoidal cells, extending laterally, even beyond the ethmoid, were described particularly well by Onodi.

Disease of the Sphenoidal Sinus

According to the studies of Zinreich, and confirmed by our own clinical experience, the sphenoidal sinus is involved in only about 16 percent of patients with chronic sinusitis. Most of the time these are not separate diseases, but contiguous edema of the mucous membranes that appears as an opacification on the tomograms. Isolated involvement of the sphenoid is nevertheless more frequent than that of the posterior ethmoid. These involvements may include mucoceles, pyoceles, and isolated mycotic infections (Figs. 5.130 to 5.134). Clinically, the most prominent findings are headache and a variable amount of secretion discharged through the sphenoidal recess into the nasopharynx. The headaches are usually central, occasionally radiating to the temples or to the crown of the head.

In most cases it is not too difficult to obtain an endoscopic view into the sphenoethmoidal recess by using a 2.7-mm 30 or 70 degree nasal endoscope. Even when it is not possible to look into the ostium of the sphenoidal sinus, changes can usually be identified that suggest the presence of sphenoidal sinus disease. The observation of highly viscous or even frankly purulent secretions or mucosal swellings of varying severity, which may completely obstruct the sphenoethmoidal recess, are all important clinical findings that suggest the presence of sphenoidal sinus disease.

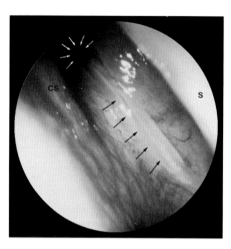

FIGURE 5.130 Note the viscous, mucopurulent secretions (*black arrows*) draining into the sphenoethmoidal recess from the ostium of a right sphenoidal sinus (*white arrows*). cs = superior turbinate and s = septum.

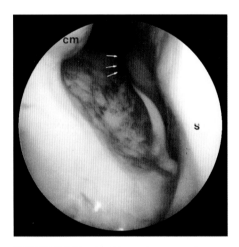

FIGURE 5.131 In this patient, purulent secretions can be seen draining from the right sphenoidal sinus through the sphenoethmoidal recess and on to the choana. Following the insertion of decongestant pledgets, the sphenoidal ostium (*arrows*) can be seen as a narrow fissure. The superior turbinate can not be seen. s = septum and cm = dorsal end of the middle turbinate.

FIGURE 5.132   This scan shows the isolated involvement of a left sphenoidal sinus. At the time of surgery, *Aspergillus fumigatus* mycosis was found. The internal carotid artery was only covered medially by a tissuepaper-thin bony lamella (*arrow*).

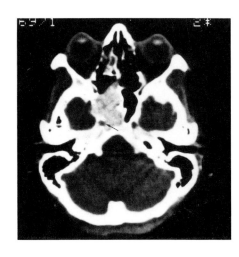

FIGURE 5.133   Note in this CT scan, the right sphenoidal sinus mucocele and the secondary edema of the mucous membrane over the intersinus septum on the left side.

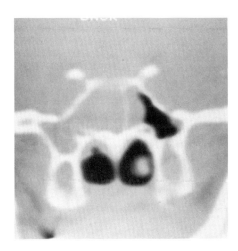

FIGURE 5.134   Note in this tomogram the small cyst on the floor of the left sphenoidal sinus.

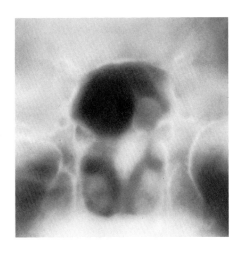

In addition to the type and extent of the disease, the points of major interest in the radiologic examination of the sphenoid are its relationship to the optic nerve and to the bulge of the internal carotid artery. During surgical procedures the surgeon must always remember that the optic canal and the bulge of the internal carotid artery may only be covered by a very thin and occasionally fragmented bony layer in the area of the sphenoid and that these two vital structures may not be well protected. In addition, the surgeon must always be aware that the internal carotid artery may bulge far into the lumen of the sphenoidal sinus (Figs. 5.135 and 5.136). Depending upon the degree of pneumatization, both the foramen rotundum and the pterygoid canal may protrude into the lumen of the sphenoidal sinus. If the bony walls of the sphenoidal sinus have been damaged, these nerves can become affected by any disease process in the sphenoidal sinus (Figs. 5.137 and 5.138). The otolaryngologist should consider the possible etiologic relationship between disease processes in the ethmoidal and sphenoidal sinuses and the wide variety of facial pains or "atypical trigeminal neuralgia" that could be cured by endoscopic means, once a proper diagnosis is made.

Isolated polyps, originating from the anterior wall of the sphenoidal sinus or from its interior and extending as choanal polyps into the nasopharynx, are extremely rare.

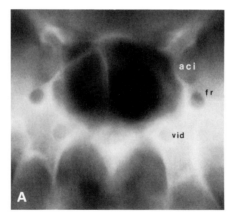 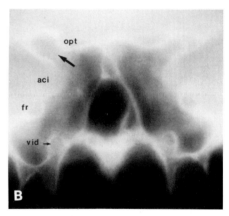

FIGURE 5.135 A and B, These tomograms show the relationship of the sphenoidal sinus to the internal carotid artery, the foramen rotundum and the maxillary nerve, and the pterygoid canal with the vidian nerve. aci = internal carotid artery; fr = foramen rotundum; vid = pterygoid canal with the vidian nerve; and opt = optic nerve.

FIGURE 5.136 The bony wall of the sphenoidal sinus shows a marked dehiscence, particularly over the bulge of the internal carotid artery. When the clinoid processes are pneumatized, the recess can be plainly seen between the bulge of the internal carotid artery and the optic nerve (*arrow*). aci = internal carotid artery.

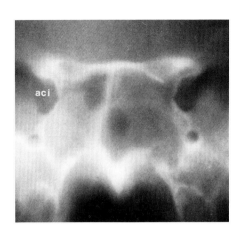

FIGURE 5.137 This CT scan shows an extensively pneumatized sphenoidal sinus that extends into the floor of the middle cranial fossa and, bilaterally, into the root of the pterygoid process. vid = vidian canal in the pterygoid processes.

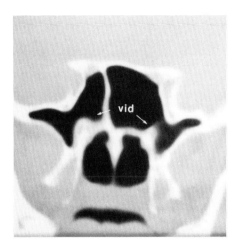

FIGURE 5.138 This extensively pneumatized sphenoidal sinus is divided by multiple septa. vid = vidian canal in the pterygoid bone.

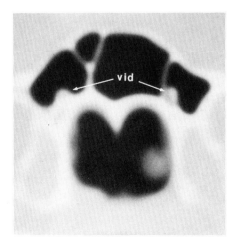

Combined Paranasal Sinus Disease on Computed Tomograms

While any of the previously described individual components of the ethmoid can be affected individually and in isolation, most commonly sooner or later the disease spreads from one key area to another until finally the larger subordinated paranasal sinuses become involved with clinical symptoms appearing at that time.

The patient in Figure 5.139 presented with a history of a chronic cold, nasal obstruction, and (most importantly) difficulty in equalizing pressure when diving. The plain films showed opacities in the maxillary and frontal sinuses, but did not allow the underlying changes in the ethmoid to be identified. Tomography, performed during one of the patient's symptom-free periods, clearly disclosed the site of the primary ethmoidal disease.

In Figure 5.139A, mucosal swelling and retained secretions can be seen in the right frontal sinus.

Figure 5.139B is a section about 8 mm posterior through the frontal recess and lacrimal fossa. One can just see the most anterior attachment of the middle turbinate and the thickened mucous membrane around the cellular septa in the frontal recess on the right.

The section shown in Figure 1.139C is 4 mm further posterior. This section cuts through the nasolacrimal duct and shows the attachment of the inferior turbinate. The most anterior portions of the bulla ethmoidalis are visible and the opacification in the frontal recess has become more pronounced.

In the section shown in Figure 5.139D, 4 more millimeters posterior, the uncinate process and the ethmoidal infundibulum appear for the first time. The mucosal swelling extends to the area between the anterior portion of the bulla ethmoidalis and the middle turbinate. The most anterior portions of the ethmoidal infundibulum appear to be clear and the right hiatus semilunaris is also clear.

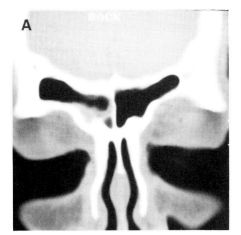

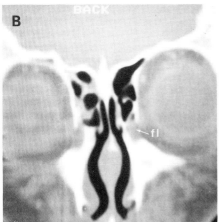

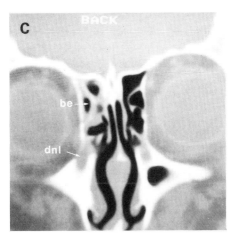

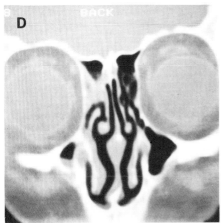

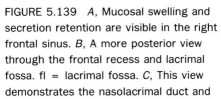

FIGURE 5.139 *A*, Mucosal swelling and secretion retention are visible in the right frontal sinus. *B*, A more posterior view through the frontal recess and lacrimal fossa. fl = lacrimal fossa. *C*, This view demonstrates the nasolacrimal duct and portions of the ethmoidal bulla. be = ethmoidal bulla and dnl = nasolacrimal duct. *D*, In this view, the uncinate process and ethmoidal infundibulum become visible.

FIGURE 5.139 continues

Four millimeters further posterior, Figure 5.139E shows not only the opacities between the bulla ethmoidalis and the middle turbinate, but the opacities in the bulla itself. The hiatus semilunaris is still clear, but the ethmoidal infundibulum is blocked anterior to the ostium of the maxillary sinus. This finding becomes particularly obvious when the two sides are compared with each other. On the left side a narrow but completely open infundibulum and a patent ostium of the maxillary sinus can be seen. For the first time the marked opacification of the anterior segments of the ethmoid becomes apparent.

This is even clearer in Figure 5.139F, another 4 mm posterior. The mucosal swelling in the bulla ethmoidalis on the right is evident although the sinus lateralis above it is still clear. This figure shows the superior turbinate for the first time and one can see that the most anterior part of the superior meatus is blocked by swollen mucous membranes.

Six mm further posterior (Fig. 5.139G), this section cuts through the center of the accessory ostium in the posterior fontanelle bilaterally. The accessory ostium is widely patent (which means that the maxillary sinus is well ventilated) and yet, there is marked mucous membrane swelling on the right side and free thick secretions were also demonstrated endoscopically. These secretions did not leave the maxillary sinus through the accessory ostium. This observation shows clearly that in diseases of the anterior ethmoid and obstruction of the infundibulum, ventilation of the maxillary sinus by itself is insufficient to produce a recovery from the disease process.

On the right side, the ground lamella of the middle turbinate can be seen, attached to the lamina papyracea representing the border between the anterior and posterior ethmoid. The superior meatus is opacified bilaterally. Figure 5.139H is at the edge of the posterior ethmoid and shows well aerated cells up to the swollen areas in the superior meatus. Further sections through the posterior ethmoid and sphenoid are unremarkable. This CT provides the surgeon with valuable information to supplement his diagnostic endocopic examination. He now knows that the center of the disease is located in the anterior ethmoid (frontal recess) around the ethmoidal bulla and in the infundibulum, and consequently, he can limit the surgical intervention to these areas. Neither the frontal nor the maxillary sinus need to be manipulated during the procedure.

At surgery, the uncinate process, which inserted far laterally on the inferior turbinate, was resected. This allowed a view of the ostium of the maxillary sinus, which was enlarged slightly at the expense of the anterior fontanelle. The ostium of the posterior fontanelle was also included in the enlarged opening to avoid a circular flow of secretions.

The secretions in the maxillary ostium were removed by suction, but the mucosa was not otherwise touched. The ethmoidal bulla was resected in its entirety and the cellular septa were removed from the frontal recess. Following this, an unobstructed view into the frontal sinus was obtained. The mucosal swelling in the superior meatus was not touched during the procedure. Inspection of the posterior ethmoid through the ground lamella showed nothing remarkable, as expected, and required no intervention in this area. Both the frontal and maxillary sinuses recovered completely and permanently following this procedure.

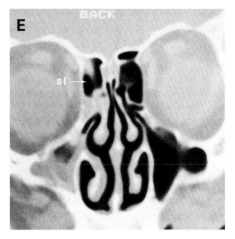
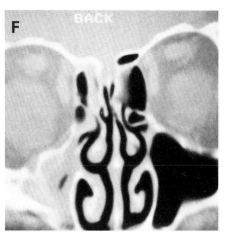
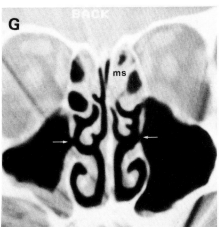
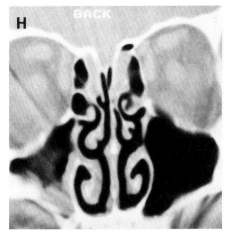

FIGURE 5.139 continued *E*, Opacities can be seen in the ethmoidal bulla, between the bulla and the middle turbinate, and in the ethmoidal infundibulum. sl = sinus lateralis. *F*, Mucosal swelling is visible in the ethmoidal bulla and the anterior superior meatus. *G*, The superior meatus is blocked by swollen mucous membranes. The *arrows* indicate patent accessory ostia in the posterior fontanelles. ms = superior meatus. *H*, This is the last tomographic cut demonstrating mucosal disease. The posterior ethmoid and sphenoid sinuses were normal.

NASAL POLYPOSIS

Polypoid changes are the most frequent pathologic manifestations in the mucous membranes that line the nasal cavity and the paranasal sinuses. In addition to "chronic sinusitis," polyposis of the nose and sinuses is the most frequent indication for surgical intervention in this area.

The etiology of polyp formation is still widely debated, and indeed, it is not yet clear whether "nasal polyposis" represents a single unified disease process of several as yet unidentified disorders. Even today, there is still no clear definition of a "nasal polyp," nor is it clear *when* an edematous change of the mucous membrane becomes a true "polyp."

Endoscopically it has been shown that with few exceptions almost all of the polyps that appear in the nasal cavity arise from the ethmoid or from its immediate anatomic vicinity.

Clinically, a wide spectrum may be seen, from circumscribed mucous membrane edema, through isolated polyps, to a massive polyposis that completely fills the nasal spaces and the paranasal sinuses. There is frequently a marked discrepancy between the patient's symptoms and the clinical findings, and it is surprising how frequently patients with marked polyposis report very few symptoms, while relatively circumscribed polypoid changes may be responsible for significant symptoms.

In uncomplicated nasal polyposis, the anterior ethmoid is almost always involved. With the exception of isolated choanal polyps (see Choanal Polyps) or adjacent to tumors, we have not seen a case of an isolated polyp arising from the posterior ethmoid.

Those cases in which no gross polyps can be seen in the nasal cavity create special diagnostic demands on the endoscopist. The small polyp, illustrated in Figure 5.108, that protrudes between the uncinate process and the attachment of the middle turbinate could not be seen either with the naked eye or with a microscope and was detected with the endoscope only after the instrument had been introduced as far as possible toward the entrance to the middle meatus. At the time of examination, there were no additional pathologic changes in the more posterior parts of the middle meatus and no secretions were visible. The plain sinus radiographs showed "normal" maxillary and frontal sinuses and there were no opacities in the ethmoid. In view of the very long history of symptoms and the presumably minor endoscopic findings, tomography was performed. This showed evident opacities in the infundibulum and in the frontal recess. At the time of surgery, surprisingly large polypoid masses were removed from this area of the ethmoid, where they had apparently been under considerable pressure, thereby contributing significantly to the patient's complaints. In this case, the minor endoscopic findings represented "the tip of the iceberg."

Even in severe polyposis, the site of origin of the polyps can frequently be identified in the middle meatus. Table 5.2 displays the findings that we have gathered in 200 patients during endoscopic examination or surgery. It is evident that the majority of the polyps originate in the narrow spaces of the (anterior) ethmoid. The most frequent sites of origin were the contact areas of the uncinate process and the middle turbinate and the ethmoidal infundibulum. Eighty percent of our patients showed polyps originating from these two areas.

In almost two-thirds of patients, polyps also originated from the anterior aspect of the ethmoidal bulla, where they obstructed the hiatus semilunaris, invaded the ethmoidal infundibulum, or protruded anteriorly between the middle turbinate and the uncinate process into the middle meatus.

In about 50 percent of the patients, polyps were found in the frontal recess. This is particularly important since in this area, in many cases, the polyps may not be visible even through the endoscope. In this situation the combination of endoscopy and tomography is particularly valuable.

Further favorite sites were the "turbinate sinus" (the space between the concavity of the middle turbinate and the medial surface of the ethmoidal bulla) (42% of all patients) and the "lateral sinus" (the variably developed space between the roof of the ethmoid above, the bulla ethmoidalis below, and the basal lamella of the middle turbinate posteriorly). The lateral sinus was most frequently affected when there was a simultaneous polypoid involvement of the posterior ethmoid (65% of patients showed a variable degree of mucous membrane engorgement in the maxillary sinus, and 23% in the frontal sinus). Except for a few cases of retention cysts, we found no instance of significant maxillary or frontal sinus pathology in which there was not also a pathologic process in the adjacent ethmoidal compartments. Polypoid changes in the sphenoidal sinus were found in only 8 percent of the patients. As a curiosity, we found three patients in whom the polyps originated from the posterior portion of the septum.

It is apparent that polyps originate much more frequently in the fissures and narrow spaces of the ethmoid, than from the ethmoidal cells themselves, or from the paranasal sinuses. Such precise identification of the site of origin is not possible if the polyposis is massive or in recurrent polyps after a preceding surgical extirpation.

The appearance of nasal polyps may vary widely from edematous, glassy, cystic to coarse and fibrous (Figs. 5.140 to 5.145). In acute rhinosinusitis, the evolution from a circumscribed edema to a subsequent polyp can be followed with the endoscope.

If polyps are visible *medial to the middle turbinate* (see Figs. 5.140 and 5.144), in our experience they usually originate from one of three sites:

1. From the mucous membrane of the olfactory fissure (which in our experience is extremely rare except in cases of diffuse polypoid rhinosinopathy).
2. From the contact area between the middle turbinate and the septum.
3. From the posterior ethmoid or from the superior meatus, from where they prolapse and thus lie medial to the middle turbinate.

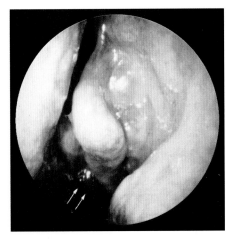

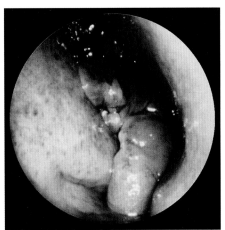

FIGURE 5.140   Nasal polyps are seen protuding from the left middle meatus. Additional polyps can also be seen deep and medial to the middle turbinate (*arrows*). At the time of surgery, these posterior polyps were seen to originate in the posterior ethmoid and had fallen anteromedially, through the superior meatus.

FIGURE 5.141   Typical appearance of a severe polyposis on the left side. The polyps protruding from the middle meatus obscure the view into the middle meatus and extend to the floor of the nose.

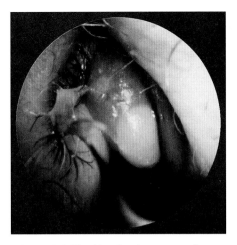

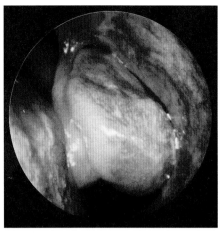

FIGURE 5.142 Nasal polyps extending to the vestibule of the nose on the right side. Histologically, the white thickened patches on the polyps showed marked squamous cell metaplasia.

FIGURE 5.143 This large, fibrous, solitary polyp originated in the left anterior ethmoid. Note how it has reduced the middle turbinate to a thin lamella.

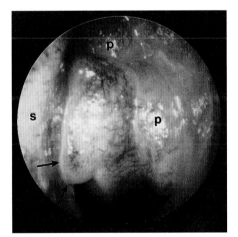

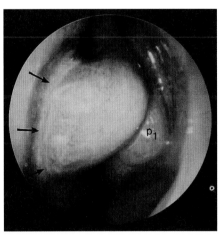

FIGURE 5.144 In this patient, there is a large concha bullosa of the left middle turbinate and polyps can be seen extruding from the middle meatus. There are also polypoid mucous membrane changes (arrows) at the area of contact between the concha bullosa and the nasal septum. p = polyps and s = septum.

FIGURE 5.145 In this patient, there is a paradoxically bent middle turbinate with polyps showing in a diseased middle meatus. The uncinate process is medially bent. The most anterior polyp (p_1) arises at the site of contact of the uncinate process with the middle turbinate. The deeper polyp (p_2) arises from the anterior surface of the ethmoid bulla. It is noteworthy that the mucosa of the middle turbinate has undergone polypoid changes in this area of its contact with nasal septum (arrows). (This picture was taken after the application of a topical decongestant.)

Polyps may prolapse into the sphenoethmoidal recess from the posterior ethmoid in a similar manner. In our experience, isolated polyps arising from the sphenoidal sinus are extremely rare.

The phenomenon of polyps originating at the site of contact of opposed mucous membranes has been well documented in many cases (Figs. 5.144 to 5.149 and see 5.38, 5.42, and 5.43).

In those patients with massive polyposis it may not be possible to advance the endoscope to the entrance of the middle meatus, especially when the polyps have already extended into the vestibule of the nose (see Figs. 5.141 and 5.142). In cases of even more severe polyposis, there may be polypoid lobular hyperplasia of the head or free margin of the middle turbinate. We have encountered this type of polypoid degeneration in about 15 percent of our patients with severe polyposis.

The degree of mucosal disease in the maxillary or frontal sinuses does not correlate with the total mass of ethmoidal polyps. Total opacification of the large paranasal sinuses may occur even in the presence of only circumscribed ethmoidal pathology.

In our experience it is not the extent of the polypoid growth in the ethmoid that determines the involvement of the maxillary and frontal sinuses, but the location of these changes. When the maxillary and frontal sinuses were opacified, we were almost always able to demonstrate pathology in the connected key sites in the lateral wall of the nose.

When considering the indications for surgical intervention, the surgeon must always remember that a significant percentage of the radiographic shadows in the maxillary sinus are simply retained secretions. These are extremely viscous and have a curved radiographic contour that frequently cannot be distinguished from cystic or polypoid changes. Assessment may be possible only at the time of surgery, through an enlarged ostium in the middle meatus or by preoperative endoscopy through the canine fossa. Not infrequently, one sees cysts and polyps extending from the ethmoid through the ostium into the maxillary sinus (see Figs. 5.176 and 5.177). In view of these facts, there is usually little need for direct surgical intervention directed primarily towards the frontal and maxillary sinuses.

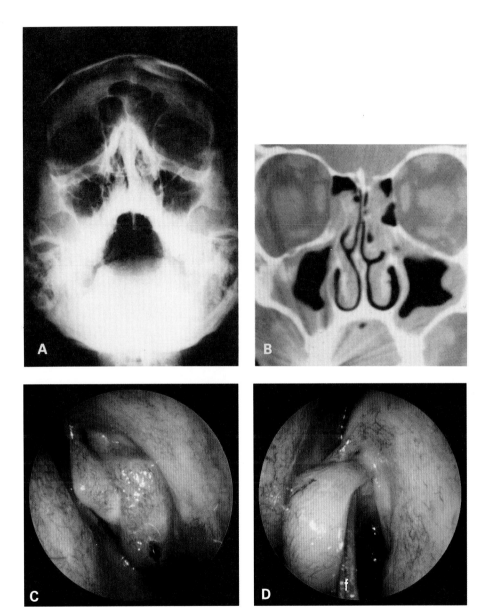

FIGURE 5.146 *A*, When the maxillary and frontal sinuses are not extensively diseased, the survey or routine plain sinus radiographs is usually unremarkable. *B*, Tomography, on the other hand, clearly shows the area and extent of the pathologic changes (both radiographs are from the same patient). These are the endoscopic findings. *C*, A large polyp can be seen extruding from the left middle meatus. *D*, When the polyp is displaced medially by a Freer elevator, the origin of the polyp can be seen. It arises by a stalk from the anterior and inferior surface of the ethmoidal bulla as well as from the topmost portion of the uncinate process.

In patients with the sinubronchial syndrome (bronchial asthma and chronic sinusitis), especially of the ASA-sensitive variety, extremely viscous secretions are usually found between the polyps. Because of their high viscosity and surface tension, these secretions frequently assume a globular shape and they cannot always be distinguished from polyps, even by endoscopy. Sometimes it is only at the actual time of extraction that the surgeon notices that the forceps have grasped a mucus plug, rather than a polyp. The production of this highly viscous secretion is a manifestation of a mucous membrane disorder of unknown etiology.

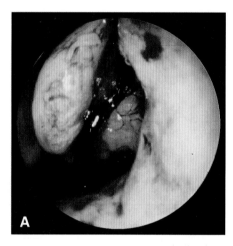 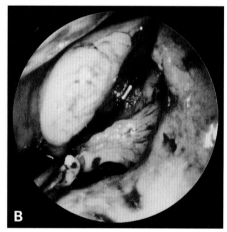

FIGURE 5.147 *A*, In a similar case as shown in Figure 5.146, after resection of the uncinate process and the removal of a few polyps from the ethmoidal infundibulum, a similar situation was present. Note the lobulated polyp arising from the anterior surface of the bulla.

This polyp filled the hiatus semilunaris and extended partially into the infundibulum. *B*, The polyp is lifted with the suction tip to demonstrate its size. Further surgery showed that the interior of the ethmoidal bulla was not diseased.

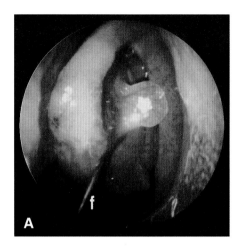 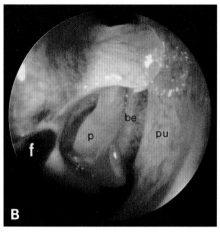

FIGURE 5.148 *A*, In this photograph, a left middle turbinate is displaced medially with a Freer elevator and the site of origin of a small polyp at the contact point between the middle turbinate and the uncinate process is demonstrated. f = Freer elevator. *B*, Advancing the endoscope revealed several additional polyps arising from the contact point between the middle turbinate and the ethmoidal bulla, the so-called turbinate sinus. f = Freer elevator; p = polyp; pu = uncinate process; and be = ethmoidal bulla.

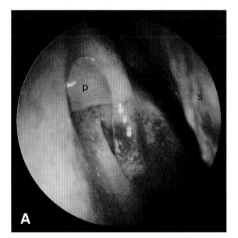 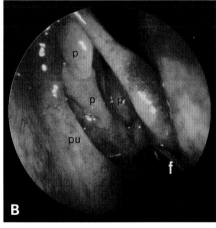

FIGURE 5.149 *A*, On the right side, the middle turbinate is slightly curled laterally and is in contact with the uncinate process. A small polyp can be seen protruding from the entrance of the middle meatus. p = polyp and s = septum. *B*, After displacing the middle turbinate medially, one can see that the "small" polyp is only the most anterior extension of a marked polypoid mucous membrane involvement that originated on the anterior surface of the ethmoidal bulla and has completely filled the hiatus semilunaris. A number of additional polyps can be seen in the turbinate sinus. pu = uncinate process; p = polyps; be = ethmoidal bulla; and f = Freer elevator.

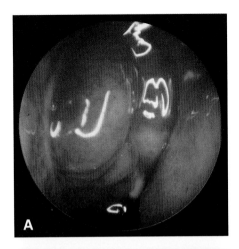

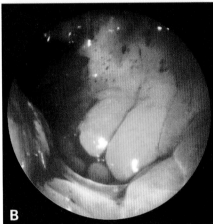

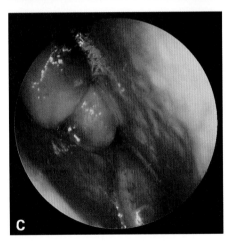

FIGURE 5.150 *A*, The endoscopic appearance of a left middle meatus in a case of severe diffuse polypoid rhinosinopathy. *B*, The view into the maxillary sinus of this patient after removal of the copious retained secretions. Note how the entire mucous membrane is polypoid and edematous. *C*, Diffuse polypoid rhinosinopathy. An intranasal view in the direction of the olfactory fissure, on the right side, anterior to the insertion of the middle turbinate. The fissure is completely obstructed. This picture was taken after extensive local (topical) decongestion.

The CT scans are frequently difficult to interpret accurately in patients with recurrent polyposis who have had previous surgical procedures and in patients with ethmoidal polyps who have a significant retention of highly viscous secretions. The chronic inflammatory stimuli and possibly the pressure from the polyps may have caused extensive destruction of the thin bony septa and cellular walls of the ethmoidal region. In addition, in older patients, there may be an ongoing decalcification. Because of the slight differences in density, the entire ENT system may be homogeneously opacified all the way to the sphenoid. This appearance may suggest the need for a radical operation, when in fact the cause of these opacities may be only a moderate polyposis with corresponding stasis and retention, which can be managed with a considerably less radical surgical intervention. This fact makes it very clear that the indications for surgical intervention in general and especially for a radical surgical procedure should not be determined exclusively on the basis of the radiologic findings (Figs. 5.151 to 5.153).

There is one specific form of nasal polyposis, "diffuse polypoid rhinosinopathy" (DPRSP), that has a distinct endoscopic appearance and that must be distinguished from the types of polyposis described above. In DPRSP the individual polyps can no longer be distinguished and the diffusely engorged polypoid mucous membrane of the middle meatus becomes confluent with the head and the free margin of the middle turbinate and with other mucosal areas. The entire mucous membrane is so swollen and engorged that it is usually impossible to identify individual landmarks. Tomography usually shows a homogeneous opacification of the entire nasal space, or at least of the ethmoidal area. The large paranasal sinuses may also be affected. Maxillary sinus endoscopy in these cases usually finds a totally diffuse swelling and polypoid degeneration of the entire mucous membrane (Figs. 5.150 and 5.151). In these patients, there is usually no evidence of an IgE-mediated, Type I allergy. Diffuse polypoid rhinosinopathy is more frequently found in patients with aspirin sensitivity, asthma, or cystic fibrosis (see Fig. 5.152).

Diffuse polypoid rhinosinopathy presents a major therapeutic dilemma:

The severe and widespread mucosal changes are hardly conducive to conservative medical therapy, and yet when treated surgically, diffuse polypoid rhinosinopathy has a high rate of recurrence with the symptoms reappearing sometimes after a few weeks. (see Chapters 9 and 13).

In diffuse polypoid rhinosinopathy, we are confronted with a disease of unknown etiology that represents a generalized involvement

FIGURE 5.151   This is a tomogram of a 68-year-old patient with ASA intolerance and bronchial asthma and long standing diffuse polypoid rhinosinopathy (DPRSP) who has not had previous surgery. No details of the bony structure of the ethmoid can be seen. There is only a hint of the middle turbinate in this tomographic section. Apparently the long period of disease has led to a partial destruction of the bony lamellae by inflammatory stimuli and pressure from the polyps. There is also significant decalcification in some areas.

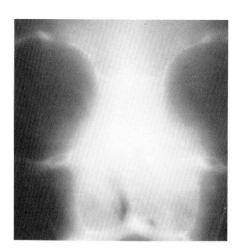

FIGURE 5.152   Note the diffuse opacification of the entire paranasal sinus system in this 7-year-old boy with cystic fibrosis. The small pocket of air in the left maxillary sinus strongly suggests that the opacification of the maxillary sinus is due to retained secretions only. The age-related, low position of the roof of the ethmoid should be noted.

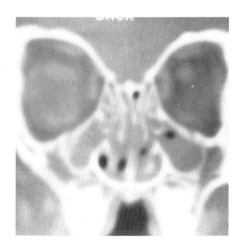

FIGURE 5.153   In this CT scan of a patient with severe bilateral polyposis, (not of the DPRSP-type) there is only minimal involvement of the maxillary sinus. The ethmoidal infundibulum was not completely obstructed (not visible in this tomographic section). Note on the right side how severely the ethmoidal fissures are involved and yet how some of the individual cells are spared (in this picture at the transition from the anterior to the posterior ethmoid).

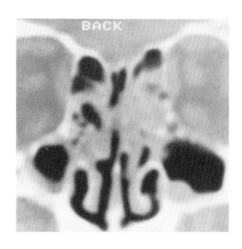

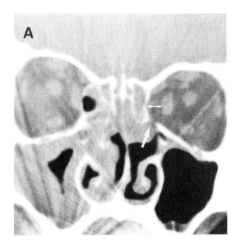

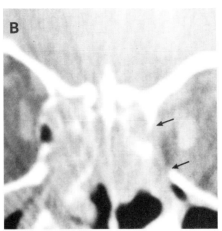

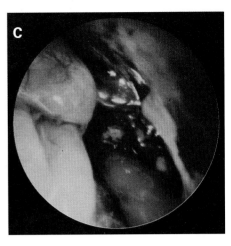

FIGURE 5.154 *A*, This is the CT scan of a patient who has undergone repeated endonasal polyp surgery during which the middle turbinate was at least partially resected. The *arrow* points to a defect produced by the surgery in the lamina papyracea. There is an "encapsulated" prolapsed piece of fat from the orbit, or a thick layer of scar tissue in the area of the ethmoid defect (note the distance between the median rectus muscle and the most proximal part of the ethmoid [*double arrow*]). *B*, In a section 5 mm further posterior, the extent of the defect in the lamina papyracea becomes more apparent (*arrows*). *C*, View into the left nostril of the patient. There is a coarse, diffuse, recurrent polyposis, embedded in tracts of scars and plaques. The middle turbinate can no longer be identified.

of the entire nasal and paranasal sinus mucosa. In our experience, the largest percentage of therapeutic failures comes from this group of patients. Even radical surgical approaches, attempted in cases of recurrent disease, have not produced a permanent cure and to date no effective medical therapy has been discovered.

A different problem of particular concern to the surgeon is presented by patients who develop recurrent polyps following previous surgery. Depending on the type and number of the previous operations, important landmarks such as the middle turbinate may be absent and the space between the lamina papyracea, the roof of the ethmoid, the cribriform plate, and the septum may be filled with dense fibrous adhesions surrounding a few polyps. In many cases even tomography cannot identify the structures that are so important for the surgeon to identify.

During repeat surgical procedures, the greatest caution is required, since the previous operation may have left significant bony defects in critical locations. Polyps on connective tissue strands may be attached to the dura of the cribriform plate or to the lamina papyracea. An attempt to remove these polyps may result in injury to these structures and the possibility of serious complications. Such preexisting bony defects may have resulted in a prolapse of the orbital contents into the anterior or posterior ethmoid. Because of their similar tissue density, such a prolapse of the orbital contents cannot be distinguished radiologically from diseased edematous mucous membranes. There is consequently a real risk of opening the orbit when attempting to remove what appears to the surgeon to be diseased mucous membrane from the area of the ethmoid (Fig. 5.154).

Choanal Polyps

Choanal polyps are a separate clinical entity. While the etiology of choanal polyps is unclear, they present a fairly uniform clinical picture. An antrochoanal polyp almost always has two components. A cystic component frequently fills most of the maxillary sinus and appears to originate from its posterolateral wall. This maxillary sinus component extends by a usually slender "stalk" through either the natural ostium of the maxillary sinus or, more frequently in our patient population, through an accessory ostium in the posterior fontanelle. This extension reaches the middle meatus where it again develops into a solid polyp that, as it enlarges, fills the floor of the nose and reaches the choana. Depending upon its size, this intranasal component of the polyp may reach the nasopharynx where it may completely obstruct the choana and occasionally become visible through the mouth, below the free margin of the soft palate.

Choanal polyps are more frequent in children and young adults. They are usually unilateral and can be diagnosed easily with the nasal endoscope. In those polyps that extend into the nasopharynx, one can easily observe the mechanical stresses to which these polyps are subjected during deglutition and talking. On endoscopy, choanal polyps seem to have an hourglass shape, with the stalk "riding" on the inferior and posterior circumference of the accessory ostium (Figs. 5.155 and 5.156). In rare cases a choanal polyp may originate from a different site, e.g., the turbinate sinus, the anteroinferior surface of the ethmoidal bulla, the sphenoethmoidal recess, or in one of our cases, from the sphenoidal sinus. In all of these patients, the maxillary sinus was not involved.

A true choanal polyp must be distinguished from patients with general polyposis, in whom the polyps extend to the choanae. Occasionally, a combination of a true choanal polyp with diffuse nasal polyposis of the ethmoid may be encountered (Figs. 5.157 to 5.160).

Choanal polyps have a high incidence of recurrence unless all of their components have been carefully and completely removed. Recurrence is particularly common when mucosal remnants are allowed to remain at the site of origin.

Figures 5.155 to 5.160 demonstrate the typical endoscopic and radiologic features of choanal polyps.

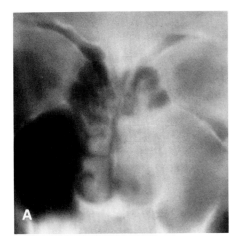

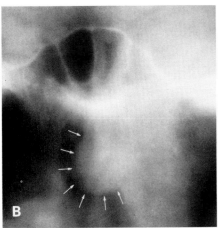

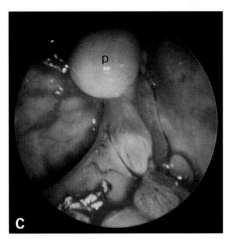

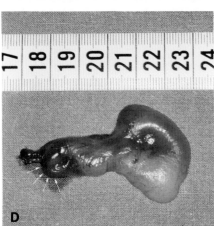

FIGURE 5.155 *A*, The typical tomographic findings in a patient with a left antrochoanal polyp. The maxillary sinus, which is homogeneously opaque, was filled by a large cyst that in this case consisted of a single chamber. The nasal passages are also homogeneously opaque because of the solid part of the polyp. *B*, The polyp extended far into the choana and produced an almost spherical shadow in this area (*arrows*). The mucosa of the left sphenoid is moderately swollen. *C*, The view into the left maxillary sinus through the canine fossa after the cystic portion of the polyp had been punctured and its contents aspirated. The cyst wall is collapsed and lies on the floor of the maxillary sinus. A relatively thin stalk extends through an accessory ostium in the posterior fontanelle. It then becomes the solid portion of the polyp and extends as far as the nasopharynx. This whole structure originated from a 5 × 5 mm area on the posterior wall of the maxillary sinus immediately adjacent to the accessory ostium. The cystic part was removed through a maxillary sinus trocar and the solid part transnasally. p = polyp. *D*, The solid portion of the specimen. The cystic part would be at the upper end of the specimen as an extension of the stalk. The part of the polyp indicated by the *arrows* had protruded through the accessory ostium into the maxillary sinus and apparently corresponds to the structure marked "p" in *C*.

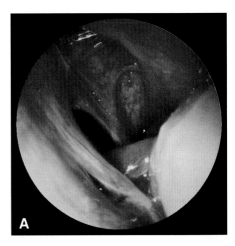

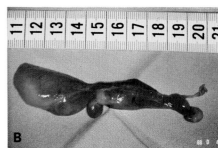

FIGURE 5.156 *A*, The stalk of a choanal polyp that extends on the right side through a large accessory ostium in the posterior fontanelle to the nasopharynx. *B*, The corresponding surgical specimen. On the right, the collapsed cystic component. On the left, the solid part of the polyp that had extended into the nasopharynx.

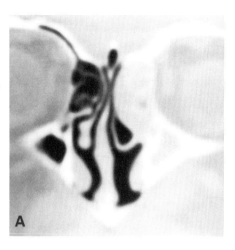

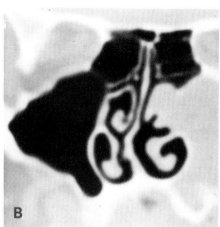

FIGURE 5.157 *A* to *C*, A CT sequence of a typical antrochoanal polyp. In addition, there is also a polypoid involvement of the anterior ethmoid (*A*).

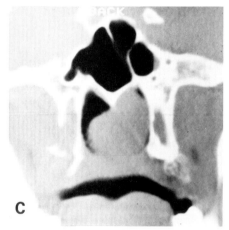

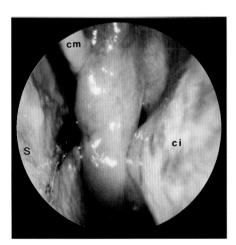

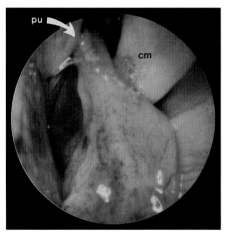

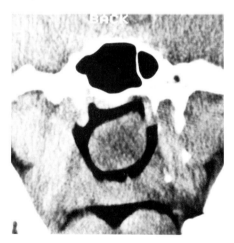

FIGURE 5.158 A single choanal polyp originates from the inferior and medial surface of the ethmoidal bulla on the left side. cm = middle turbinate; s = septum; and ci = inferior turbinate.

FIGURE 5.159 This choanal polyp had only a small cystic component in the maxillary sinus and extended through the natural ostium, the infundibulum, and the hiatus semilunaris into the nasopharynx. The stalk appears from behind the uncinate process (*arrow*). pu = uncinate process and cm = middle turbinate.

FIGURE 5.160 A large choanal polyp originating from the left sphenoethmoidal recess without involving any of the sinuses.

Etiology of Nasal Polyps

A complete discussion of all of the etiologic theories of the nasal polyps is beyond the scope of this book, as the proposed theories are too numerous and controversial. Our knowledge about the details of the influence of external or internal stimuli on the manifold biochemical regulatory mechanisms of the human nasal mucous membranes are still rudimentary. Only one common denominator can be taken as proven in the etiology of nasal polyps: mucosal edema.

Whatever its underlying etiology, the first manifestation of nasal polyps is a circumscribed or general thickening and swelling of the mucous membranes. If the etiologic factors continue to act, the next step is the formation of broadly based, more or less circumscribed, semispherical, sausage-shaped or strand-like area of mucosal edema from which the polyps evolve.

These areas of mucosal edema are usually tear-shaped for several reasons. Because of gravity, and like water in a balloon, dependent edema accumulates and the polyp tends to become wider at the bottom. Those polyps originating in the narrow spaces of the ethmoid are constrained by their anatomic boundaries and follow the path of least resistance into the middle or inferior meatus. In this area, the bony constraints are no longer present and thus the distal end of the polyp can enlarge, free of external pressure.

The suction and the relative negative pressure generated by respiration, sneezing and particularly swallowing may be of significance as an additional mechanical component. In those polyps that extend into the choana, the considerable traction and shear pressure acting on it during swallowing can be observed through the endoscope. Through the formation of a thick, edematous "body" and of a long, thin "neck," a "throttling effect" may be created, which significantly inhibits retrogression of the polyp.

A number of vasoactive substances were studied in an attempt to establish the etiology of the mucous membrane. These included the arachidonic acid metabolites, the prostaglandins, leukotrienes, bradykinins, and the "H" substances, histamine, serotonin, SRS-A (slow reacting substance of anaphylaxis) and more recently, the peptidergic neurotransmitters. In addition to a number of neurotransmitters, CGRP (calcitonin-gene-related peptide) and substance "P" are also present in human nasal mucous membranes. On stimulation of the polymodal nociceptors in the nasal mucosa, there is not only a sensation of pain, mediated by substance "P" along an afferent, orthodromal impulse to the cortex, but substance "P" is also liberated by a so-called antidromal impulse in the effector organ in the mucous membrane. Substance "P" produces local vasodilation and leakage of plasma into the tissues. This results in the so-called "neurogenic edema" (for a detailed description of the axon reflex, see Chapter 12). A fact that may possibly be of significance in the etiology of polyp formation is that substance "P" immunoreactive nerve fiber receptors of the nasal mucous membrane react not only to noxious stimuli, such as infection, toxins, chemical agents (cigarette smoke), and thermal stimulation, but *also* to pressure. Such pressure may be generated during intensive contact between apposed mucous membranes in the narrow spaces in the lateral wall of the nose. At the present time while we don't know what additional factors may be required, we do know that the liberation of certain neuropeptides can initiate a cascade effect and trigger the release of histamine and related substances from the mast cells and from the basophils. These substances all contribute to the increase of edema.

Even though the biochemical relationships are not entirely understood, our daily clinical experience, and the frequency with which polyps arise at sites of contact, strongly suggest the importance of contact in the etiology of the majority of polyps. It seems likely that this may be one of the principal reasons for the success of functional endoscopic surgery. A planned and circumscribed elimination of the contact areas or narrow spaces leads to a regression and disappearance of polypoid changes in the remaining mucous membranes of the ethmoid and large paranasal sinuses, even though these were not subjected to surgery.

Diffuse polypoid rhinosinopathy obeys other and little known mechanisms. Under light microscopy the difference from a "normal" polypoid mucous membrane involvement is obvious. There are massive, dense, mononuclear infiltrates with eosinophils representing the majority of the inflammatory cells. There are frequently eosinophil aggregates that resemble granulomata (see Fig. 5.214). It is usually not possible to demonstrate Type I allergy in these patients.

In patients with aspirin sensitivity, nasal polyps, and bronchial asthma, electron microscopy demonstrates the complete absence of a crystalloid substance that is normally found in the granules of the eosinophils. In patients with "normal" nasal polyps, this change was either minimal or not found at all. How much importance can be placed on this degranulation remains to be elucidated by further research. This clinical entity has also been labelled "NARES" (*non*allergic *r*hinitis with *e*osinophilia).

When we speak of nasal polyposis, we must realize that we are not dealing with a single disease entity, but that there are at least two, and probably more, clinically and pathophysiologically distinct diseases. This must be considered when planning therapy and when evaluating different treatment modalities. Until we have better knowledge, we must distinguish between "normal," primarily inflammatory, polyposis and "diffuse, polypoid rhinosinopathy." Diffuse polypoid rhinosinopathy consists histologically of a dense, partly granulomatous, primary eosinophilic infiltrate with degranulation demonstrable by electron microscopy degranulation. It is further characterized by having a high and early recurrence rate.

ENDOSCOPY OF THE MAXILLARY SINUS

Indications

Maxillary sinus endoscopy (maxillary sinuscopy) has proven extremely useful in evaluating diseases of the maxillary sinus. When correctly performed, this procedure is well tolerated by the patients with few risks and only minor complications. Endoscopy of the maxillary sinus is indicated when there is any suspicion of a specific or malignant disease process that requires biopsy under direct vision. Microbiological cultures can be taken (under anaerobic conditions if necessary) with special equipment and certain foreign bodies may be removed from the sinus.

Maxillary sinuscopy is usually a diagnostic procedure that provides correlation of clinical symptoms and the radiographic findings, particularly when the latter cannot be clearly interpreted. In cases of symptomatic cysts, isolated polyps, or foreign bodies, the diagnostic approach is usually combined with therapeutic manipulations. Cysts may be punctured, and their contents aspirated. Cyst walls, isolated polyps, and foreign bodies can be removed and inspissated material can be aspirated and examined. We are very conservative with maxillary sinuscopy in children and rarely find an indication to perform this technique in children younger than 8 or 9 years in cases of inflammatory diseases of the sinuses. The exceptions to this are usually children who present with antrochoanal polyps in whom the maxillary portion of that polyp (which usually is cystic) is opened and removed via an endoscopic approach through the canine fossa.

Due to the degree of development of the child's dentition and the degree of pneumatization of maxillary sinus we do not perform maxillary sinuscopy via the canina fossa before the age of 9 years to avoid potential damage to the tooth germs. In these cases we perform an inferior meatal approach similar to that for sinus irrigation and for this purpose, specially designed trocars with an outer diameter of 3.0 mm are available that can be used with the 2.7 mm endoscopes. In general, maxillary sinuscopy is the most accurate diagnostic technique for all disease processes that affect the lumen or the mucosa of the maxillary sinus.

Instrumentation

Little instrumentation is needed to perform maxillary sinuscopy. The most important tool is the trocar with its sleeve (Fig. 5.161), which has an outer diameter of 5.0 mm and accepts the various 4.0-mm endoscopes. We prefer the shovel-like type of trocar sleeve, which has several advantages over the blunt type. Various polyethylene catheters should be at hand to puncture cysts and for aspiration purposes. A 10-milliliter syringe with a polyethylene catheter attached (which should be no longer than the trocar sheath) can be used to either instill saline solution to dissolve thick inspissated material into the sinus and facilitate its aspiration or to instill topical vasoconstrictors in the case of mucosal bleeding. Additional topical anesthetics may similarly be administered if required for biopsy purposes.

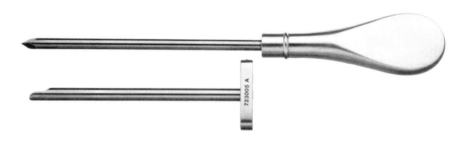

FIGURE 5.161　Trocar with sheath, outer diameter 5.0 mm. Note the shovel-like mouth of trocar sheath.

The biopsy forceps (Fig. 5.162) can be used to take biopsies, open and/or remove cysts, and to remove small polyps and inspissated material. The biopsy forceps can also be used to palpate various conditions of the mucosa, determine the consistency of the mucosa, check for a bony destruction in case of malignancy, and help distinguish between polyps and minimally edematous mucosa over bony prominences in the sinus walls.

The ideal endoscope for the initial diagnostic approach to the maxillary sinus is the 4.0-mm 30 degree endoscope. This endoscope usually provides a clear view of most of the sinus, with the exception of the anterior wall. The area of the maxillary ostium is almost always visible with the 30 degree lens. With the 70 and 120 degree 4.0-mm endoscopes, even the most remote corners and the anterior wall, through which the maxillary sinus was entered, can be investigated. The 0 degree straight forward endoscope helps to aim the canula directly at those areas where further manipulation is required.

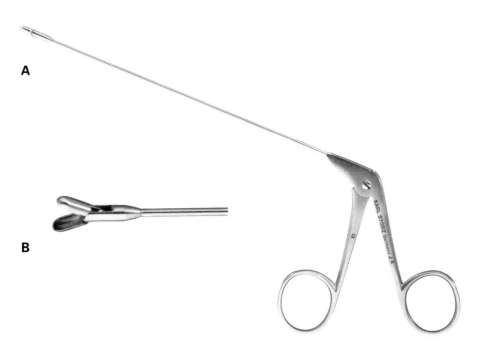

A

B

FIGURE 5.162 A, Biopsy forceps to be used through trocar sheath. B, Close-up view of forceps mouth.

A

B

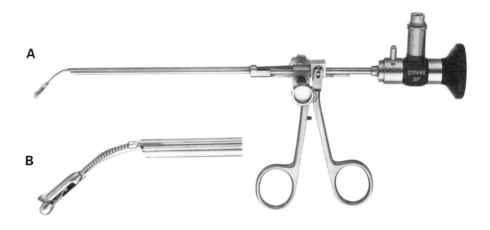

FIGURE 5.163 *A* and *B*, Optical biopsy forceps with 2.7-mm 30 degree endoscope. For insertion through the trocar sheath, the flexible part of the forceps is maximally retracted. After insertion, the flexible forceps can be advanced gradually downward into the visual field of the 30 degree lens.

Technique

With the exception of children maxillary sinuscopy is routinely performed under local anesthesia. The patient lies on his back on the table with a firmly and stably supported head. We prefer this position to the sitting or reclining position, which are less comfortable for the patient.

Initially we place a well squeezed out cotton pledget that has been soaked in a mixture of 2 percent Pontocaine (5 parts) and adrenaline 1:1,000 (1 part) into the oral vestibule over teeth 3 and 4 (the canine and the first premolar). Cocaine solution or flakes may be used for this purpose as may xylocaine spray. After a few minutes, the swab is removed and the canine fossa infiltrated, using an 18-gauge needle, with 4 to 5 milliliters of a 1 percent lidocaine solution with epinephrine 1:200,000. The bony depression of the canine fossa can usually be easily palpated and identified. It is important that the injection should reach the maxillary periosteum and preferably some anesthetic should also be infiltrated near the infraorbital nerve and towards the piriform aperture of the nose.

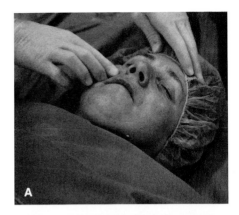

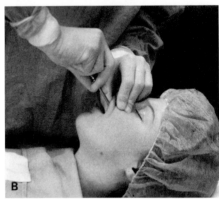

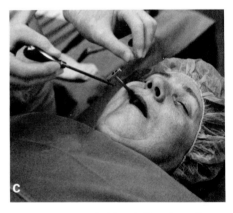

FIGURE 5.164 *A*, After infiltration of 4 ml of a local anesthetic into the canine fossa, a gentle massage helps to spread the anesthetic through the soft tissues and into the infraorbital foramen. *B*, Inserting the trocar into a left maxillary sinus. *C*, After penetrating the facial wall of the right maxillary sinus, the sheath is kept in place, while the trocar is withdrawn.

After about 2 minutes, during which time a gentle massage helps to spread the local anesthetic evenly through the soft tissues of the canine fossa (Fig. 5.164), the trocar is inserted through the mucosa of the canine fossa. It is helpful for orientation if one finger rests at the inferior margin of the orbit. No incision is made in the mucosa. The tip of the trocar is inserted into the lateral aspect of the canine fossa high above the space between the roots of the canine tooth and the first premolar inferior and lateral to the infraorbital foramen. Firstly, with a gentle rotation of the entire trocar the mucosa is pierced and then the orientation of the trocar in the lateral aspect of the canine fossa is reconfirmed. A constant to-and-fro rotating movement is applied to the trocar, which is advanced through the anterior wall of the maxillary sinus (Figs. 5.165 and 5.166).

The thickness of the bony maxillary wall varies between individuals and as such, the pressure to perforate it must be adapted to the individual case. Sometimes the bone appears to be paper thin and the trocar slips effortlessly into the maxillary sinus. In other cases the bone offers marked resistance and considerable rotation pressure must then be applied to penetrate the wall. When having to apply increased pressure, one must be prepared to *stop immediately* when the trocar passes through the anterior bony wall, in order to avoid damage to the posterior wall of the sinuses and to structures within the sinus.

The surgeon should have studied the appropriate radiograph prior to the procedure in order to keep the dimensions and the topographic relations of the individual maxillary sinus in the mind's eye during insertion of the trocar. The trocar should be aimed towards the maxilloethmoidal angle, which is the medial, posteriosuperiorly located corner of the maxillary sinus. In this direction one usually finds the largest diameter of the sinus and minimizes the risk of iatrogenic damage. Under no circumstances should the trocar be aimed toward the floor of the orbit.

FIGURE 5.165 Schematic drawing of the twisting, to-and-fro movement when inserting the trocar. Note the index finger of the left hand palpating the inferior margin of the orbit. The tip of the trocar was pierced through the mucosa high in the oral vestibule in the projection of the line between teeth 3 and 4 well above their roots.

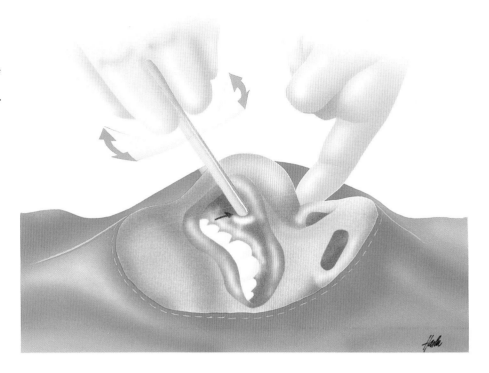

FIGURE 5.166 Schematic drawing demonstrating the arc of rotation of the trocar sheath that can be used with this approach without discomfort for the patient.

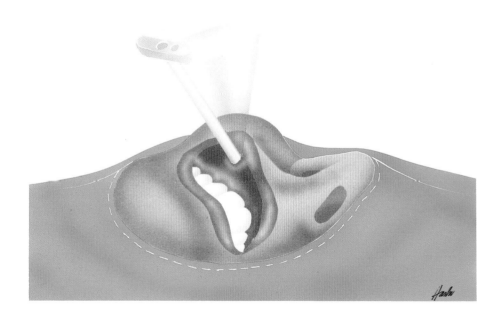

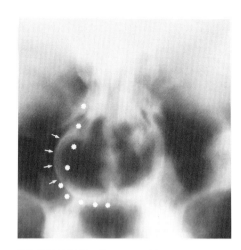

FIGURE 5.167 Tomographic cut demonstrating a far laterally bulging medial wall of the maxillary sinus (*arrows*). The lateral contour of the soft parts of the outer nose is indicated by the line of asterisks.

The piriform aperture and the bony medial sinus wall in the inferior meatus (Fig. 5.167) sometimes protrude more laterally than would be expected from the outer configuration of the nose. The bony margins of the piriform aperture, therefore, should be identified by palpation prior to insertion of the trocar.

One should avoid insertion of the trocar close to the piriform aperture in order to avoid perforating the medial wall of the maxillary sinus and ending up in the inferior meatus of the nose.

With experience, the surgeon inserting the trocar through the anterior wall of the maxillary sinus is able to identify the different phases of the perforation. Firstly there is the minimal resistance when sliding through the mucosa, which has been thickened by the injection of local anesthetic. This is then followed by firm resistance when the tip of the trocar reaches the bone. One then identifies the increasing resistance, when the bone is "drilled through" during the twisting to-and-fro movement of the trocar and finally one recognises the gradual decrease in resistance when the pointed tip of the trocar begins to

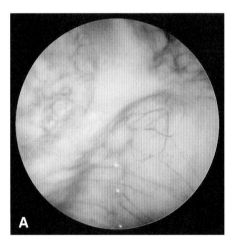

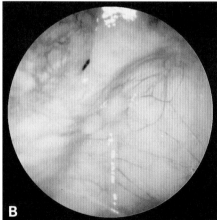

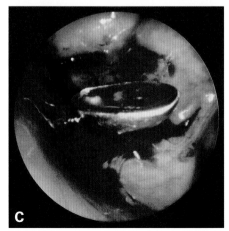

FIGURE 5.168 *A*, Left maxillary sinus, looking from the canine fossa toward the area of the natural ostium, which is blocked. *B*, During the Valsalva maneuver, the ostium opens a little bit and thus can be identified. *C*, Under direct visual control, a bent spoon can be inserted via the middle meatus into the natural ostium and the latter consequently enlarged at the expense of the anterior fontanelle.

enter the sinus. The trocar should be removed from the canula only after the opening of the latter has been fully inserted into the sinus lumen. If when inserting the endoscope through the canula one finds that only half of the trocar lip has entered the sinus, the trocar should be replaced inside the canula and the puncture completed (Fig. 5.169). The canula should not be forced through the anterior wall without the trocar in place.

Despite the bulky looking instruments, this procedure is usually well tolerated by patients. Due to the infiltration of local anesthetic containing a vasoconstrictor, there is usually little bleeding. The main advantage of this technique compared to the approach via the inferior nasal meatus is the wider range of mobility of the trocar sleeve. Without additional stress to the patient, the trocar sleeve can be rotated, and consequently all corners of the maxillary sinus may be inspected.

This range of rotation is helpful when surgical manipulations are required within the sinus because wherever one can point the canula, one can reach instruments (see Fig. 5.166). Only if the bone of the anterior maxillary wall is thick are the movements of the trocar sleeve restricted. Pain may also restrict movements of the trocar sleeve if the initial puncture was performed too close to the dental roots.

Any mucosal bleeding within the sinus can usually be stopped by appropriate aspiration and instillation of decongestants and/or vasoconstrictors through the trocar sleeve. If required, additional topical anesthetics may be instilled through the trocar prior to biopsies or other manipulations.

If a surgical endonasal procedure is planned in a patient and a maxillary sinuscopy is indicated, we always start with the latter. In some cases it is helpful to leave the trocar sleeve in situ after maxillary sinuscopy until the surgery in the middle meatus has been completed and the natural maxillary ostium has been widened via the middle meatus approach. The widened ostium can, thus, be checked from both sides. If during surgery, difficulties arise in locating the maxillary sinus ostium from the middle meatus, direct visualization through the maxillary sinus toward the medial maxillary wall can be helpful. Moreover, the natural ostium of the fontanelles in the middle meatus may be palpated by this route (Fig. 5.168). Finally, in cases where inspissated material (e.g., fungal disease) must be removed from the sinus or isolated polyps need to be resected, the trocar sleeve is a helpful instrument that allows the surgeon to manipulate in the maxillary sinus from both sides.

Manipulation in the Maxillary Sinus

To perform a biopsy, the trocar sleeve with the 0 degree lens is aimed towards the appropriate area. The trocar sleeve is then firmly held in place, the lens removed, the biopsy forceps inserted and the biopsy taken ''blindly.'' With some experience, one finds that this is a faster and more effective procedure than using the optical biopsy forceps. The same aiming technique can be used to take microbiology cultures.

To open maxillary sinus cysts we use the following technique (Figs. 5.169 to 5.171). The canula is directed towards the cyst and if possible pressed against the cyst wall so that the cyst bulges into the lumen of the canula (see Fig. 5.169). Depending on the thickness of the cyst wall, we sometimes succeed in opening the cyst with the twisting movements of the canula. If not, the tip of a polyethylene catheter is cut to a point and with this harpoon-like instrument, the cyst wall can usually be pierced (see Fig. 5.170). The cyst contents are then aspirated and the cyst wall collapses. With this technique of aiming the canula under visual control directly towards the cyst, multiple maxillary cysts can be opened sequentially. If the collapsed cyst walls cannot be aspirated, they can be grasped with the fixation forceps and removed (Fig. 5.171). Through the canula, excellent optical control can be achieved (Fig. 5.172). Only occasionally do we use the optical biopsy forceps to remove remnants of the cyst wall under direct vision, as the angulation that can be achieved with the flexible forceps is usually inadequate (Fig. 5.163).

Foreign bodies, depending on their size and composition, can be removed through a maxillary sinuscopy trocar in many cases. As illustrated in Figure 5.179, aberrant root filling material was found in that sinus. The material was too large to be transported through the natural ostium, but it was possible to ''shovel'' the debris onto the lip of the canula and then remove it with an aspirator. In other cases with larger foreign bodies, we succeeded in breaking the material down into smaller portions, which then could be aspirated through the canula. This technique, of course, is insufficient if the material is too hard to split into smaller parts.

If inspissated material proves too viscous to be aspirated, it sometimes helps to instill a few drops of a mucolytic or saline solution and to wait for a few minutes before reaspirating.

The diameter of the suction catheter should be such as to always allow some air to pass into the maxillary sinus between the canula and the suction catheter. If the suction catheter completely fills the lumen of the canula, negative pressure in the maxillary sinus results if suction is applied when the sinus ostium is blocked. This can be very painful for the patient.

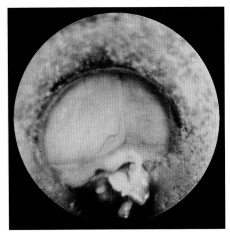

FIGURE 5.169 In the left maxillary sinus, two cysts bulge into the trocar sheath inserted via the canine fossa. Note that the sheath has not yet completely entered the sinus and therefore needs to be advanced after reattachment of the trocar core, before any manipulations start.

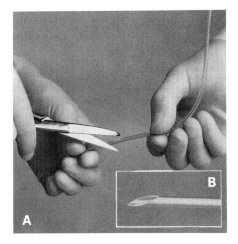

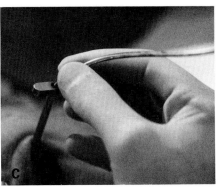

FIGURE 5.170 *A,* A polyethylene catheter has been cut with scissors. *B,* The end is cut at an angle to form a point. *C,* The catheter is then inserted through the trocar sheath to puncture the cyst and aspirate its contents.

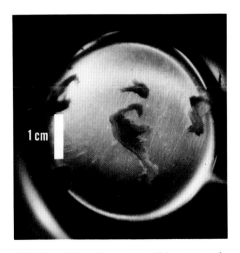

FIGURE 5.171 The cyst wall is removed with the biopsy forceps.

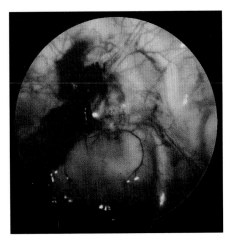

FIGURE 5.172 View into the sinus after complete removal of the cyst. Only a minor mucosal lesion indicates the origin of the cyst.

If there are isolated pendulated (stalked) polyps on the walls of the sinus that may be difficult to reach via the middle meatus, we proceed as follows.

The stalk of the polyp can usually be cut easily or "shaved off" the sinus wall with the trocar sleeve leaving the polyp free within the maxillary sinus. The polyp can then be pushed toward the widened maxillary sinus ostium (with the help of the trocar sleeve) where it can be grasped with a suitable instrument and removed via the middle meatus.

In general, we do little surgery within the maxillary sinus. We do not consider diffuse polyposis of the sinuses or an empyema to be an indication for maxillary sinuscopy. We would not operate on an isolated asymptomatic maxillary sinus cyst as long as it is not blocking the ostium or radiographically is not suspicious of any other disease. If a patient has endoscopic surgery to the lateral nasal wall anyway and maxillary sinus cysts are present, we will, however, try to open these during the same procedure.

At the end of the endoscopic or therapeutic procedure, the trocar sleeve is pulled out of the sinus with the same twisting movement. The mucosal defect in the oral vestibule usually does not require a suture. The defect usually closes airtight within the next 2 days. During this period, the patients are advised not to blow their noses to avoid subcutaneous emphysema.

Complications

As mentioned above, maxillary sinuscopy is well tolerated by the vast majority of patients. Discomfort may be experienced by patients who have had previous Caldwell-Luc procedures. The scars in the area of the facial window in the canine fossa usually are more sensitive to pressure and pain. There are surprisingly few problems with permanent dysesthesia or other irritations of the infraorbital nerve following maxillary sinuscopy. Occasionally patients complain about a temporary numbness in the upper lip or of the frontal teeth on the side of the surgery. This however, usually disappears within a few days.

We have only had a handful of patients among thousands who complain of persisting dysesthesia attributable to irritation of the infraorbital nerve. In our experience it is important to penetrate the facial wall of the maxillary sinus as far laterally in the canine fossa as possible. In this area there are anastomotic nerve branches between the rami buccales superiores of the facial nerve (the so-called "pes anserinus minor") and the infraorbital nerve. Consequently, a lesion to one nerve fiber in this area bears less risk of permanent sensory deficit.

More commonly we have seen emphysema of the soft tissues of the cheek, when patients unintentionally blew their noses in the first few hours after the sinuscopy. None of these, however, has lead to any persistent problem. The emphysema will resorb within a few days after the patient has been told not to blow his nose. Depending on the individual situation, an oral antibiotic may be required in some of these cases. If maxillary sinuscopy is performed in cases of an acute sinusitis with empyema, there is a risk of infection of the soft tissue of the cheek. For this reason, we do not perform maxillary endoscopy routinely in these cases.

Early in our experience after we had instilled antimycotic ointments and solutions into ethmoidal or maxillary sinus operative cavities (cases of mycotic sinusitis) via the middle meatus on the first and second postoperative days, a number of patients developed painful and long lasting granulomatous infiltrations of the soft tissue of the cheek. This had apparently occurred because the antimycotic ointment reached the soft tissues of the cheek through the still patent trocar perforation in the canine fossa.

Currently we postpone the instillation of antimycotic substances into the operative cavities until the fifth or seventh postoperative day. Since we started this protocol, we have not seen this complication.

When withdrawing the trocar sheath out of an infected maxillary sinus, care must be taken that no infectious material is "implanted" into the perforation channel as this could lead to a sublabial abscess. In particular the tip of the sheath must be cleansed by suction and we prefer to have a suction catheter inside the trocar as it is withdrawn in such cases.

There are several possibilities for "false passages." As previously mentioned, the lateral wall of the nose can bulge a surprising distance into the maxillary sinus and this configuration cannnot be predicted from the external shape of the nose. This creates the risk of a false passage into the inferior meatus. If the puncture of the anterior maxillary wall is created too low, there is a risk to the roots of teeth, particularly to the canine and first premolar. In children, care must be taken not to damage dental germinal centers. Radiographs should be carefully checked for unerupted teeth and for the dimensions of the individual maxillary sinus. For this reason we normally do not perform the canine fossa approach before the age of 9 years, depending on the development of the sinus (see Figs. 5.194 and 5.195).

If excessive force is used when inserting the trocar through the anterior wall (especially if the bone is thick and hard), break through and damage to the structures of the posterior maxillary wall may result from failure to stop immediately after penetrating the anterior wall.

Potentially one could enter into the retromaxillary fossa and damage the structures therein, producing consequent hemorrhage and a risk of infection. We have not encountered damage to the posterior wall in our series of patients and we think that good technique is critical in avoiding such a problem.

We maintain that it is important that the patient lie on his back on a firm table, as this gives the best support to his head and allows the surgeon to aim and direct the trocar to the correct and desired angle and position.

If one uses sheer force and does not insert the trocar with the twisting and rotating movement, the anterior wall of the maxillary sinus might infracture and pieces of bone might be displaced into the maxillary sinus. In such circumstances, if the bony fragment is small and still adherent to normal mucosa, no further treatment is usually required. If, however, larger bony fragments without mucosal attachment are free in the lumen of the maxillary sinus and if it is evident that they are too large to be transported out through the natural ostium, these splinters must be removed.

Bleeding with maxillary sinuscopy is rare and mostly indicates acute inflammation or tumors of the maxillary sinus. A few drops of blood due to the trocar insertion usually allow for an elegant examination of the mucocilary transport, as the blood-stained maxillary sinus mucus is transported towards the natural ostium (see Chapter 2).

Endoscopic Findings

In this section, some clinically important and some unusual endoscopic findings in the maxillary sinus are demonstrated.

Symptomatic cysts are the most common indication for maxillary sinuscopy. It should be noted that the size of a maxillary cyst does not necessarily correlate with the severity of the symptoms it produces.

Figure 5.173 shows a maxillary retention cyst that was smaller than a pea in size and yet produced longstanding midfacial pain. Plain radiology was unable to demonstrate this small cyst. Tomography, however, revealed the tiny cyst located on the canal of the right infraorbital nerve. Figure 5.174 shows the endoscopic appearance of the yellowish-white cyst located along the course of the infraorbital nerve on the roof of the maxillary sinus not far from the natural maxillary ostium. An incidental finding was an accessory ostium in the posterior fontanelle. After removal of the cyst through the trocar sleeve, the course of the infraorbital nerve was identified. The midfacial pain of this patient disappeared following removal of the cyst.

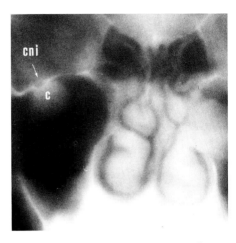

FIGURE 5.173 Tomographic view of a maxillary retention cyst on the canal of the right infraorbital nerve. cni = infraorbital nerve canal and c = cyst.

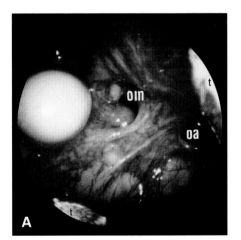 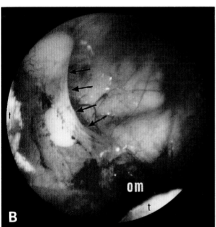

FIGURE 5.174 *A*, Endoscopic appearance of the cyst (see Fig. 5.173) near the maxillary ostium and an accessory ostium. om = maxillary sinus ostium; oa = accessory ostium; and

t = trocar. B, After cyst removal, the course of the infraorbital nerve was visible (*arrows*). om = maxillary sinus ostium and t = trocar.

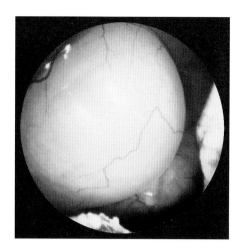

FIGURE 5.175 A large cyst found within the left maxillary sinus.

Figure 5.175 demonstrates the endoscopic finding of a larger cyst that was present in the patient's left maxillary sinus and which originated from the area of the posterior nasal fontanelle. This larger cyst was easily removed through the trocar sleeve after first having been punctured and its contents aspirated.

A similar case is demonstrated in Figure 5.176. Here a relatively small sized cholesterol cyst was located close to the infraorbital nerve at the roof of a left maxillary sinus near the anterior wall of the sinus. The course of the nerve can be seen. The bony canal was dehiscent and the nerve was only covered by mucosa. Figure 5.176B shows the sinus through a 70 degree lens following the removal of the cyst.

The patient in Figure 5.177 was to undergo an operation for anterior ethmoidal disease. His problems resulted in part from a large overpneumatized ethmoidal bulla. When performing maxillary sinuscopy to investigate the almost spherical soft tissue mass at the roof of his left maxillary sinus, we were surprised to find completely normal mucosa with no pathology at the roof of the sinus. As the tomography had only been performed the day prior to the endoscopy, it seemed very unlikely that a cyst or a polyp had vanished in such a short period of time.

FIGURE 5.176 A, A cholesterol cyst near the infraorbital nerve, which was covered by mucosa only. B, After cyst removal.

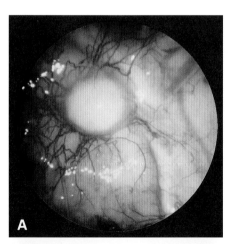

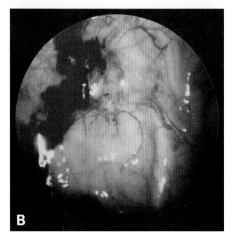

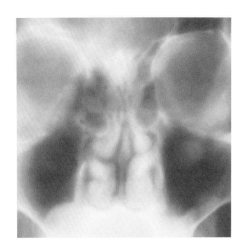

FIGURE 5.177   Tomogram showing opacity at the roof of the maxillary sinus.

Only by accident were we able to unveil the secret of this phenomenon. Time and time again we have seen balls of mucus of up to 5 millimeters in diameter being transported over an apparently normal mucosa. Figure 5.178 demonstrates a mucus ball at the roof of a right maxillary sinus inspected via the enlarged window in the middle meatus some weeks after surgery. The mucus ball in these cases consisted of a highly viscous but nonpurulent mucus. The sphere apparently results from the surface tension either of the thick mucus itself or the overlying gel layer of the "normal" mucus blanket. In any event, the adhesion between the normal mucus layer and the isolated ball of mucus must have been strong enough to prevent the mucus ball from dropping by gravity down to the floor of the sinus. Whether this phenomenon is due to a localized abnormality of the mucosal glands or is the result of some other pathologic process is unknown. As long as these mucus balls can be transported out of the sinuses, they do not appear to have any pathologic significance.

The ability of the ciliary beat and the adhesive forces of the mucus layer to transport relatively heavy items upwards to the natural ostium of the maxillary sinus is nicely demonstrated in Figure 5.179. A small metal cylinder of dental root filling material that had reached the maxillary sinus has been transported all the way up to the natural ostium. As it was too large to pass through the ostium it was retained there, causing irritation to the ostial mucosa. After removal of the foreign body through the trocar sleeve this mucosal irritation around the ostium can be clearly seen. The weight of this foreign body was 3.5 grams.

Cysts in the maxillary sinus can originate from many different areas: retention cysts can arise from almost any area of the maxillary sinus mucosa. Those cysts resulting from dental problems are usually located on the floor of the sinus in the alveolar recess.

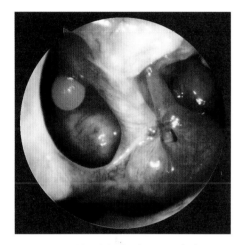

FIGURE 5.178   A ball of mucus being transported along the roof of a right maxillary sinus.

FIGURE 5.179   *A*, Dental filling material transported to the maxillary sinus ostium. This cylinder was too large to go through the ostium, so it remained and caused irritation. *B*, The extent of the irritation is visible after removal of the foreign body.

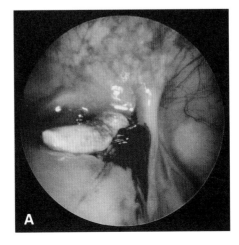
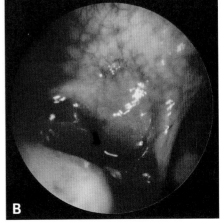

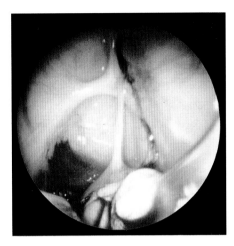

FIGURE 5.180 Cysts in the maxillary sinus.

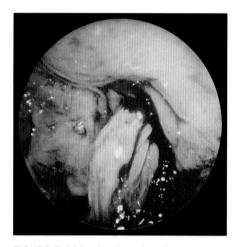

FIGURE 5.181 Cystic polyps in the maxillary sinus.

Not all the cysts within the maxillary sinus arise from the mucosa of the sinus. Cysts (Fig. 5.180) and cystic polyps (Fig. 5.181) can expand into the maxillary sinus from the anterior ethmoid. The thin stalk of a cyst that collapsed after having been punctured can be seen clearly entering the right maxillary sinus through its natural ostium. There was infundibular disease present in this case and the stalk of the cyst could be traced back to diseased mucosa in the semilunar hiatus and the anterior face of the ethmoidal bulla. The same was true for the cystic polyp, which more or less completely filled the right maxillary sinus. These findings are further examples of ethmoidal disease spreading into the maxillary sinus.

Figure 5.182 demonstrates intramucosal petechial hemorrhage in the right maxillary sinus of a diver who had decompression problems as a result of anterior ethmoidal disease. Minor nose bleeding is not an unusual experience for divers, especially if they dive with concurrent sinus problems. The bleeding is usually the result of an inability to equalize the pressure differences between the sinuses and the nasal cavity.

In a case of more extensive bleeding into the maxillary sinus, we may encounter the situation shown in Figure 5.183. In this patient a blood clot is about to be transported out of a right maxillary sinus 3 days after a blowout fracture. Maxillary endoscopy in this case was performed to evaluate whether there was a need for the surgical repositioning of prolapsed contents of the orbit. As the patient had no double vision, there was no herniation of orbital contents at sinuscopy, and the orbital floor proved to be relatively stable, no surgery was indicated. Besides the pear-shaped blood clot in the lumen of the sinus, the massive intra- and submucosal bleeding at the roof of the sinus can be seen clearly.

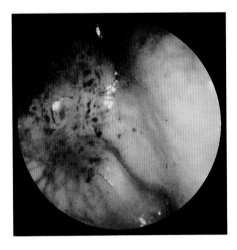

FIGURE 5.182 Intramucosal petechial hemorrhage in the right maxillary sinus of a diver with decompression problems.

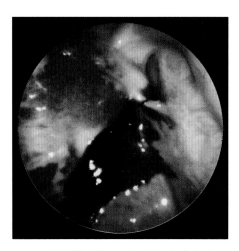

FIGURE 5.183 Extensive blood clots in a maxillary sinus being transported out 3 days after a blowout fracture.

The patient whose left maxillary sinus is demonstrated in Figure 5.184 was seen after an indwelling tube had been inserted at another center via the inferior meatus into the maxillary sinus for treatment of "chronic maxillary sinusitis." This procedure had brought no relief. In contrast, the patient suffered from increasing pain when irrigations and instillations were performed. Behind the eminentia lacrimalis, the shaft of the indwelling tube can be seen for a few millimeters before the tube enters the swollen and inflamed posterior wall mucosa. Attempts to irrigate through this tube with saline solution caused bulging of this mucosal area and intense pain to the patient. When trying to retract the tube via the inferior meatus, we found that the T-shaped distal end had been implanted into the mucosa of the posterior wall (Fig. 5.184B). Consequently, irrigations did not reach the lumen of the sinus but instead lifted the mucosa from the bony wall (Fig. 5.184C). It took considerable force to remove this indwelling tube. Figure 5.184D shows the tube that was removed from the maxillary sinus of this patient.

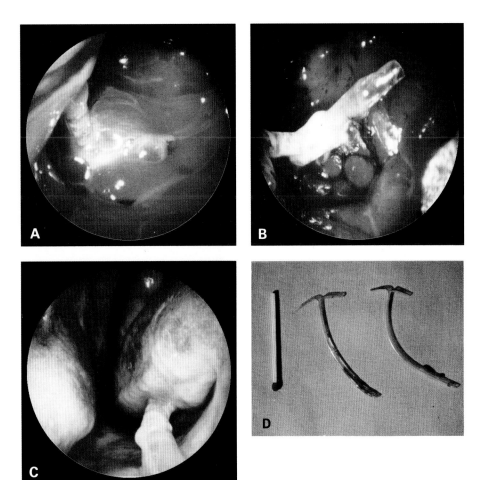

FIGURE 5.184 *A*, A patient with an indwelling tube for treatment of chronic maxillary sinusitis from another center still had pain from irrigations and instillations. The mucosa bulged as irrigation fluid lifted it from the bony wall. *B*, The T-shaped proximal end was embedded in the mucosa. *C*, The indwelling tube in situ in the left inferior nasal meatus. *D*, The tube after removal from the patient.

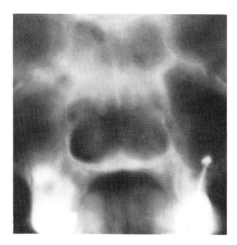

FIGURE 5.185   A tomogram of a patient with dental filling material in the maxillary sinus.

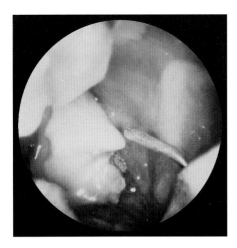

FIGURE 5.186   The patient in Figure 5.185 viewed endoscopically revealed the oro-antral fistula as well as inflamed mucosa, a probe entering via the fistula, and pus surrounded food particles.

The tomogram in Figure 5.185 shows a patient in whom root filling material was pressed into the maxillary sinus. The dentist's attempt to remove this material resulted in an oro-antral fistula with a secondary maxillary sinusitis. This situation is shown in Figure 5.186, where a probe enters the left maxillary sinus through the fistula. The sinus mucosa is inflamed and there is pus around food particles that have entered the sinus through the fistula.

Figure 5.187 shows an *Aspergillus fumigatus* fungal ball in a right maxillary sinus. There is currently no active inflammation. The fruiting heads of the *Aspergillus* can be seen on the surface of the fungal ball. There was one streak of whitish, thickened secretion, which contained fruiting heads and fungal spores, running from the floor of the sinus (not visible in this picture) to the natural ostium. A second streak of mucus entered the maxillary sinus via an accessory ostium in the anterior fontanelle and was transported upwards toward the natural ostium where it left the sinus, only to enter again through the accessory ostium. This is an example of mucus recirculating between an accessory ostium and the natural ostium.

Figure 5.188 demonstrates the CT scan of another patient in whom dental root filling material has gone astray in a left maxillary sinus. The radiographic density measurement (2560) clearly defines the radiopaque material as metal. The mucosa around the foreign body appears to be swollen. The endoscopic findings are shown in Figure 5.189. Endoscopy was performed several weeks after the CT scan when the patient started to develop symptoms from his maxillary sinus. The mucosa is now extensively inflamed and the root filling material that protrudes into the sinus cavity is covered with pus.

The initial irritation of the mucosa is said to be caused by the disinfecting chemicals that are added to this type of dental filling material. In our experience, aberrant root filling material within the maxillary sinus predisposes a patient to fungal sinusitis and, for this reason, we recommend its removal even when the patient is free of symptoms.

Fungal growth is occasionally seen on other inspissated material in the maxillary sinus. Figures 5.190 and 5.191 show how fungi can grow on antibiotic ointment which has been instilled into the maxillary sinus for therapeutic purposes (usually following maxillary sinus irrigations).

We have seen a case in which a cherry-sized polyp or cyst was tightly filled with antibiotic ointment. In this patient the ointment apparently had been instilled either directly into a cyst or polyp or between the posterior wall mucosa and the underlying bone, leading to the formation of a "false" cyst or polyp.

Figure 5.192 demonstrates fungal growth (*Aspergillus fumigatus* and *niger*) on top of a soft, bulging mass of tissue in the alveolar recess of a right maxillary sinus. A biopsy revealed an underlying squamous cell carcinoma of the maxilla.

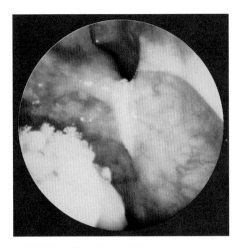

FIGURE 5.187 *Aspergillus fumigatus* fungal ball in a right maxillary sinus.

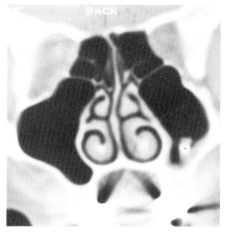

FIGURE 5.188 Another patient with dental filling in the maxillary sinus has a CT scan that demonstrates the radiopaque material to be metal (M = 2560).

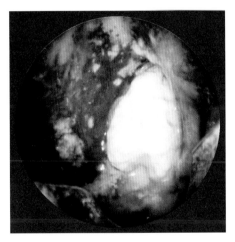

FIGURE 5.189 Endoscopy of the patient in Figure 5.188 weeks after CT scan demonstrates extensive inflammation and pus-covered dental filling material.

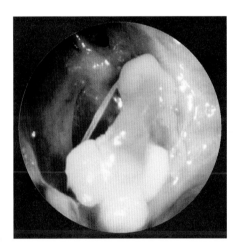

FIGURE 5.190 Fungal growth on antibiotic ointment.

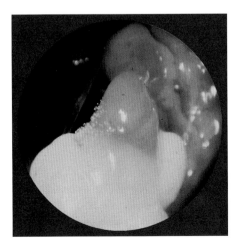

FIGURE 5.191 Fungal growth on antibiotic ointment.

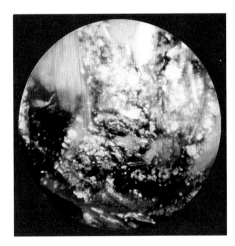

FIGURE 5.192 Fungal growth on a tissue mass that was revealed at biopsy to be squamous cell carcinoma.

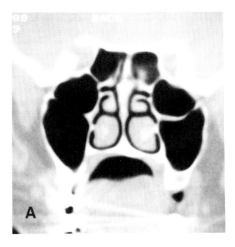

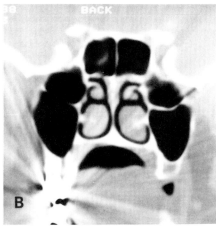

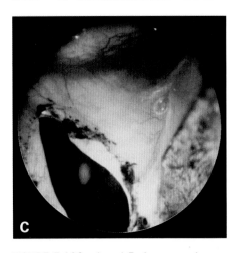

Septations of the maxillary sinus as seen on the CT scans in Figure 5.193 are rare. In this unusual case there was a complete septation of the left maxillary sinus with both compartments having their own ostia and draining into the middle meatus. On the right side the partition was incomplete with a more or less horizontal fold arising from the posterior wall of the sinus towards the lumen. Vertical septations have also been described in literature although we have never encountered this rare finding. If maxillary sinus disease occurs, it will be necessary to provide ventilation to both compartments by removing the bony or membranous septa to reestablish normal drainage.

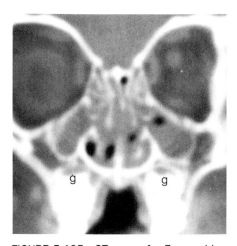

FIGURE 5.194 Right maxillary sinus: protrusion of the roots of second molar teeth through the alveolar recess. The mucosa appears normal. If the trocar sheath (*arrow*) is inserted too close to the maxillary sinus floor and advanced too far posteriorly, the tips of the dental roots might be injured in such a case.

FIGURE 5.193 *A* and *B*, An unusual finding of complete septation of the left maxillary sinus. *C*, The endoscopic finding in this patient. The trocar has entered the first chamber of the maxillary sinus and the septation to the second chamber has been perforated. There is a small retention cyst visible in the back wall of the second chamber. Note circular transport pattern of blood-stained mucus around the perforation in the septating wall.

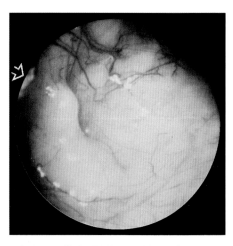

FIGURE 5.195 CT scan of a 7-year-old boy with cystic fibrosis. The floor of the maxillary sinus is between 5 (left side) and 8 (right side) millimeters above the lowest level of the floor of the nose. g = dental germs in the alveolar recess contacting the floor of the maxillary sinus.

HISTOLOGIC FINDINGS

It is not the purpose of this book to discuss the entire spectrum of all the possible histologic changes of the mucous membranes in the paranasal sinuses. The complexities of immunohistochemical and electron microscopic investigations can only be mentioned briefly. Emphasis is placed on those histologic changes that can be identified regularly by light microscopy on biopsy specimens of diseased ethmoidal mucosa.

In contrast to the histologic findings in primary, acute sinusitis, which is dominated by inflammatory edema, lympho- and leukocytic infiltrates, and increased vascularization, the light microscopy in chronic, recurrent sinusitis reveals a predominance of glandular changes, in addition to the edema. Acute or chronic inflammatory infiltrates and changes in the surface epithelium are secondary findings. Surgical specimens routinely show an extraordinary increase in glandular acini and an edematous enlargement of the secretory portion of the gland and of the excretory duct. The mucous membrane may be several times thicker than normal and it may be almost entirely replaced by glandular convolutions (Fig. 5.196) that create the appearance of an intramucosal retention mucocele. These glands, and to a lesser degree the vessels, may be surrounded by more or less pronounced round cell infiltrates. If the disease has an allergic component, plasma cells and eosinophils predominate.

There are frequently small (up to pea-size) cysts, which are filled with inspissated and occasionally calcified secretions (Fig. 5.198). These cysts consist of both secretory end pieces and excretory ducts. In the case of dilated encysted excretory ducts, the wall of the cyst is composed of markedly flattened ductal epithelium. In the secretory part, stasis of the secretions leads to a gradual flattening of the mucus-producing cells.

Light microscopy can no longer differentiate between the intracellular secretory granules and the mucous material in the center of the cyst. The nuclei, initially round or oval, migrate to the base of the cells and become almost completely flat (Figs. 5.196A and 5.197 to 5.202). This process, which is initiated and furthered by the increasing stasis of secretions, can be followed to its endpoint, i.e., the complete encystment of the secretory portion. At this point, there is no longer any functional, glandular epithelium visible on light microscopy and the serous crescent is absent. In many of these retention cases, surprisingly, a wide and open glandular excretory duct (see Fig. 5.197) is present. In addition to the presumptive block through contact between the opposing mucous membrane surfaces, the etiology of these findings must also be because of an increase in the viscosity of the secretions.

FIGURE 5.196 *A*, Infundibular mucous
membrane in chronic rhinosinusitis. Note
the numerous distended glands. There is
retention of secretions and the incipient
cystic dilation of the terminal ducts and
the end pieces of the glands are clearly
visible. HE stain. Magnification: 60 ×.
B, Note the extravasation of mucus
between the distended glands. HE stain.
Magnification: 60 ×.

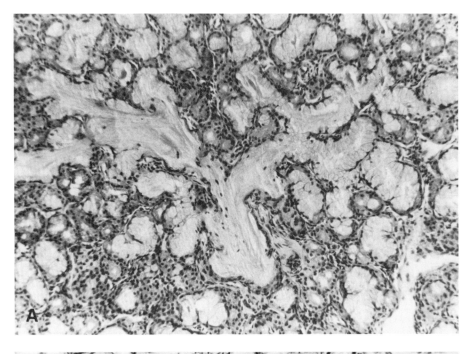

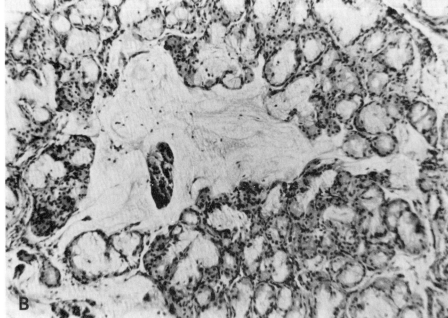

FIGURE 5.197 Note the retained secretions in the terminal duct and end-piece of the glands, even though the terminal duct is patent. HE stain. Magnification: 40×.

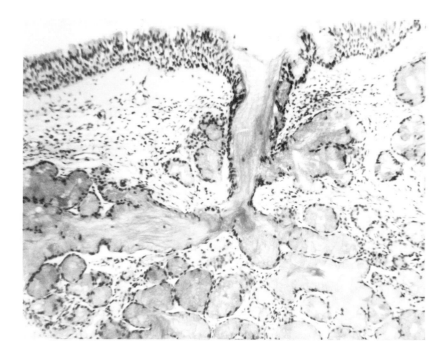

FIGURE 5.198 There are major cystic changes in the terminal ducts. The ducts are filled with inspissated and partially calcified secretions. The epithelium of the duct is markedly thin. PAS stain. Magnification: 25×.

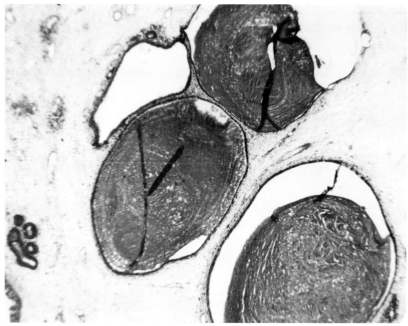

Even the pressure of the mucus still produced in the acini is insufficient to move these secretions through the duct. This leads to retention and to the formation of the cysts described above.

Another frequent finding that may affect large areas of the surface of the mucous membrane is goblet cell metaplasia. In these areas, the epithelium is frequently inverted and these invaginations may develop into cysts, filled with retained secretions (see Figs. 5.199 to 5.202).

A frequent complication of cyst formation and mucus retention is the extravasation of mucus into the surrounding tissues. This in turn leads to granulomatous reactions with macrophages surrounding and invading the granulomata. The extravasated mucus may also develop into cystic structures in which endothelium or a continuous epithelial surface can no longer be distinguished (Figs. 5.196B and 5.203).

Mucous membrane polyps, arising primarily at the site of intimate contact between opposing mucous membrane surfaces are histologically typically uniformly edematous with occasional myxoid or cystic changes. These polyps rarely contain any significant vessels and glandular convolutions are rare. The surface of the polyp, particularly at the areas of contact with another mucous membrane surface, may show squamous epithelial metaplasia on the free surface that faces the nasal lumen.

FIGURE 5.199 Marked, circumscribed goblet cell metaplasia, above an edematous mucosal stroma. Invagination and cystic degeneration of the epithelium. Note, adhering to the epithelium, the tenacious mucus that was not loosened by the fixation, embedding, and sectioning of the tissue. The upper half of the slide shows unremarkable respiratory epithelium above edematous mucosa. PAS stain. Magnification: 60×.

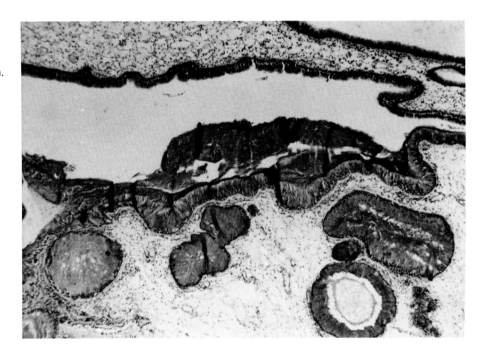

FIGURE 5.200 Goblet cell metaplasia with the production of highly viscous, solidly adherent mucus. The epithelium is invaginated into the edematous mucosa and shows the formation of retention cysts. PAS stain. Magnification: 85×.

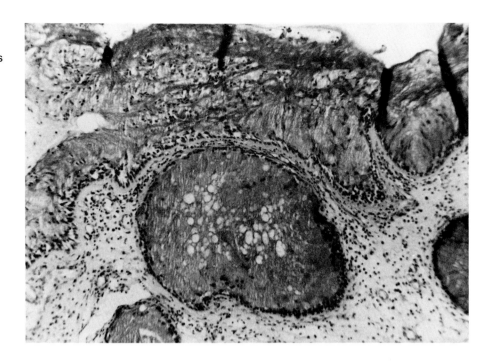

FIGURE 5.201 Goblet cell metaplasia with marked epithelial invagination and retention cyst formation. Incipient inflammatory infiltrates. PAS stain. Magnification: 60×.

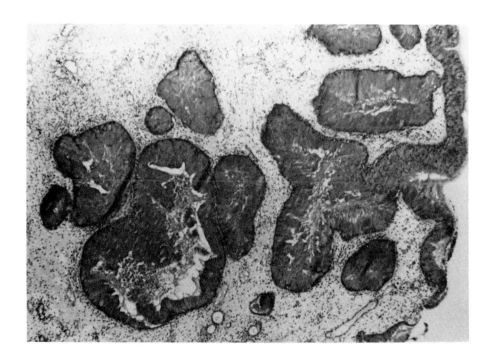

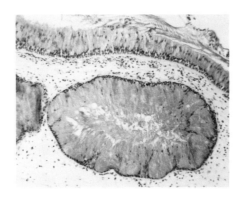

FIGURE 5.202 Detail of the invaginated and encysted goblet cell epithelium. The nuclei are displaced against the periphery of the cell by the increasing pressure of the secretions. Light microscopy no longer shows cellular walls between the goblet cells. PAS stain. Magnification: 100×.

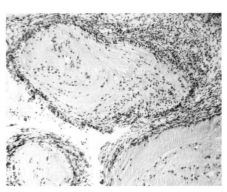

FIGURE 5.203 Extravasated mucus in incipient cyst formation. The mucus pools are surrounded by a layer of macrophages, with a number of cells having migrated to the center of the pool. The epithelial walls can no longer be demonstrated clearly. HE stain. Magnification: 85×.

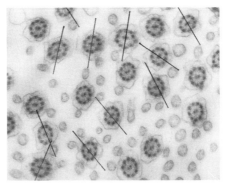

FIGURE 5.204 Electron-microscopic findings: Dyscoordination of the direction of the ciliary sweep. The ciliary axes deviate by as much as 60 degrees. Magnification: 30,000×.

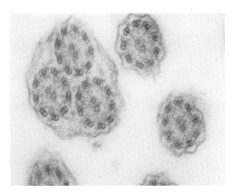

FIGURE 5.205 Compound cilium. Magnification: 92,700×.

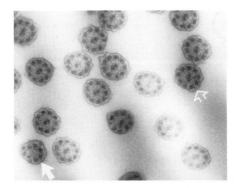

FIGURE 5.206 Abnormal cilia: 9 + 3 (*open arrow*). Absent central axonema, an external tubule, malposition in the external 9-ring (*white arrow*). Magnification: 45,900×.

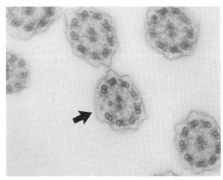

FIGURE 5.207 Abnormal cilia: 8 + 3. Magnification: 92,700×.

Numerous ciliary abnormalities have been identified in electron microscope studies of mucous membrane biopsies from diseased ethmoids (Figs. 5.204 to 5.213). The significance of these changes in individual cases was, however, difficult to assess. We encountered the following deviations from the customary 9+2 pattern:

9+2+1:   An additional subfiber lies outside of the ring of nine

9+2+2:   Two microtubules lying outside the ring of nine

8+3:   Eight peripheral doublets surround three central microtubules

8+2+1:   The peripheral circle consists of eight doublets that surround a central microtubule. There is a subfiber outside the ring of eight

10+3:   A circle of ten peripheral doublets surrounding three central microtubules

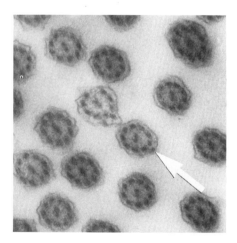

FIGURE 5.208   Abnormal cilia: 9 + 2 + 1.

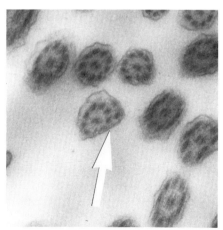

FIGURE 5.209   Abnormal cilia: 9 +2 + 2.

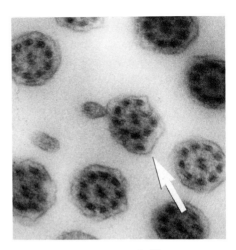

FIGURE 5.210 Abnormal cilia: 9 + 2 + 1.

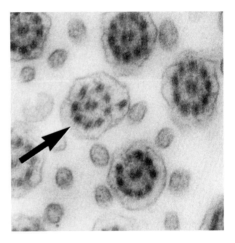

FIGURE 5.211 Abnormal cilia: 8 + 2 + 1.

There was frequently an absence of several subfibers that could not be explained on the basis of the fixation of the cilia in a given direction and the ensuing reciprocal displacement of the fibers (Fig. 5.213). Compound cilia were also a frequent finding. In these, several normal 9+2 systems were surrounded by a common cytoplasm and a common membrane (see Fig. 5.205).

A significant divergence in the direction of the ciliary sweep was found, particularly in those patients with mycotic infections. The axis of the ciliary sweep would diverge by as much as 70 degrees (see Fig. 5.204). Deviation of the ciliary axis and consequently the direction of the ciliary sweep between 6 and 25 degrees are considered physiologic variations that can still accomplish effective ciliary motion and the transportation of secretions in a given direction.

The picture found on light microscopy in diffuse polypoid rhinosinopathy is quite different. Dense inflammatory primarily eosinophilic and plasmacellular infiltrates are found around the glands, around the vessels, and also in the edematous stroma. In the stroma, aggregations of eosinophils are found that are reminiscent of granulomata (Fig. 5.214). This picture is so typical of patients with bronchial or aspirin intolerance asthma, that our histopathologists refer to them as "asthma granulomata." In eosinophil aggregations like these, the degranulation phenomenon described by Sasaki, Takasaka, et al could be demonstrated.

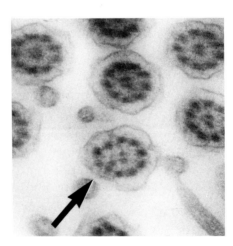

FIGURE 5.212 Abnormal cilia: 10 + 3.

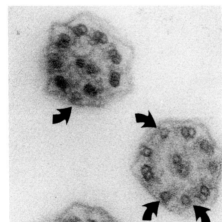

FIGURE 5.213 Abnormal cilia: Absent subfibers (arrows).

A number of the histologic changes described above may result in a thickening of the mucous membrane. The increase in the number of glandular acini, the retention of secretions, the formation of cysts, and the extravasation of mucus with its ensuing granuloma formation are particularly important in this respect. If these changes take place in the key narrow areas of the anterior ethmoid and particularly if these areas are further narrowed by one of the anatomic variations described above, the negative effects this may have upon the sinuses is obvious.

FIGURE 5.214 Histologic findings in diffuse polypoid rhinosinopathy. *A*, Dense infiltrate with eosinophils and other mononuclear cells, mostly in the area of the basilar membrane. There is goblet cell metaplasia in the epithelium. *B*, Almost concentric mass of eosinophils and plasma cells, the so called "asthma granuloma." The spreading of the basilar membrane is obvious. *C*, The entire, grossly thickened mucous membrane has been taken over by infiltrates. *D*, There are dense infiltrates primarily around the clogged excretory ducts of the glands. HE stain. Magnification: 25×. *E*, A higher power view of the dense infiltrate in the area of the basilar membrane. Note the goblet cell metaplasia. *F*, A higher power view of the perivascular infiltrates. HE stain. Magnification: 160×.

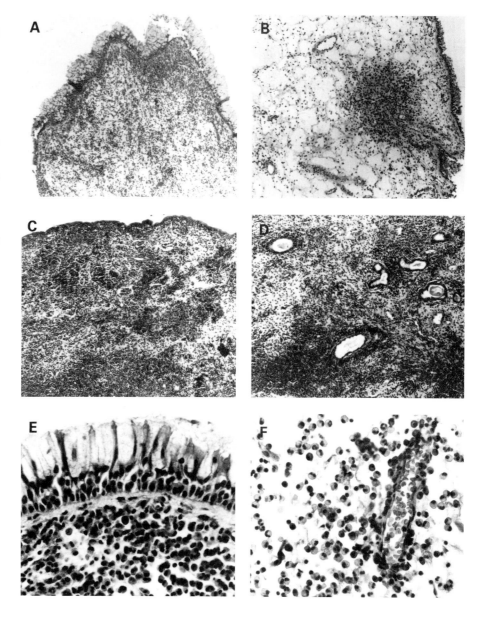

DIFFERENTIAL DIAGNOSIS

A variety of specific and nonspecific infections as well as benign and malignant neoplasms may affect the nose and paranasal sinuses. These different diseases may produce typical and diagnostically pathognomonic changes as well as atypical nonspecific changes in the mucous membranes.

Messerklinger, in his book *Endoscopy of the nose* has assembled a representative collection of the endoscopic appearances and differential diagnoses of a large number of these diseases. A careful review of this outstanding work is recommended for all who engage in nasal endoscopy. At this time we wish to discuss some of the differential diagnostic aspects of endoscopy that may be of value in separating malignant diseases from the chronic inflammation.

It is not always possible to identify specific diseases as clearly as the mucous membrane changes in sarcoidosis (Fig. 5.215). Frequently the changes are so subtle that there appears to be no indication for a biopsy before initiating medical therapy or even performing surgery. This was the case in Figure 5.216 where a relatively benign clinical appearance concealed a highly active tubercular lesion. It is particularly important in mycotic infections to remember that fungi can appear not only as harmless parasites on encrusted secretion, but also may appear frequently on the ulcerated surfaces of malignant growths (see Chapter 11, Mycoses). For this reason, the mucous membrane under a mycotic growth must be carefully examined and a biopsy should be taken.

Radiographically, once there is tissue destruction and diffuse invasion, malignant processes usually have a characteristic appearance. It should be remembered, however, that chronic inflammatory processes may also produce local destruction or at least simulate it on the X-ray film. This is particularly true ot the mycotic diseases ot the paranasal sinuses, which may be misinterpreted on radiography as a malignant process on the basis of real or presumptive destruction of the lateral wall of the nose.

The clinical symptoms are not helpful in distinguishing between invasive and chronic inflammatory processes, particularly in the early stages. A moderately symptomatic "chronic cold" may mask a carcinoma of the lateral wall of the nose. Blood-stained secretions, on the other hand, should *always* be considered a serious indication of a hidden malignancy.

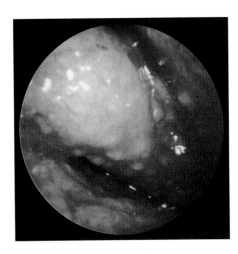

FIGURE 5.215 The typical mucous membrane changes in a right inferior turbinate in a case of sarcoidosis.

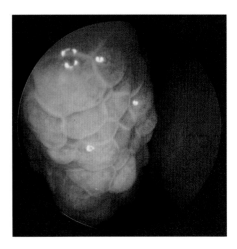

FIGURE 5.216 Mucous membrane tuberculosis (in a case of open pulmonary tuberculosis). Right inferior turbinate.

In neoplastic changes of the interior of the nose, the surrounding mucosa frequently becomes edematous, so that the ensuing, frequently significant polyp formation may completely obscure the underlying malignancy. For this reason, even in cases of apparent obvious nasal polyps, every attempt should be made to carefully inspect all areas of the nose that can be reached with the endoscope. In the patient in Figure 5.217, an extensive nasopharyngeal carcinoma was hiding behind a massive "typical" polyp in the right side of the nose. The carcinoma was identified only after the endoscope had been passed beyond the polyps that extended to the choana and after the last polyp was retracted into the nasal passage with an aspirator (Fig. 5.217B). In the same patient, posterior rhinoscopy only showed a polyp extending into the nasopharynx.

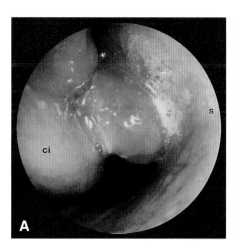 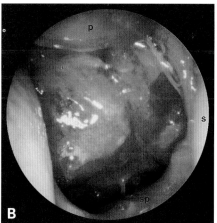

FIGURE 5.217 *A*, Right nasal cavity. Large glassy polyps extend to the floor of the nose and to the nasopharynx. ci = inferior turbinate and s = septum. *B*, After the polyps were retracted, a diffuse swelling in the nasopharynx becomes visible. On biopsy this proved to be a carcinoma of the nasopharynx. p = polyp and s = septum.

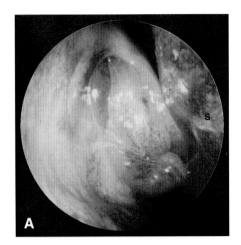

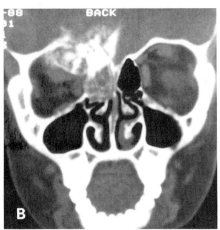

FIGURE 5.218 *A*, Note the "typical" polyps in the right middle meatus. The middle turbinate has become thinned by pressure from the polyps and is pressed against the septum. s = septum. *B*, The CT scan of the patient shows extensive destruction of the frontal bone by an esthesioneuroblastoma that has already invaded the skull, the orbit, and the ethmoid.

Figure 5.218 shows the case of an 8-year-old boy who came to the hospital because of a "persistent cold." The complaints began only a few weeks prior to the visit and were so slight that they did not alarm either the child or his parents. He was brought to the hospital only after the secretions became tinged with blood. Endoscopically we found the typical appearance of a diseased middle meatus with an unremarkable polyp protruding from it. The CT scan, however, showed an extensive and destructive neoplasm (histologically a neuroblastoma) that had extensively invaded the skull and destroyed the frontobasal area.

Figure 5.219 shows a large squamous carcinoma of the maxillary sinus on the right side. Endoscopically, the bulging of the lateral nasal wall can be seen, indicating that it has already been extensively invaded by carcinoma (arrows). On CT, the extensive destruction of the lateral wall of the nose and the posterior wall of the maxillary sinus area clearly visible. Also, the extension of the tumor can be followed into the retromaxillary space.

Granulating lumpy changes must always raise suspicion of a malignancy, particularly if they bleed easily on contact. This led to the unmasking of a squamous carcinoma that was infiltrating the ostium of a left maxillary sinus (Fig. 5.220).

The tight bulging of the medial infundibular wall on the left side of the nose in Figure 5.221 concealed a fibrosarcoma of the middle meatus. Endoscopically, the findings could easily have been mistaken for a chronic disease of the anterior ethmoid or for a mucocele. Eventually, the tense vascular pattern suggested the presence of a neoplastic process.

A very similar picture was presented by a rare leiomyosarcoma of the ethmoid, which can be seen bulging from the left middle meatus in Figure 5.222. The tense and increased vascular markings are again evident on the surface of the tumor.

FIGURE 5.219 *A*, The lateral wall of this right middle meatus is diffusely infiltrated and bulges medially. The middle turbinate is pressed against the septum. Biopsies taken from the whitish mucosal area (*arrows*) revealed the presence of a squamous cell carcinoma. s = septum. *B*, The CT scan shows destruction of the lateral wall of the nose and extension through the posterior wall of the maxillary sinus. The site of origin of the tumor can no longer be identified.

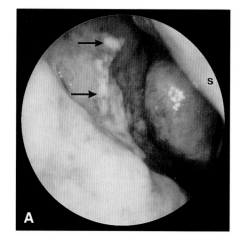

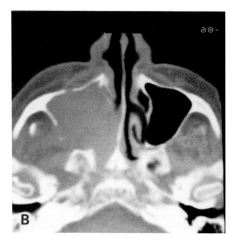

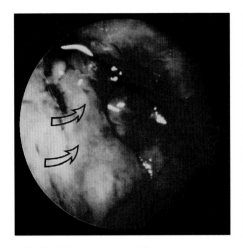

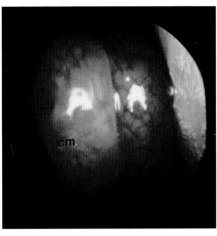

FIGURE 5.220   Left maxillary sinus endoscopy showing a maxillary sinus ostium that is severely constricted by granulating lumpy mucous membrane changes. The air bubble shows the location of the ostium. The infiltrations are particularly prominent over the lacrimal eminence (*arrows*). Histologically this was a squamous cell carcinoma.

FIGURE 5.221   View into a left middle meatus. The medial infundibular wall is bulging with an increased number of dilated vessels on its surface. Histologically this was diagnosed as a fibrosarcoma. cm = middle turbinate.

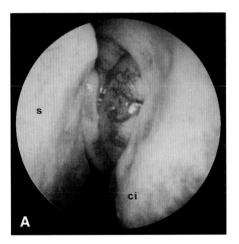

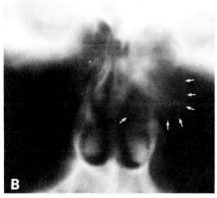

FIGURE 5.222   *A*, The almost spherical bulge with increased dilated vessels in this left middle meatus is a leiomyosarcoma. s = septum and ci = inferior turbinate. *B*, The tomographic findings. The spherical, well circumscribed tumor can be easily identified (*arrows*).

Inverted papillomas present their own very special problems. Not uncommonly, inverted papillomas can not be distinguished macroscopically from "normal" nasal polyps. Even the radiographic findings are confusing unless there is already clear evidence of destruction and invasion. The patient in Figure 5.223 had endoscopic surgery for typical massive nasal polyps without any difficulties (Fig. 5.223B). The polypoid mass had a relatively circumscribed root in the ethmoidal infundibulum. Much to our surprise, histologic examination of the surgical specimen revealed a fully developed inverted papilloma that had almost completely replaced some of the polyps and had just begun to appear on the surface of others (Fig. 5.223C). It is evident that the inverted papilloma does not always demonstrate the typical small granular to furrowed surfaces that are visible on the surgical specimen in Figure 5.223D.

Our procedure in the case of an inverted papilloma is as follows:

If the diagnosis is made only postoperatively, as in the above case, and the patient was operated on for "nasal polyposis," an ongoing thorough endoscopic follow-up is instituted. If the tumor was completely removed, there is usually no need for further therapy. Potential recurrences can be recognized and treated promptly. The rational basis for such an approach is that histologically there was no evidence for any malignant degeneration in the removed neoplasm. If the diagnosis of an inverted papilloma is made preoperatively, further intervention depends on the size of the tumor. If endoscopically a relatively circumscribed base can be identified, we select an endoscopic surgical approach. If, however, the tumor shows evidence of destructive or invasive growth, there is no longer any indication for primary endoscopic intervention.

If there is a malignant degeneration in the tumor, we use the endoscopic approach to obtain a biopsy and confirm the diagnosis. Resection of the tumor is then performed by one of the well proven external approaches and the extent of the resection is determined by the findings.

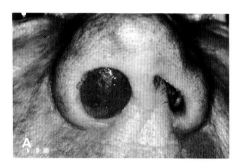
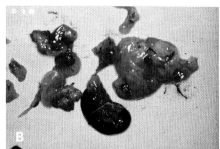
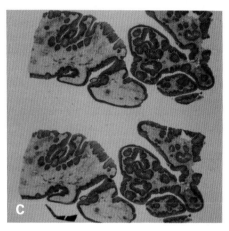
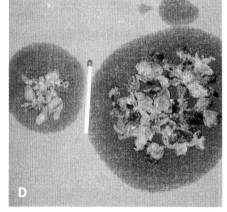

FIGURE 5.223   *A*, The preoperative view of a presumably typical, large nasal polyp. *B*, The surgical specimen. *C*, This proved to be an inverting papilloma with no malignant features. This patient had polyps on the left side as well, but these showed no evidence of papilloma formation. *D*, Typical lobular structure of the inverted papilloma is seen in this surgical specimen.

SUMMARY AND CONCLUSIONS

The anterior ethmoid is the central component of the ostiomeatal unit and as such has a key function in both the normal and the pathophysiology of the paranasal sinuses. The frontal and maxillary sinuses communicate with the middle meatus by way of a narrow and complex system of clefts in the anterior ethmoid. The frontal recess and the ethmoidal infundibulum can be regarded as "vestibules" or prechambers for the large paranasal sinuses located behind them. As long as these narrow spaces are healthy, they are of key importance in the drainage of these large paranasal sinuses.

The mucosal surfaces in these prechambers are frequently separated by less than 1 mm over an extensive area and make it possible to transport abnormal secretions through these bottle necks, since the ciliary sweep can attack the film of secretion from both sides. In the ostia, the cilia can work on the secretions from all sides. If, however, the mucosal surfaces in these narrow areas are compressed against each other, for whatever reason, to such an extent that the cilia can no longer move, then ciliary transport comes to a halt at this area of intense contact. Their ventilation and drainage may become impaired or even cease completely. This results in inadequate ventilation and consequently in decreased pO_2 and pH. Impaired ciliary transportation may also lead to the retention and thickening of the secretions to such an extent that the ciliary transport comes to a halt at this area of contact. Depending upon the location and the extent of such changes, the paranasal sinuses may become secondarily involved.

Due to these retained secretions, circumscribed points of contact in the lateral nasal wall frequently become circumscribed foci of infection that may remain free of clinical symptoms for a long time. In superinfection, however, there may be progressive involvement extending by a cascade effect from the circumscribed focus to the surrounding areas, particularly the ethmoidal infundibulum and the frontal recess. From there the involvement may extend to the paranasal sinuses and present with the clinical appearance of a recurrent frontal and/or maxillary sinusitis.

The anterior ethmoid may show a large number of anatomic variations that may additionally narrow the already normally constricted spaces in the ostiomeatal unit. These anatomic variations may predispose the patient to recurrent infections, particularly if the variations occur in combinations. Under these conditions it takes only a slight swelling of the mucous membranes, from whatever cause, to block the narrow area completely.

There are many ways in which pathogens reach the large paranasal sinuses through the nose, even when their ostia are almost completely obstructed. Because of the way the nasal valve is structured, almost 90 percent of the inhaled air stream is directed toward the insertion of the middle turbinate where it then proceeds medially and laterally to the middle turbinate. As a consequence, the majority of the dust particles and pathogens in the air stream are deposited onto the mucosal surfaces of this area. It is no accident that the adenocarcinoma of woodworkers develops in the anterior ethmoid at the entrance to the middle meatus where the majority of the inhaled carcinogens are deposited.

Particles deposited at the entrance to the middle meatus may in certain disease states remain there and they may even be transported into the paranasal sinuses, as shown in Chapter 2. The transportation of secretions is directed *toward* the frontal sinus from the frontal recess and toward the maxillary sinus through the accessory ostia in the nasal fontanelles.

These pathogens frequently find ideal conditions for growth in these diseased and constricted spaces. This is particularly true when decreased ventilation produces almost anaerobic conditions in the sinuses.

The clinical symptoms may include, in addition to obstructed nasal breathing, a feeling of fullness or pressure between the eyes, headaches and secretions in the nasopharynx, i.e., the typical findings in frontal and maxillary sinusitis. The mucosal changes found in these sinuses are in most cases not the direct cause of the disease, but are only secondary manifestations of the primary disease of the anterior ethmoid segments. Recognition of these changes is the primary function of endoscopic and radiographic diagnosis.

Constriction of the clefts and air cells of the anterior ethmoid by anatomic variants, mechanical factors, inflammatory and/or allergic mucosal changes, and disturbances in the mucociliary transport may result in a vicious cycle from which medical therapy alone no longer provides recovery. Mucociliary activity may be significantly reduced or entirely abolished by the pressure of opposing mucous membranes pressed into intimate contact because of inflammation and swelling. Goblet cell and squamous epithelial metaplasia may produce areas with reduced ciliary activity and thus promote disturbances in transport and the retention of abnormal secretions. Areas with extensive goblet cell metaplasia produce a highly viscous secretion that can only be transported with difficulty (or even not at all) by the healthy mucosa of the adjacent areas.

Inside the paranasal sinuses, certain factors, such as lowered pH, O_2 deficiency, and increased pCO_2 promote the formation of increased and viscous secretions. These secretions, which are rich in protein and glucose, provide a favorable medium for colonization by bacteria and fungi.

Tenacious secretions block the excretory ducts of the glands and are responsible for the retention of mucus, cyst formation, and the extravasation of mucus. This extravasation produces granulomatous reactions that further thicken the mucous membranes, which further contributes to the obstruction of the narrow spaces and/or the ostia of the paranasal sinuses. Through a mechanism that is not entirely clear, polyps originate, in many cases, from the swollen mucosa at the points of contact and these polyps may completely occlude the entire ethmoid area.

These findings and observations led to the development of an endoscopic surgical approach that attempts to achieve a cure by small and locally limited intervention by following an exact diagnostic recognition of the basic changes in the key areas of the ethmoid. With this technique, the ventilation and drainage of the large paranasal sinuses is reestablished by physiologic means. It is fascinating to observe how, even after such minimal interventions, the most massive mucosal changes in the paranasal sinuses clear up within a few weeks without any surgical intervention in the sinuses themselves. The regenerative ability of the mucosa of the paranasal sinuses is apparently much greater than has previously been assumed. The impressive achievements of this target-oriented functional endoscopic surgery on the lateral nasal wall fully justify our assumptions that with few exceptions, the inflammatory changes in the frontal and maxillary sinuses are secondary to disease in the anterior ethmoid and lateral wall of the nose.

The detailed and systematic endoscopic diagnosis of the lateral nasal wall and the target oriented functional endoscopic surgery based on the results of the diagnostic examination are the great accomplishments of the Messerklinger Technique. A combination of endoscopic examination and conventional and computed tomography has proven most successful for the comprehensive diagnosis of chronic inflammatory diseases of the paranasal sinuses. Neither anterior nor posterior rhinoscopy nor conventional radiography of the paranasal sinuses can provide the necessary information about the point of origin of the disease process. It is precisely this accurate diagnostic information that enables us to determine which therapeutic modality is possible or necessary and also enables us to avoid radical surgery in most instances.

Chapter 6

INDICATIONS FOR ENDOSCOPIC SURGERY

The indications for endoscopic sinus surgery are derived from a combined assessment of the patient's history, the results of the endoscopic diagnostic examination, and the tomographic films. Opacities on the radiographs without related clinical symptoms are an indication for further diagnostic exploration and evaluation in order not to miss a hidden malignancy. Once a malignancy has been excluded, *no surgical procedure* should be planned if the patient is asymptomatic. In this event, we discuss the findings with the patient and explain symptoms, which, for instance, large cysts of the maxillary sinus might produce someday, and explain that surgical intervention would be necessary only then. Exceptions are mycoses, mucoceles, and other conditions that can be *expected* to produce problems sooner or later and thus may be indications for surgical procedure even in the absence of symptoms.

The most important and frequent indications for endoscopic sinus surgery in our patient population are summarized in Table 6.1, although this is by no means a complete list. We should emphasize those indications in which there seems to be no relationship between the patient's history and involvement of the paranasal sinuses, particularly when the survey radiographs are unremarkable. In this context, headache of unknown etiology (see Chapter 11), some eustachian tube problems, increased or pathologic secretions in the nasopharynx (postnasal drip), and tearing should be mentioned. Anosmia can be of rhinogenic origin without any rhinoscopic or radiographic basis. Some facial neuralgias may originate in the ethmoidal sinus, although they are allegedly related to such problems as a deviation of the nasal septum. It is in these patients that good tomography or CT is especially important.

TABLE 6.1 Range of Indications for Functional Endoscopic Surgery

Polyposis	Eustachian tube problems
Obstructed nasal respiration	Postnasal drip
Recurrent and chronic sinusitis	Continuing complaints after Caldwell-Luc
Epiphora (tearing)	procedure or intranasal fenestration
Anosmia	procedures
Chronic headaches	As adjuvant therapy in allergies
Mucocele of any paranasal sinus	Sinubronchial syndrome
Retention cysts	Bronchial asthma
Mycoses (noninvasive)	Recurrent pharyngitis
Orbital complications of acute sinusitis	Some phonation disturbances
Septal spurs	Special cases of snoring

It is not surprising that many patients undergo endoscopic sinus surgery for the treatment of "nasal polyps." The mucosa of the ethmoidal and other paranasal sinuses is limited in its response to inflammatory stimuli. Circumscribed swellings, edema and, finally, polyp formation predominate. Polyp formation can be regarded as a nonspecific reaction to a variety of inflammatory, allergic, chemical, toxic, thermal, or mechanical stimuli. It may be the result of the simultaneous influence of a number of these factors upon circumscribed or extensive areas of the mucous membranes, with a variety of etiologies producing a similar, clinical morphologic appearance. Consequently, the diagnosis of nasal polyps is more of a description of the localized findings rather than a definition of the type or etiology of a specific disease entity.

Simple nasal polyps should be distinguished from diffuse polypoid sinusitis on the basis of clinical appearance and behavior (see Chapter 5). Diffuse polypoid sinusitis is apparently the result of a generalized mucous membrane disease rather than a more or less circumscribed area of diseased mucus membrane (mucosal disease versus diseased mucosa).

On the basis of the diagnostic information provided by the combination of the endoscopic examination and the CT, one can obtain a large number of individual surgical indications that are significantly more specific than could be expressed by the classic catchall term of "sinusitis."

In principle, every inflammatory disease of the nose or paranasal sinuses or those diseases in this area as the result of anatomic variations that require surgical correction can be addressed with the Messerklinger technique.

We also use the endoscope in the treatment of small neoplasms in the area of the paranasal sinuses, in the closure of CSF fistulas, in performing dacryocystorhinostomies according to the technique described by West, and for a variety of other procedures in the paranasal sinuses and the nasopharynx (blow-out fracture of the orbital floor, orbital decompression in endocrine orbitopathy, removal of foreign bodies from all sinuses, choanal atresia, etc.). These techniques offer considerably expanded areas of utilization in which the endoscope is preferable to the microscope. These are not a component of the Messerklinger technique per se and are therefore not further mentioned in this discussion.

It is our opinion that, in general, a surgical procedure is justified only when it is justified by the symptomatology, when medical therapy is not successful, or when the changes are of such a nature that medical therapy is doomed to failure.

CONTRAINDICATIONS

The Messerklinger technique is not designed for the surgical approach to extensive invasive processes in the area of the paranasal sinuses (Figs. 6.1 to 6.3) or the skull base. Extensive bony changes such as a broadly based osteoma are also not suitable subjects for this technique. Coarse bony postinflammatory stenoses of the ostium of the frontal sinus are rare findings that may stretch the usefulness of endoscopic technique to its limits. Enlargement of the ostium of the frontal sinus after an osteitic process is not a suitable procedure for the instruments developed for the Messerklinger technique and cannot be performed under local anesthesia.

If the area of the frontal recess and the ostium of the frontal sinus can no longer be identified accurately from the nose because of scarring or ossification following previous surgery, a two-pronged approach is possible. Through a burr-hole in the anterior wall of the frontal sinus (e.g., as in the Beck procedure) a 30 or 70 degree lens can be introduced into the frontal sinus and thus the endonasal approach can be visually controlled from above. In such cases with osteal stenosis or obstruction, we leave a polyethylene drain in place for 3 to 6 months after appropriate surgical enlargement of the ostium.

If, in an orbital extension of an acute sinusitis, there is even the slightest indication of an incipient central complication (e.g., meningitis, subperiosteal or epidural abscess, or cavernous sinus thrombosis) or if there is evidence of osteitis or osteomyelitis of the frontal bone with sequestration (see Fig. 6.1A), a primary endoscopic procedure according to the Messerklinger technique is contraindicated (see Chapter 9). The same holds true for orbital complications in which there is an acute visual or visual field loss or blindness. In these situations, and especially when there is sequestrum formation or an intracranial complication, we prefer a traditional, anterior approach.

In mucoceles in the area of the frontal sinus (ordinarily an ideal indication for a functional endoscopic procedure) one must always remember that the mucocele may be chambered or that there may be a second mucocele located so far laterally that it can not be reached endoscopically over the frontal recess. In these rare cases an anterior approach may be necessary.

The exceptional cases in which we open the *maxillary sinus* through the canine fossa in inflammatory diseases are:

1. In some mycoses when the mycotic mass completely fills the maxillary sinus and cannot be broken up into smaller fragments or be removed satisfactorily through an enlarged ostium via the middle meatus or when there is a suspicion of an invasive mycotic infection.
2. In some cases of previous radical maxillary sinus surgery when the recess is scarred and compartmentalized and where it can no longer be reached and opened endoscopically with any degree of confidence (see Fig. 6.2).

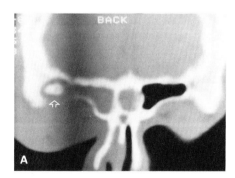 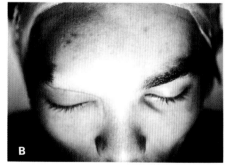

FIGURE 6.1 *A*, This is the tomogram of a patient with recurrent right frontal sinusitis, following previous external surgery. A sequestered piece of bone (*arrow*) and the soft tissue swelling can be clearly seen. *B*, This is the clinical photograph of the same patient immediately prior to surgery. The scar from the previous external operation can be seen below the partially shaved eyebrow. A doughy, fluctuant swelling (Pott's puffy tumor) can be seen on the forehead extending from the glabella almost to the hairline. In this clinical situation, an endoscopic procedure was not indicated.

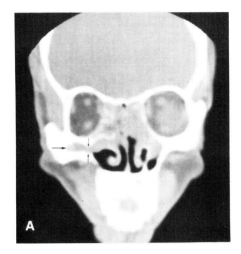
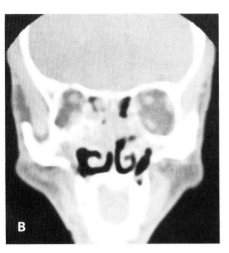

FIGURE 6.2 *A* and *B,* This patient had undergone repeated, bilateral Caldwell-Luc and fenestration procedures. The bony defects in the facial wall of the maxillary sinus and the marked deformities of the remaining bony walls can be clearly seen. On the right side a laterally extending, deep recess has formed (*arrows*). This recess contained an encapsulated empyema that could not be reached with an endoscope.

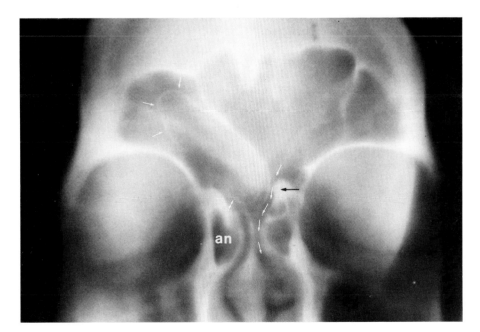

FIGURE 6.3 The bulla frontalis (frontal bulla). The bulla frontalis is an anterior ethmoidal air cell that can extend into the frontal bone and appear as though it were the frontal sinus. In this case the air cell of a bulla frontalis (*white arrows,* patient's right side) extends into the right frontal sinus. Well pneumatized agger nasi air cells severely constrict the frontal recess on both sides. The *row of arrows* marks the path from the ostium of the frontal sinus, through the frontal recess, and past the agger nasi cell. The *black arrow* points to a small osteoma near the ostium of the left frontal sinus. This patient suffered from recurrent frontal sinus empyemas and frontal headaches. This patient was not treated endoscopically. an = agger nasi cell.

CONSERVATIVE ENDOSCOPIC MANAGEMENT

The pathophysiologic mechanisms leading to an acute frontal or maxillary sinusitis were discussed earlier. Most cases of acute sinusitis require no surgical management.

Even during the conservative management of an empyema of the frontal or maxillary sinus we may resort to the endoscope (Fig. 6.4). In most cases of acute frontal sinusitis, even if there is already an obvious air-fluid level, the placement of epinephrine and Pontocaine pledgets may decrease the swelling of the frontal recess and thus permit spontaneous drainage from the frontal sinus (Figs. 6.4 and 6.5). Under endoscopic guidance, these pledgets can be placed with accuracy. With a slender biopsy forceps or a bayonet forceps, they can be advanced with gentle pressure under the middle turbinate into the frontal recess and left there for 20 to 30 minutes. This form of therapy is employed 2 to 3 times each day in addition to the appropriate antibiotic and anti-inflammatory medical therapy. In this way even severe cases of acute sinusitis can be cured. It is most impressive to see the stream of pus that emerges from the engorged and inflamed nasal passages after the placement of a decongestant pledget into the ethmoidal area, particularly into the frontal recess (see Figs. 6.4 and 6.5). The endoscopist can usually see very clearly *where* the source of the (secondary) frontal sinus pathology lies.

Using this technique, we have not needed to employ the Beck burr-hole technique during the last 15 years for the treatment of acute frontal sinusitis.

In acute recurrent or drug therapy resistant frontal sinus disease, we make an attempt to identify the underlying changes in the middle meatus and in the frontal recess with endoscopy and CT and promote a cure by surgical means. The timing of the surgical intervention depends entirely on the clinical course of the disease. If there is no response to the therapy described above, then we open the frontal recess after 2 to 3 days, provided that there are no complications. If pain persists in spite of therapy, we may act even sooner.

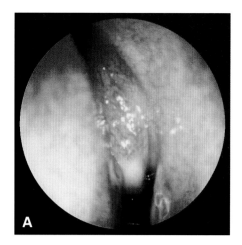

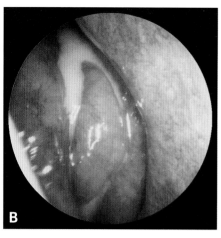

FIGURE 6.4 *A,* This is the left middle meatus of a patient with pansinusitis. The uncinate process is folded sharply medially and is in close contact with the middle turbinate. No purulent secretions can be seen, even though the nose was sprayed with Pontocaine and a vasoconstrictor. *B,* After the 15-minute application of a decongestant pledget, directly into the middle meatus, a profuse flow of pus can be seen coming from the anterior ethmoid.

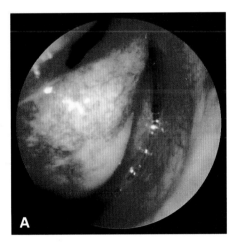

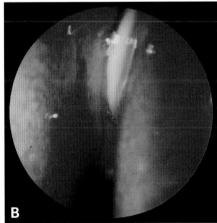

FIGURE 6.5 *A,* The left middle meatus of a patient with an acute frontal sinusitis and an air-fluid level. There is a concha bullosa in the left middle turbinate. The mucosa covering the lateral surface of the concha bullosa is engorged by inflammatory edema at the site of contact with the uncinate process. No significant purulent secretions can be seen. *B,* After the application of a topical decongestant in the frontal recess, the emergence of pus from this area can be seen clearly (30 degree lens, upward view).

Frontal sinus surgery from the outside for inflammatory disease may be required only for the reasons discussed above under "Contraindications." Under no circumstances is an air-fluid level or an uncomplicated empyema (Figs. 6.6 and 6.7) a sufficient indication for a primarily external approach and quite particularly not for a radical procedure, such as an obliteration of the frontal sinus (see Figs. 6.4–6.7).

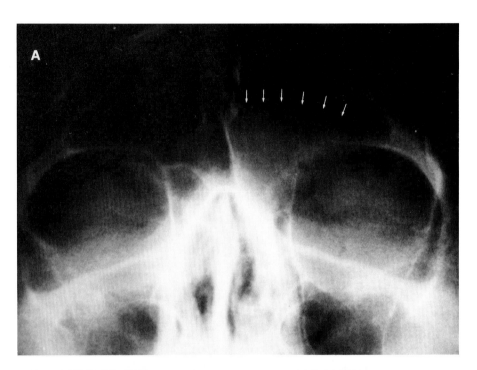

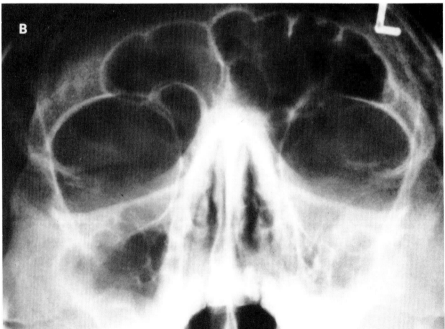

FIGURE 6.6 These are the radiographs of the patient shown in Figure 6.4. *A*, pretreatment film, note the air-fluid level in the left frontal sinus (*arrows*). *B*, After conservative therapy the frontal sinus cleared completely.

A similar goal-oriented local therapy is also very useful in the treatment of acute maxillary sinusitis. We may perform an initial maxillary sinus puncture and irrigation through the inferior meatus in acute primary sinusitis, depending on the clinical findings and the severity of the case. Subsequently, therapy consists of the placement of local decongestant and anesthetic pledgets into the middle meatus. This usually eliminates the need for serial punctures. By following this approach we have not yet found a need to insert an indwelling catheter in the maxillary sinus.

In acute purulent sinusitis accompanied by severe pain, it is advantageous to use not only a topical vasoconstrictor, but also a topical anesthetic, e.g., 2 percent Pontocaine. This provides relief for the patient, particularly if the first application produces only a slight or transient improvement in drainage. It is always amazing to see the enormous amounts of retained purulent secretions that can emerge from the middle meatus and from the sinuses after a 20-minute application and the great relief that the patient obtains from this simple procedure.

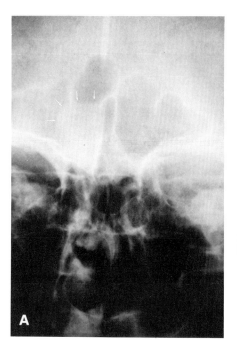 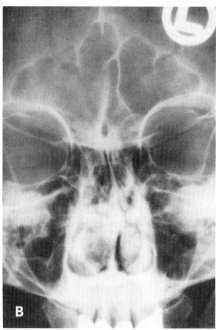

FIGURE 6.7 These are the radiographs of an 81-year-old patient with acute *right* frontal sinusitis, before (*A*) and after (*B*) conservative endoscopic management. After the direct placement of decongestant pledgets into the frontal recess, the purulent secretion in the right frontal sinus (*arrows*) completely disappeared.

Chapter 7

SURGICAL TECHNIQUE

SURGICAL PRINCIPLES

While a total sphenoethmoidectomy can be performed with the Messerklinger technique, one of the major advantages of this technique is that because of the initial, precise diagnosis (even in severe cases) such an extensive resection is only rarely necessary. On the basis of a step-by-step advance, which is always adapted to the specific pathologic findings, the surgeon can usually identify and differentiate severe pathologic mucosal changes in the ethmoid and sphenoid areas from collateral edema, which requires no surgical removal.

Accurate diagnosis remains the basic principle of the Messerklinger technique even during the surgical procedure. In this way, the surgical procedure can be limited to the *absolute minimum*. Since most diseases of the paranasal sinuses originate in or are dependent upon the ethmoid, the surgical procedure is focused on this area. Even in those cases with massive involvement of the frontal or maxillary sinuses, correction of the ethmoid disease usually results in recovery of the larger sinuses within a few weeks, even though these sinuses have not been touched. In most cases, the ostium of the frontal sinus does not need to be touched and fenestration of the maxillary sinus into the inferior meatus is not necessary. When required, the natural ostium of the maxillary sinus in the middle meatus can be enlarged at the expense of the adjacent fontanelles. In comparison to fenestration into the inferior meatus, an enlarged natural ostium is much less likely to become stenotic (see Chapter 13).

Every attempt should be made to achieve the desired results with the least traumatic functional procedure and to spare the patient from unnecessary "routine" radical procedures. This is facilitated by applying a tissue-sparing and mucosa-preserving surgical technique and by using special instruments. The enormous regenerative potential of even massively diseased mucosa is always impressive.

The goal of the surgical procedure is not the creation of a large smooth cavity connecting all of the paranasal sinuses. The aim is to remove the obstructing anatomic variations and to resect only the most severely diseased mucosa in these key locations. The mucosal lining should be preserved wherever possible. Under no circumstances should extensive bony surfaces be denuded of their mucosal covering. It is not necessary to remove remnants of bony walls or septa with a diamond drill.

The Messerklinger technique does not provide a surgical cure for all inflammatory paranasal sinus disease. As indicated in Chapters 5, 9, and 13, there are some polypoid paranasal sinus diseases in which none of the currently available surgical techniques can provide a definite cure. Since, however, in these cases even radical procedures do not assure a better long term result, we feel confident in using the Messerklinger technique, which produces at the least similar results with much less morbidity and less intra- and postoperative stress on the patient.

INSTRUMENT MANIPULATION

Endoscopic surgery is primarily a one-handed procedure in which the instruments are introduced alongside and parallel to the endoscope. One of the surgeon's hands, usually the left one, handles the endoscope, while the other hand manages the instruments and the suction tip (Fig. 7.1). Initially, this "one-handedness" may appear as a handicap. The experienced surgeon does not view this as a problem and the potential difficulties are more than compensated for by the remarkable clarity of the endoscopic image, the outstanding depth perception, and the ability to move the endoscope freely within the nasal cavity (Fig. 7.2). This mobility provides an excellent "spatial sensation" that permits outstanding orientation, which can be enhanced by the surgeon's ability to look around corners with a variety of angled lenses.

The insertion and manipulation of the endoscope, which is held like a pencil with three fingers, is made easier by the development of special handles. These handles also help compensate for the rotational force of the light cable, the observer side arm, or a camera. With these special handles, the angled lenses can be more easily rotated around

FIGURE 7.1   The typical position of the hands in endoscopic surgery. For details, see text.

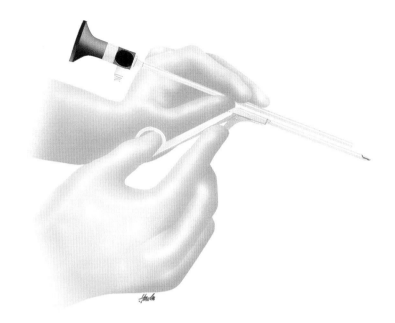

FIGURE 7.2   The range of motion of the instrument around the endoscope.

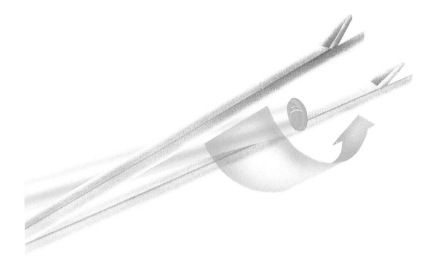

their long axis, without danger of losing the view and without the surgeon developing a cramped feeling (see Figs. A.3 and A.4). Nasal specula or other holding devices are not required for either diagnostic or surgical procedures.

As shown in Figure 7.1, the endoscope is held in the middle of its shaft with the thumb, index, and middle fingers. The little finger and the edge of the left hand rest very gently on the bridge of the patient's nose or cheek to guide the endoscope. The endoscope is always introduced into the nasal vestibule under *direct vision*. This technique prevents incidental injury and avoids the nasal hairs, which may become coated with debris, mucus, or bloodstained secretions, thereby keeping the lens free from dirt and deposits. It is usually not necessary to cut the hairs in the nasal vestibule.

The introduction of the 30 degree lens requires some skill, while the introduction of the 70 degree lens requires considerable skill, since the latter no longer permits a forward view along the long axis of the scope. The surgeon can use the trocar sleeve to assist in the insertion of the 70 degree endoscope (Fig. 7.3). This is accomplished by first advancing the trocar sleeve to the desired depth with the zero or thirty degree lens, which is then removed from the trocar sleeve. The 70 degree lens is then inserted into the sleeve.

A   **B**   **C**

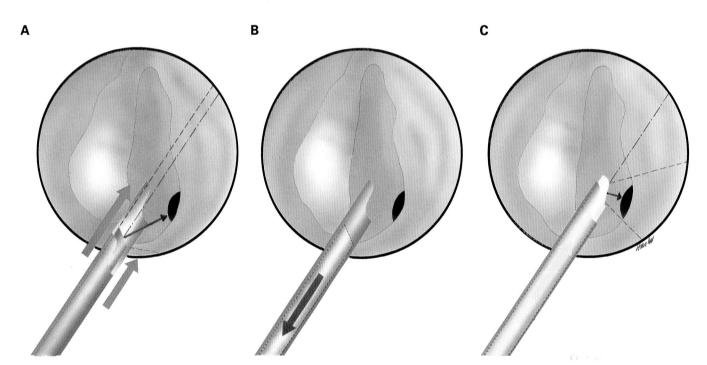

FIGURE 7.3 The technique for introducing a 70 degree lens into the middle meatus under narrow and difficult conditions. *A,* A 0 or a 30 degree endoscope is inserted into the trocar sheath (*blue*), which is then introduced into the middle meatus under direct vision. The trocar sheath is then carefully advanced under the middle turbinate (*blue arrows*). *B,* The trocar sheath is then stabilized with the left hand and the endoscope is withdrawn (*red arrow*). *C,* The 70 degree endoscope is then carefully advanced through the fixed trocar sheath (*yellow arrow*). After passing beyond the tip of the trocar sheath, an unimpeded view can be obtained of the target structure (in this case a look at and through the maxillary ostium).

A right-handed surgeon *always* introduces the surgical instruments along the right side or underneath the scope. As shown in Figures 7.2 and 7.4, this assures the greatest mobility for the instrument without obstructing the surgeon.

During the introduction of an instrument into the nasal cavity, it is advanced parallel to the endoscope, using the shaft of the endoscope as a guide to advance the instrument. This is the best way to avoid accidental damage to the skin of the nasal vestibule and injury to the mucosa of the anterior nasal passages. We recommend that the left eye be used as the "guiding" eye for the endoscope allowing the right eye to control the introduction of the operating instruments without the surgeon taking his or her eye away from the endoscope. When *changing instruments* it is advisable to take the guide eye away from the scope, or to open the right eye, so that the new instrument can be introduced under direct vision, thereby preventing accidental injury to the nose. With experience the surgeon becomes able to introduce instruments blindly by advancing them alongside the endoscope and guiding them into the nasal vestibule with the fingers of the left hand. All changes of instruments should be accomplished expeditously and carefully, but without haste.

FIGURE 7.4 The typical posture during endoscopic surgery.

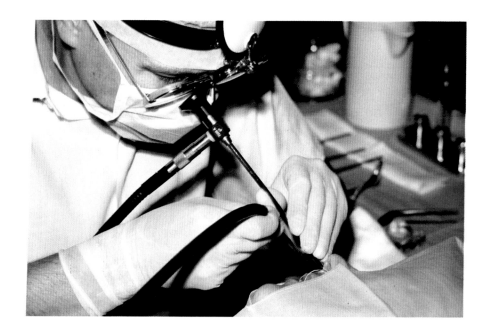

The smallest mucosal laceration may cause enough bleeding to make the rest of the procedure extremely difficult. The guiding principle of *atraumatic surgery* must be kept in mind at all times. The same care should be devoted to the introduction of instruments in the nose as is used in middle ear surgery.

Because of the clarity of the optical image and the wide angle effect of the nasal endoscope, there is an initial temptation to get as close as possible to the target area. During endoscopic sinus surgery, especially if the posterior ethmoid or the the sphenoid sinus must be reached, this can result in the formation of a tunnel or "channel," in which (while the individual details are extremely clear) unfortunately the general overview is lost. This increases the risk of the surgeon losing his or her depth perception and *underestimating* the depth of penetration into the nose. The endoscope should always remain as far as possible behind the instrument. This means that the anatomic landmarks necessary for proper orientation must always be kept in view. Even when the surgical procedure involves the middle meatus, it is not always necessary to enter it with the endoscope.

The most anterior insertion of the middle turbinate is the most important landmark for judging the depth of entry into the nose and the angle of the advancing instrument relative to the skull and the lamina cribrosa. This is of particular importance when a precise identification of the anatomic structures is no longer possible because of the extent of the disease, e.g., diffuse or recurrent polyposis.

The following procedure has proven helpful in providing a rough estimation of the depth of penetration. The index finger is placed on the shaft of the instrument at the level of the anterior nasal spine when the tip of the instrument is inside the nasal cavity and the distance to its end can be estimated. All of our suction tips are marked in centimeters and therefore, the depth of an intranasal instrument can be determined by laying the suction catheter alongside the instrument that is inside the nose. It is also useful to check the position and the angle of the endoscope and of the instruments and their relationship to the skull and the orbits by taking the eye away from the lens and looking at the set-up. This technique is useful in providing a rough orientation, but it can never replace a precise identification of the anatomic landmarks.

The CT scan provides the surgeon with an excellent method of determining all of the important distances preoperatively. The most important distances and angles are those between the anterior nasal spine and the frontal recess, the roof of the ethmoid, the basal lamella, and the anterior wall of the sphenoid sinus (see Chapter 4, Fig. 4.14).

With practice, the surgeon should gain an excellent feel for the spatial relationships by the relative motion of the endoscope and the instrument or by moving with the advancement and retraction of both. When working in the ethmoid, this freedom of changing the direction of the view and of the approach combined with the superb visibility provided by the nasal endoscope gives this technique a definite advantage over the operating microscope in our hands.

Initially one may encounter some difficulty in avoiding contact between the lens of the endoscope and the mucosa or with secretions or blood. Such contact requires frequent withdrawal, cleaning, and reintroduction of the endoscope. Again, basic atraumatic procedure is the principle to follow.

The suction tip should always be introduced *without suction* until the tip appears in view through the endoscope to avoid blood being drawn from the depth of the field, not only into the suction tip, but also onto the lens of the endoscope.

When endoscopes are switched during the procedure, the endoscope not in use should be immersed in a cotton lined container of warm sterile saline. This prevents lens damage and the drying of blood and secretions on the lens (see Fig. 8.2B). Before each introduction, the lens is treated with antifog solution, which is not wiped off, but left as a thin layer on the lens. The excess solution is usually lost during the passage through the vibrissae.

Before introduction into the nose, the endoscopes should be warmed to prevent condensation of the moist exhaled air forming on the lens of the scope.

If it becomes necessary to enter the middle meatus with the endoscope and if the entrance is very narrow, the instrument or a more slender suction tip can be used to carefully displace the middle turbinate medially, thereby allowing the endoscope to be introduced into the meatus. At the least, a good view can be obtained with this maneuver. In doing this, great care must be exercised not to injure the mucous membrane on the head of the middle turbinate.

We do not use the commercially available suction-irrigation endoscopes, as they are too bulky. Entry into the middle meatus with these instruments is frequently impossible without injuring the head of the turbinate. In addition, the use of irrigation in the prone, nonintubated patient is not permissible, since the irrigating solution would run directly into the pharynx.

In Chapter 8 the need for the surgeon to be in a relaxed posture is emphasized. The resting of both elbows on a Mayo stand or on a small table is useful in preventing fatigue.

SURGICAL TECHNIQUE AND OPTIONS

In the following, the individual steps of functional endoscopic sinus surgery are illustrated on a cadaver. The steps shown are not necessarily the routine steps, but include all of the steps that are technically possible with this approach.

While the Messerklinger technique is suitable for the performance of a total sphenoethmoidectomy, the general idea is to avoid routine radical procedures even in cases of massive disease.

The preferred endoscope for the surgical procedure is the zero degree (straight forward viewing) instrument. The 30 or 70 degree nasal endoscopes are used only in special situations, e.g., involvement of the frontal recess, enlargement of the natural ostium of the maxillary sinus, or in procedures within the latter.

The zero degree nasal endoscope has many significant advantages, especially for the inexperienced endoscopist. The zero degree endoscope is the only instrument in which the surgeon sees along the same line as is being worked on, corresponding exactly to the direction of the shaft, i.e., the long axis of the instrument (Fig. 7.5). When using a rigid endoscope, the beginner instinctively feels that the endoscope points in the direction of the image seen and that the instrument used is also located along the same axis. This is only true for the zero degree nasal endoscope. Even a slight angulation, such as the 30 degree lens can confuse the beginner and make the anatomic and topographic orientation difficult. This is particularly true when the anatomic landmarks have been destroyed by the disease process or removed during a procedure.

The angle between the endoscope and the surgical instrument can not be appreciated when looking through the endoscope. As shown in Figure 7.6, the impression can be generated that the action is along the long axis of the instrument, i.e., that the action is at the basal lamella of the middle turbinate, when in fact the roof of the ethmoid has already been reached. For this reason we strongly urge all beginners in endoscopic techniques to use the zero degree endoscope as much as possible for all of the surgical steps and to use the angled endoscopes only for the few specific indications given above, and then only after the important topographic landmarks have been identified.

FIGURE 7.5 Only with the 0 degree endoscope does the instrument point exactly in the same direction as the shaft of
the endoscope and in the same direction
as the view seen (a).

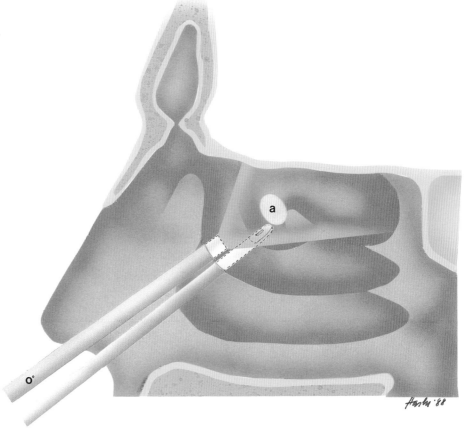

FIGURE 7.6 Even with a 30 degree endoscope, one no longer looks in the
direction in which the instrument points
(a), but depending on the orientation of
the lens, [in this case anterocranially (a′)].
As a result, the beginner may suffer from
the misconception that he is working with
the instrument in the same direction in
which the endoscope points (a, b). The
surgeon is actually working at a considerable angle from this direction, because of
the angulation of the endoscope lens
(a′, b′). The angled lenses should only be
used *after the key anatomic landmarks*
(roof of the ethmoid, anterior ethmoidal
artery, etc.) *have been unmistakably identified*.

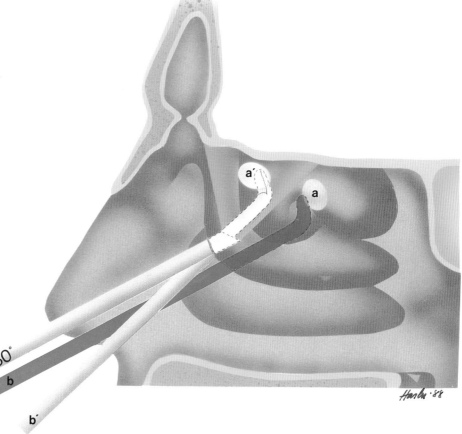

Figure 7.7 represents the starting position in a right nasal cavity. The zero degree nasal endoscope has been introduced through the naris, passed through the nasal vestibule, and advanced to a position 1.5 cm anterior to the insertion of the middle turbinate without touching the septum or the lateral nasal wall. The endoscope directly views the front of the middle turbinate, its insertion into the lateral wall of the nose, and the anterior aspect of the middle meatus. The free posterior margin of the uncinate process and behind it a portion of the anterior surface of the ethmoidal bulla can be seen.

Since most sinus disease involves the anterior part of the ethmoid, the first step in most operations is the opening of the ethmoidal infundibulum by resecting the uncinate process. The medial wall of the ethmoidal infundibulum is formed by the uncinate process and its mucous membrane covering. The uncinate process is resected by inserting a curved knife blade carefully into the uncinate process just below the insertion of the middle turbinate (Fig. 7.8). The insertion of the uncinate process on the lateral wall of the nose is transected in a convex arch from anterosuperior to posteroinferior. In this process, the tip of the sickle knife usually does not extend more than 3 or 4 mm through the uncinate process into the ethmoidal infundibulum. It is of utmost importance that the knife be advanced through the uncinate process at a shallow angle (i.e., in a plane parallel to the medial wall of the orbit). Under no circumstances should the sickle knife proceed so far laterally and advance so far as to injure the lamina papyracea of the orbit. If the infundibulum is flat or atelectatic, there is a considerable danger of such an injury. We always attempt to hold the handle of the knife parallel to the lateral wall of the nose after its tip has penetrated the uncinate process.

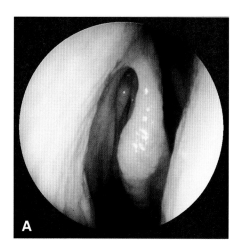

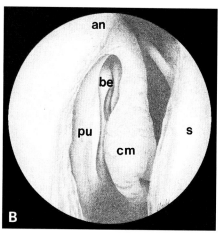

FIGURE 7.7 *A*, The view through a 0 degree endoscope into a right middle meatus. For a more detailed description see the text. *B*, A schematic drawing of

A. cm = middle turbinate; pu = uncinate process; be – ethmoidal bulla; an = agger nasi; and s = septum.

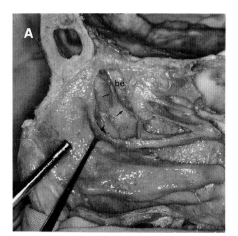

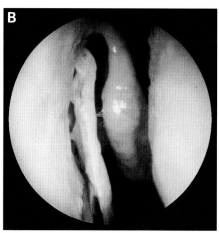

FIGURE 7.8 *A*, A right lateral nasal wall. The middle turbinate has been fenestrated so that the underlying structures can be seen. *Arrows* indicate the free posterior margin of the uncinate process. The hiatus semilunaris is located between the arrows and the anterior surface of the ethmoidal bulla. In this case, the bulla lamella extends to the skull base (*white arrow*) and separates the frontal recess

from a potential lateral sinus. The sickle knife cuts around the anterior insertion of the uncinate process. *B*, An endoscopic view of the same situation. The uncinate process was incised from above downward with the sickle knife. Note the shallow angle of the blade to the lateral nasal wall (to avoid penetrating the lamina papyracea).

In Figures 7.8 and 7.9, a window has been cut into the middle turbinate so that subsequent surgical steps can be shown from the medial side.

The uncinate process is then carefully displaced medially so that the surgeon can look into the ethmoidal infundibulum (Fig. 7.10). The anterior wall of the ethmoidal bulla can be seen at the bottom and any pathologic changes in this area can be identified.

The superior insertion of the uncinate process is then carefully grasped with Blakesley-Weil forceps, without injuring the adjacent middle turbinate, and the bony insertion is separated from the lateral nasal wall by a twisting motion of the forceps. The inferior insertion of the uncinate process is then grasped with the Blakesley-Weil forceps and separated with a similar twisting motion so that the uncinate process can now be removed in its entirety.

After the uncinate process has been circumferentially incised, it should not be simply pulled out with the forceps, since this can lead to uncontrolled tears of the mucous membrane. This can occur particularly at the insertion of the middle turbinate and lead to troublesome hemorrhage and to the creation of opposing raw wound surfaces (e.g., between the lateral wall of the nose and the lateral surface of the turbinate). Even a few drops of blood in this area can make inspection into the frontal recess very difficult.

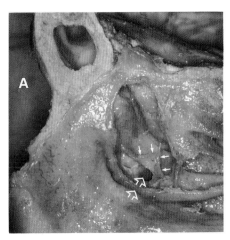
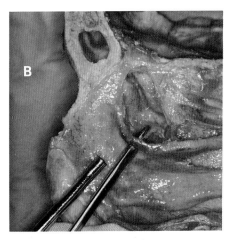
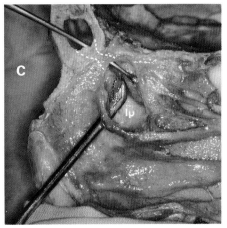

FIGURE 7.9 *A*, A view through the fenestrated middle turbinate. The anterior insertion of the uncinate process has been incised and displaced medially and superiorly (*small arrows*). The ostium of the maxillary sinus, hidden on the floor of the ethmoidal infundibulum, can now be plainly seen (*open arrows*). *B*, Resection of the uncinate process. For a detailed description see the text. *C*, After resection of the inferior 2/3 of the uncinate process, one can see the lamina papyracea just above the ostium of the maxillary sinus. Note in this specimen how the ethmoidal infundibulum terminates superiorly in a blind pouch (the recessus terminalis). This happens because the uncinate process deviates laterally and inserts onto the lamina papyracea. The tip of the upward angled forceps dips into the recessus terminalis. The outline of the recessus terminalis is marked with *black dots*. A sound has been placed through the ostium of the frontal sinus, into the frontal recess. The *broken white line* shows the outline of the floor of the frontal sinus, with its funnel-shaped constriction toward the ostium of the frontal sinus and the adjacent, also funnel-shaped, enlargement of the frontal recess. The resulting hourglass configuration is evident. lp = lamina papyracea.

294

Figure 7.11 shows the appearance after resection of the uncinate process: the wide passage made into the anterior ethmoid can be seen clearly. The ethmoidal infundibulum no longer exists since its medial wall, the uncinate process, has been removed. The anterior surface of the ethmoidal bulla limits the view posteriorly. Remnants of the insertion of the uncinate process can still be seen superiorly and inferiorly. These remnants can be removed if indicated by the pathology present.

FIGURE 7.10 *A*, The endoscopic appearance after the uncinate process has been incised. The uncinate process is pushed medially with the sickle knife so that an unrestricted view is gained through the ethmoidal infundibulum to the anterior surface of the ethmoidal bulla. *B*, A drawing of the endoscopic situation. be = ethmoidal bulla; pu = uncinate process; and s = septum.

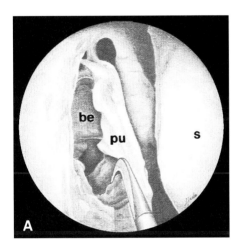 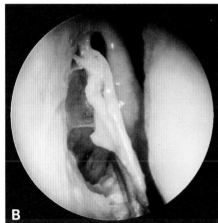

FIGURE 7.11 *A*, Endoscopic view of the appearance after the major portion of the uncinate process has been removed. *B*, A schematic drawing. There are a few small remnants of the uncinate (*open arrow*) covering the ostium of the maxillary sinus. The ethmoidal bulla is now exposed. The path to the lateral sinus (*single arrow*) posterosuperiorly through the hiatus semilunaris is medial to the bulla. The path to the frontal recess is now open anterosuperiorly (*curved arrows*). The frontal recess can be explored *without* resecting the bulla. be = ethmoidal bulla.

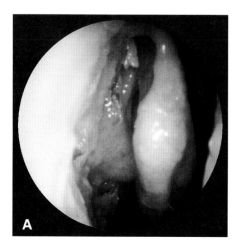 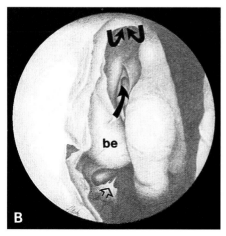

The anterior insertion of the uncinate process into the lateral wall of the nose cannot always be clearly identified. Occasionally the uncinate process can be identified by careful palpation. As mentioned previously, the anterior line of insertion of the uncinate process, in many cases, follows the projection of the anterior edge of the middle turbinate on the lateral wall of the nose. Unfortunately this is not a reliable landmark. When in doubt, it is safer to begin the resection at the posterior edge of the uncinate process, (since this can almost always be clearly identified) and to resect the uncinate process anteriorly from this point by removing strips.

Depending upon the pathology, the uncinate process may consist of very solid bone or it may be thinned out by inflammation or polyp formation so that its bony layer is almost nonexistent. When this happens there is almost no resistance to the sickle knife and the "uncinate process" consists of only a double layer of mucous membrane.

Depending upon the extent and location of the disease within the ethmoid, the surgical steps described above may prove sufficient. The infundibulum has been opened, can easily be inspected, and the surgeon can then determine if further procedures in the area of the frontal recess or the ostium of the maxillary sinus are required.

The ostium of the maxillary sinus frequently becomes visible after the uncinate process has been resected. If the ostium cannot be seen after resection of the uncinate process, it is either closed by diseased mucous membrane, and/or it may be hidden behind a posteroinferior remnant of the uncinate process. This remnant can be identified by palpation with a small angled spoon and then removed. The ostium may be located by pressing on the lateral nasal wall with an instrument in the region of the anterior or posterior fontanelle. The appearance of small bloody bubbles may indicate the location of the natural ostium.

If the frontal sinus is involved, then after the uncinate process has been resected, the way is open to the frontal recess. If, on the basis of the preoperative examination and tomogram or as a result of the intraoperative findings it becomes apparent that the ethmoidal bulla is also involved or that the resection *must* proceed to the posterior ethmoid or even to the sphenoid, these steps should be performed before the frontal recess is opened. This avoids even minimal bleeding, which flows backward by gravity from the frontal recess into the posterior ethmoid or sphenoid in the supine patient and complicates the surgical procedure unnecessarily.

The technique for opening the frontal recess is described, therefore, following the procedures for opening the posterior ethmoidal and sphenoidal sinuses.

If the ethmoidal bulla or the space between the medial wall of the bulla and the lateral surface of the middle turbinate (the "turbinate sinus") is diseased, the next step is the resection of the ethmoidal bulla (Fig. 7.12). Resection of the bulla is also indicated when a healthy bulla is so large that it completely fills the turbinate sinus, has extensive contact with the middle turbinate, or if the bulla extends anteriorly overlapping the hiatus semilunaris and thus blocking the ostium of the maxillary sinus.

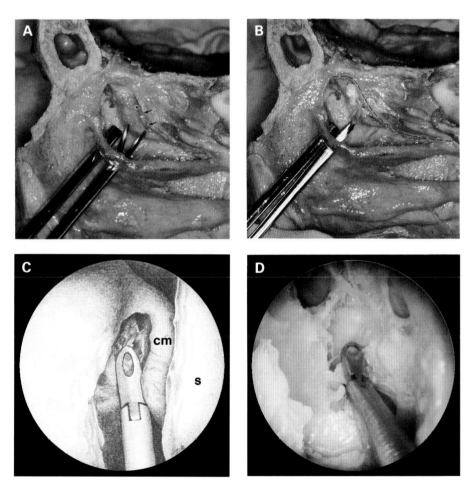

FIGURE 7.12 *A,* The anterior surface of the ethmoidal bulla is forced inward with a straight cup forceps. The *arrows* point to the cleft of the superior hiatus semilunaris and to the lateral sinus that is still hidden behind the remnants of the middle turbinate. For purposes of demonstration, the window in the middle turbinate had been enlarged. Note how far anteriorly and superiorly the path to the frontal recess and to the ostium of the frontal sinus goes. For the position of the endoscope selected for this preparation, the angle to the target is almost 90 degrees. *B,* The bulla is opened and is being removed. The *dotted line* shows the course of the ground lamella of the middle turbinate. In this case it corresponds to the edge of the chosen window. *C,* A drawing of the endoscopic view of the resection of the bulla. On first entering the bulla it is important to stay as far medially as possible. cm = middle turbinate and s = septum. *D,* The removal of the smaller cellular septa and the remnants of the bulla from the ground lamella and the roof of the ethmoid. The roof of the ethmoid can be seen as a pale yellow structure, directly above the forceps. At 11 o'clock, the passage through the frontal recess, in the direction of the frontal sinus, can be seen (see also Fig. 7.15A).

The bulla is opened by gently pushing in the anterior surface of the bulla in a medial direction with a delicate Blakesley-Weil forceps. If the lumen is identified, the entire bulla can be resected step by step. Excessive force should not be used; the septa and the mucous membrane should not be torn or pulled out vigorously, but instead removed gently with a rotatory motion of the forceps. It is important to remove the medial wall of the bulla, which can be adherent to the middle turbinate or even hidden behind the "overhang" of the turbinate.

The ethmoidal bulla should always be opened as far medially as possible and the resection should be continued only if a clear lumen can be identified or if some other disease process is found within the bulla. It is important to remember that the ethmoidal bulla is not always pneumatized. There may only be a bony ridge (called the "torus lateralis" by Grünwald and referred to in the latin-american literature as the "promontorio"). The bulla may also be small or absent. In these circumstances, the trochlea of the orbit may be hidden behind a bulge in the lateral wall of the nose, and if this bulge is opened, the orbit is entered. This is usually not a serious complication, provided that the bulging orbital fat is not mistaken for mucosa and aggressively removed (see Chapter 13).

Above and slightly anterior to the bulla may be one to three usually distinct smaller ethmoidal cells. A variably large space, the sinus lateralis, extends between the bulla and the roof of the ethmoid medial to the lamina papyracea, lateral to the middle turbinate and posteriorly between the bulla and the ground lamella of the middle turbinate (see Chapter 3).

If it is desirable to clean off the roof of the ethmoid, the location of the anterior ethmoidal artery can usually be demonstrated. This artery usually runs just below the roof of the ethmoid in a bony canal (that is occasionally dehiscent) across the anterior ethmoid on its way from the orbit to the olfactory fossa in the anterior skull base (for the precise anatomy of the anterior ethmoidal artery see Chapter 3).

After removal of the ethmoidal bulla and any of its adjacent cells (which is necessary only when these cells are diseased), the operative field is bordered medially by the middle turbinate, laterally by the lamina papyracea, superiorly by the roof of the ethmoid and posteriorly by the ground lamella of the middle turbinate (Fig. 7.13).

If there is no sign of posterior ethmoid disease, but the frontal recess and sinus are diseased, their operative treatment is begun.

A

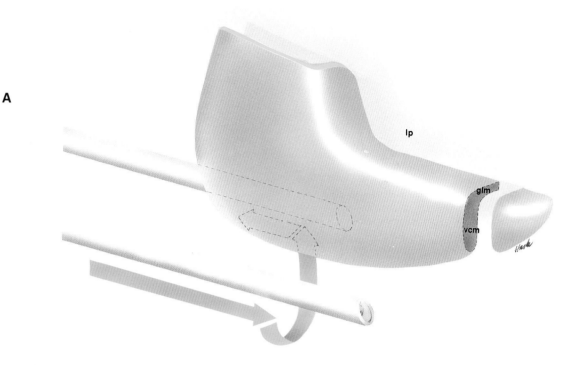

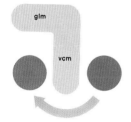

FIGURE 7.13   *A*, This is a schematic drawing of a right middle turbinate and its ground lamella. The insertion of the horizontal posterior portion, as well as of the middle frontal segment on the lamina papyracea can be seen. The insertion of the anterior third is separated from the lamina papyracea and inserts vertically onto the base of the skull, at the lateral edge of the lamina cribrosa, exactly across from its lateral lamella. A small segment has been excised from the posterior end of the middle turbinate to demonstrate the norizontal part of the ground lamella, which forms the roof of the middle meatus in its posterior aspect. lp = lamina papyracea; glm = ground lamella of the middle turbinate; and vcm = the vertical portion of the middle turbinate. *B*, View of the resected edge of the middle turbinate showing the ground lamella and vertical portion of the middle turbinate relative to the positioning of the endoscope (end-on view). glm = ground lamella of the middle turbinate and vcm = vertical portion of the middle turbinate.

B

If the posterior ethmoid is also involved, it is now approached through the ground lamella of the middle turbinate. The ground or basal lamella divides the anterior and posterior ethmoid. Dehiscences and perforations of the ground lamella are the most common route through which disease spreads from the anterior to the posterior ethmoid.

After the ethmoidal bulla has been removed, the course of the ground lamella can usually be easily followed with the endoscope. Commencing at the posterior end of the middle turbinate, as the horizontal insertion of the middle turbinate, it forms the roof of the middle meatus. Posterior to the ethmoidal bulla, the ground lamella curves superiorly into an almost vertical plane (approached sagittally by the endoscope) and inserts laterally into the lamina papyracea and occasionally even onto the medial wall of the maxillary sinus. Thus, it reaches the skull. At this point its insertion extends medially for the last 1.5 to 2 cm and forms the vertical insertion of the middle turbinate at the skull.

Identification of the ground lamella may be made difficult by pathologic changes or anatomic variations. If there is a prominent lateral sinus, it extends between the posterior surface of the ethmoidal bulla and the ground lamella. If the lateral sinus is small or nonexistent, the posterior wall of the bulla frequently fuses to the ground lamella. In this case, perforation of the posterior wall of the ethmoidal bulla opens directly into the posterior ethmoid or the superior meatus.

Identification of the ground lamella is made even more difficult by the fact that the lamella is not always a smooth flat bony plate. Posterior ethmoidal cells may cause the lamella to bulge markedly anteriorly, i.e., into the lumen of the anterior ethmoid. Similarly, anterior ethmoidal cells, particularly with an irregularly shaped lateral sinus, can dent the lamella in the direction of the posterior ethmoid. If such a cell is opened during the procedure on the anterior ethmoid, identification of the ground lamella and the beginning of the posterior ethmoid may become very difficult.

If the posterior ethmoid must be opened, the ground lamella should be perforated as far medially and inferiorly as possible. The best place is 3 to 4 millimeters cranially from the point where the ground lamella turns superiorly from its horizontal course as the roof of the posterior one-third of the middle meatus just behind the ethmoidal bulla (Fig. 7.14). The ground lamella is carefully pushed inward and the lumen behind it is identified before the opening is enlarged as needed (Fig. 7.15). Under no circumstances should the entire ground lamella be removed, since this destabilizes the middle turbinate.

FIGURE 7.14 This is a lateral schematic view of a middle turbinate and its ground lamella. The turbinate is shown here separate from the lamina papyracea. The ethmoidal bulla has already been removed (*the ghosted white contour*). The ground lamella is being perforated with the straight cupped forceps, 3 to 4 mm above the point at which it turns upwards from its posterior horizontal course.

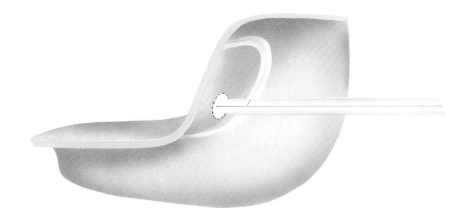

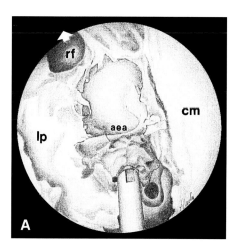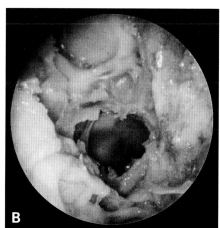

FIGURE 7.15 *A*, The appearance after perforation of the ground lamella. After the perforation is made to identify the posterior ethmoid (the round opening at 5 o'clock on the right below and alongside the forceps), additional portions of the ground lamella are removed. rf = frontal recess; lp = lamina papyracea; aea = anterior ethmoidal artery; and cm = middle turbinate. *B*, This endoscopic picture shows the appearance after the hole in the ground lamella has been enlarged.

There is now an unobstructed view into the posterior ethmoid, and the roof of the ethmoid can be clearly identified. The dangers of inadvertent injury are largely eliminated once the roof of the ethmoid has been clearly identified anterior and posterior to the anterior ethmoidal artery, and the artery itself has also been identified. If indicated, it is now possible to remove additional cellular septa and disease in the immediate vicinity of the ethmoidal artery at the skull base.

The posterior ethmoid is now freely accessible and the surgeon can determine if some mucosa needs to be resected. When working in the posterior ethmoid, the surgeon must always keep in mind that a markedly pneumatized posterior ethmoid may be in intimate contact with the optic nerve laterally. The lamina papyracea, as the lateral border of the inferior ethmoid, extends posteriorly into a triangular shaped plate that corresponds to the apex of the orbit. In a surprisingly large number of patients, the extension of the tip of this triangle posteriorly shows a bulge in the posterior ethmoid under which the optic nerve runs.

The zero angle endoscope should have been at a 45 degree angle to the palate when the infundibulum was opened (Fig. 7.16). Now, just before the anterior wall of the sphenoid sinus, the endoscope should be at a 30 degree angle to the palate. This change in the orientation of the endoscope allows us to follow the path along the skull base.

If the sphenoidal sinus must be opened, the surgeon must remember that the path through the ethmoid does *not* lead to the anterior wall of the sphenoidal sinus in the region of its natural ostium, but farther superiorly and laterally. In cases of isolated involvement of this sinus, its natural ostium can be approached through the sphenoethmoidal recess, medial to the turbinates, via the nasal cavity. There are cases of pneumatization in which the cells of the posterior ethmoid extend far laterally from the sphenoid and may even extend over it as Onodi cells, (see Chapters 3 and 13). Onodi cells are usually pyramidal in shape, with the base of the pyramid facing anteriorly (toward the surgeon). Under no circumstances should the anterior wall of the sphenoidal sinus be sought behind such a lateral extrusion of the posterior ethmoid because of *the close proximity to the optic nerve*.

FIGURE 7.16 *A*, A schematic drawing of the endoscopic procedure. The path of the instruments is shown as a *grey arrow*, assuming that an advance to the sphenoid is necessary or that the frontal recess needs to be entered for some manipulation anterior to the bulla and in an anterosuperior direction. *B*, This schematic drawing illustrates the change in angulation of the endoscope required as it advances into the ethmoid. Initially, the endoscope is introduced at an angle of about 45 degrees to the hard palate, this angle decreases as the instrument is advanced posteriorly. Depending upon the anatomic conditions, the final angle of the endoscope at the anterior wall of the sphenoid sinus is in the range of 15 to 25 degrees to the hard palate.

A

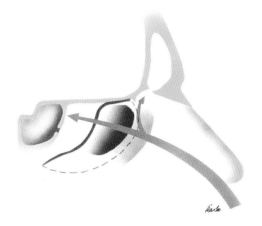

B

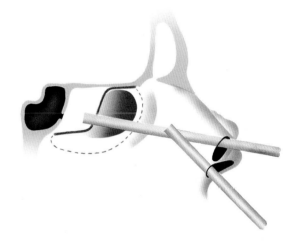

When the anterior wall of the sphenoidal sinus must be opened, it must be done as far *medially and inferiorly* as possible. The anterior sphenoid wall can be indented with a delicate bent spoon, the lumen of the sphenoid sinus identified, and finally, as much of the anterior wall can be removed as is required for the proposed procedure (Fig. 7.17).

In any operation on the posterior ethmoidal or sphenoidal sinus, it is particularly important for the surgeon to study the tomograms preoperatively and to become thoroughly familiar with the spatial relationships between the optic nerve, the internal carotid artery, and the sphenoidal sinus. The greatest care must be taken when working near the lateral wall and the roof of the sphenoidal sinus. In any attempt to perforate or remove septa in the sphenoidal sinus, the surgeon must be certain that these septa are not adjacent to the canals of the internal carotid artery or the optic nerve.

FIGURE 7.17 *A*, The tip of the 0 degree endoscope has passed through the ground lamella of the middle turbinate (resected here for demonstration purposes) and is located in the posterior ethmoid. The anterior surface of the sphenoid sinus is carefully depressed with a bent spoon. Note the position of the spoon, with the bend *downward*. The *triangular arrow* indicates the position of the anterior ethmoidal artery. *B*, An endoscopic view with a 0 degree endoscope through an operatively opened left sphenoid sinus. The course of the optic nerve, coming from the apex of the orbit and underneath the somewhat posterior course of the internal carotid artery, can be seen clearly. 1 = optic nerve and 2 = internal carotid artery. *C*, In these delicate maneuvers, minor details may become important. Thus, for instance, the window in the jaws of the Blakesley-Weil forceps may permit a view through the jaws of the forceps, if the endoscope is brought close to the fenestration. *D*, This is not possible in the otherwise similar Takahashi forceps.

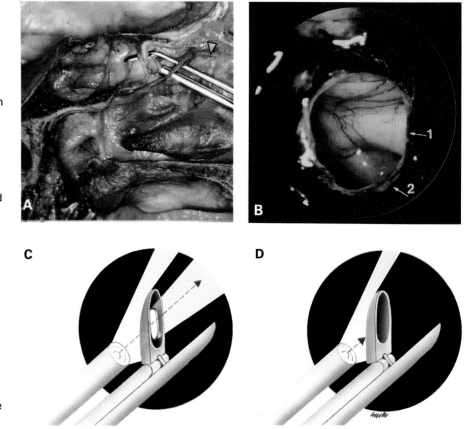

If the sphenoidal sinus is not or only minimally diseased, the bulge of the optic nerve canal is usually visible on the lateral wall just below the roof. (Occasionally the bulge of the optic nerve may have already been seen in the posterior ethmoid.) Below the optic nerve, the more or less prominent bulge of the internal carotid artery can be seen in its course in the cavernous sinus (see Fig. 7.17). The distance between the carotid artery and the optic nerve is determined by the degree of pneumatization of the sphenoidal sinus. The surgeon must remember that in 25 percent of patients, the bone over the carotid artery is "clinically" dehiscent. This means that while in histologic sections, a paper thin layer of bone may be found over the artery, no considerable resistance is felt by the palpating instrument. Cutting instruments, curettes, or punch forceps should be used extremely carefully in this area, especially in revision procedures where scars may be present.

For opening the frontal recess, we use a delicate angled Blakesley-Weil forceps and the 30 degree nasal endoscope (Fig. 7.18). Figure 7.19 shows the direction in which the instrument is advanced. The angled forceps can usually be advanced superiorly, below the insertion of the middle turbinate, and the involved mucous membrane and cellular septa removed. The exact technique depends in each case upon the extraordinarily variable anatomic configuration of this area (see Chapter 3). It is usually possible to view the frontal sinus without having to manipulate the ostium itself after the cranial extensions of the uncinate process have been removed.

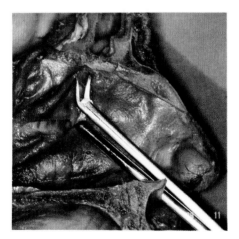 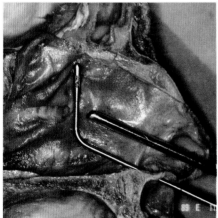

FIGURE 7.18   For work in the frontal recess we prefer to use a 30 degree lens and a variety of curved Blakesley-Weil forceps. This illustration shows how the frontal recess may be treated without requiring resection of the ethmoidal bulla. For purposes of demonstration, the middle turbinate is deflected upward. A superior remnant of the uncinate process is being removed with the upbiting forceps.

FIGURE 7.19   A variety of upturned forceps, which are available with a variety of angles and with both horizontal and vertical jaws are also suitable for this purpose.

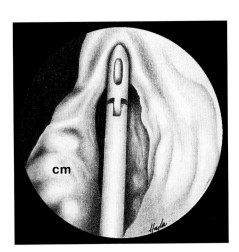

FIGURE 7.20 If the agger nasi is pneumatized, it may become necessary to open it or as in this illustration to dissect it along the insertion of the middle turbinate in order to reach the frontal recess more easily. This may result in oozing from the terminal branches of the ethmoidal artery that run inferiorly in the mucosa of this region. For this reason, we try to avoid this procedure. cm = middle turbinate.

In cases of extensive pneumatization and involvement of the agger nasi (Fig. 7.20) or when the uncinate process bends laterally and inserts onto the lamina papyracea (with the formation of a terminal recess of the infundibulum), localization of the ostium of the frontal sinus may be difficult. In the first case, the incision to resect the uncinate process can be carried further superiorly, beyond the insertion of the middle turbinate. From here it is possible to clean the agger nasi cells, and also obtain a better view of the anatomy of the frontal recess. If the uncinate process and the agger nasi extend far medially, the path to the ostium of the frontal sinus may be a very narrow slit located medially between the uncinate process and the middle turbinate. Thin, angled forceps have been found useful for working in this area, since they can grasp both horizontally and vertically. This is important since the cellular septa may be oriented in either direction (see the Appendix).

Depending upon the degree of pneumatization of the frontal sinus, the axis through the ostium of the frontal sinus and the frontal recess may be angled fairly far forward. This means that the path for the surgeon is first posterosuperiorly under the insertion of the middle turbinate and then anterosuperiorly to the ostium of the frontal sinus (Figs. 7.19 and 7.21). When conditions are very restricted and the ethmoidal infundibulum ends in a terminal recess, work in this area may be the most difficult of the entire procedure. In these cases the frequently slit-like entrance to the frontal recess lies much more medial, i.e., closer to the middle turbinate, than expected. While working in this area it must always be kept in mind that one is close to the thinnest and most fragile portion of the anterior skull: the medial precipice of the ethmoid in the area of the exit of the anterior ethmoidal artery. If it is difficult to identify the ostium of the frontal sinus and yet pathologic conditions require that this be done, the surgeon should always try to visualize the anterior ethmoidal artery in order to dissect forward from this area in a retrograde fashion. In front of the anterior ethmoidal artery there is usually a small extension of the ethmoid roof that can open into a supraorbital recess (Fig. 7.21). If the recess is deep, it may be mistaken for the frontal sinus. As a rule, however, the sinus is usually anterior to the recess (see Chapter 3). Under no circumstances should any pressure be exerted superiorly or medially with any instrument introduced into the frontal recess.

Occasionally it is impossible to place both the endoscope and the instrument under the medial turbinate simultaneously and thus be able to look and work at the same time. In such a case the surgeon may try to remove a part of the insertion of the middle turbinate from the lateral wall of the nose with an angled Blakesley forceps. The disadvantage of this maneuver may be a slight hemorrhage that further impedes the view (see Fig. 7.20). With experience it becomes possible to look into the frontal recess with the angled lens, identify the part to be removed, withdraw the endoscope a few millimeters, and make room for the introduction of the instrument. After removal of the tissue or bony segment, the endoscope is again advanced and the recess is again inspected. This procedure requires the greatest caution and may be the most demanding that the surgeon ever encounters.

Occasionally the path to the frontal sinus is indicated by the presence of abnormal secretions. Tiny bubbles appearing in the blood droplets during surgery on the frontal recess may also be of assistance.

A good view of the inside of the frontal sinus can be gained now with a 30 or 70 degree endoscope. In cases of isolated cysts or polyps, the sinus can be entered through the ostium and the disease can usually be removed through the ostium. Disease located laterally within the frontal sinus usually cannot be approached via this route.

We do not routinely enlarge the ostium of the frontal sinus. In patients with an isolated frontal recess problem, the last surgical steps can be performed after the uncinate process has been resected and without touching the ethmoidal bulla or any of the other deeper structures.

FIGURE 7.21 Once the anterior ethmoidal artery has been identified, the 30 degree lens usually shows a small recess that is present directly in front of the artery. This recess is easily mistaken for the route to the frontal sinus, particularly if it widens into a supraorbital recess. Typically, the actual route to the frontal sinus is farther anterior, separated from this recess by a bony ridge. aea = anterior ethmoidal artery; 1 = a small recess directly anterior to the anterior ethmoidal artery; and 2 = the actual route to the frontal sinus.

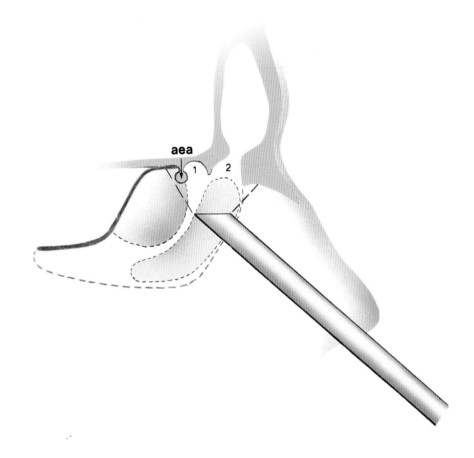

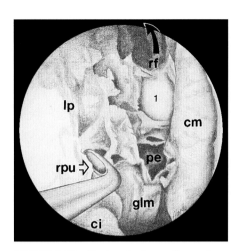

FIGURE 7.22 To locate the ostium of the maxillary sinus, we first identify the remnants of the uncinate process with a bent spoon. The ostium is usually found laterally and below, between these remnants and the almost always identifiable insertion of the bulla lamella. The safest technique is to stay so far inferiorly as to "ride" on the bony insertion of the inferior turbinate. cm = middle turbinate; lp = lamina papyracea; rf = frontal recess with path to the frontal sinus (*arrow*); pe = view into the posterior ethmoid through a perforation in the ground lamella; rpu = remnants of the uncinate process; glm = horizontal portion of the ground lamella serving as a roof to the posterior third of the middle meatus; ci = inferior turbinate; and 1 = "dome" of the roof of the ethmoid

If the disease process requires it, the next step is the localization and enlargement of the natural ostium of the maxillary sinus. If the ostium has not yet become visible, then it is either closed or covered by diseased mucous membrane, or it is hidden by a posteroinferior remnant of the uncinate process (Fig. 7.22). The best way to find the ostium of the maxillary sinus is by carefully palpating with a bent spoon, along the bony insertion of the inferior turbinate. This either leads into the ostium itself or into one of the fontanelles. The surgeon should never palpate too far superiorly (in order to avoid breaching the orbit through the lamina papyracea). Frequently, small bubbles emerging from between folds of mucosa, from between polyps, or from a pool of blood, reveal the site of the ostium.

Once identified, the ostium can be enlarged with a bent spoon, a small curette, or a pair of forceps. The appropriate instrument is introduced into the ostium and gently pulled anteriorly and inferiorly in the direction of the anterior fontanelle, at the expense of which the ostium is enlarged. In the area of the fontanelle there is no bone between the mucosa of the maxillary sinus and that of the middle meatus and thus the enlargement of the ostium can be accomplished with ease. The ostium can be trimmed to the desired shape with a reverse cutting punch forceps. If accessory ostia are present in one of the fontanelles, then the accessory ostium and the natural ostium should be united to avoid the circular transportation of secretions as described in Chapter 2. Anteriorly, the bony nasolacrimal duct limits the enlargement of the ostium. This bone is considerably harder than any other in this area and thus is easy to identify. It must be remembered, however, that the reverse cutting punch forceps are strong instruments that can remove even this hard bone.

With the appropriate instruments (angled suction tip or a special malleable forceps) under guidance of a 30 or 70 degree nasal endoscope, some procedures can be performed inside the maxillary sinus through its natural or enlarged ostium (Fig. 7.23). These procedures may include the removal of an isolated large symptomatic cyst or pedunculated polyp, or the evacuation of retained secretions. We usually do not touch extensive polypoid changes. Figure 7.23 shows the position of the enlarged ostium in the middle meatus and the excellent view that it permits into the maxillary sinus. The course of the infraorbital nerve is clearly visible. Enlargement of the natural ostium of the maxillary sinus is *not* a routine component of endoscopic ethmoid surgery.

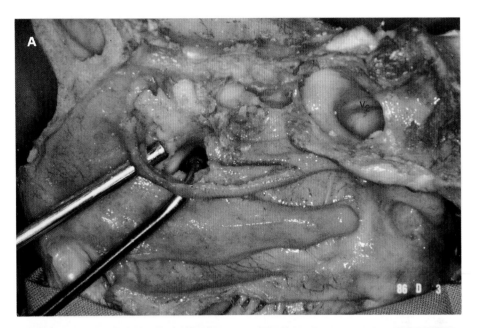

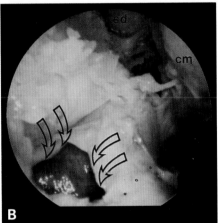

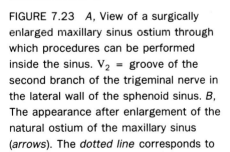

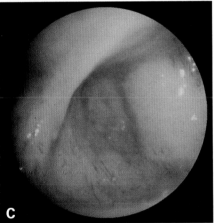

FIGURE 7.23 *A*, View of a surgically enlarged maxillary sinus ostium through which procedures can be performed inside the sinus. V_2 = groove of the second branch of the trigeminal nerve in the lateral wall of the sphenoid sinus. *B*, The appearance after enlargement of the natural ostium of the maxillary sinus (*arrows*). The *dotted line* corresponds to the line of insertion of the inferior turbinate. *C*, View into the maxillary sinus through the natural ostium with a 70 degree lens. The course of the infraorbital nerve can be seen clearly, curving inferiorly from the roof of the maxillary sinus to the infraorbital foramen on the anterior wall of the sinus.

309

In a bimeatal procedure (as described by Hellmich in a similar fashion for the inferior meatus) work in the maxillary sinus can be undertaken from two sides. For instance, a trocar sheath left in the maxillary sinus following a preliminary endoscopic exploration through the canine fossa, can now be used to remove single polyps from the wall of the sinus. The polyp is manipulated by the trocar sheath toward the ostium, where it can be grasped with the suction tip or angled forceps and removed. We use this approach especially for the removal of mycotic masses.

In this way a total sphenoethmoidectomy can be performed by the Messerklinger technique without resecting the middle turbinate (Fig. 7.24). We rarely perform such a total sphenoethmoidectomy, but when we do, we see no need to remove the entire mucous membrane. Only the clearly pathologic manifestations, like polyps, are removed and the moderate collateral edema in the sphenoid mucosa is left. We take great care, however, to assure that the connections between the compartments are patent. With the Messerklinger technique it is not necessary to perform "cosmetic surgery," i.e., there is no need to smooth and polish the roof of the ethmoid with a diamond drill or to totally remove all of the cellular septa. This would only create uncovered bony surfaces, which in turn cause a delayed healing

FIGURE 7.24 This schematic drawing illustrates the four primary lamellae that must be crossed in an almost frontal plane on the way to the sphenoid sinus: 1 = uncinate process; 2 = anterior wall of the ethmoidal bulla (*pink*); 3 = ground lamella of the middle turbinate; and 4 = anterior wall of the sphenoidal sinus. Between *3* and *4*, an additional ground lamella of the superior (and occasionally of the supreme) turbinate may be encountered. These structures are not always present and do not have the clinical significance of the ground lamella of the middle turbinate. 5 = frontal recess; 6 = lateral sinus; 7 = ostium of the frontal sinus; 8 = ostium of the maxillary sinus; 9 = ostium of the sphenoidal sinus. The frontal recess (*5*) and the lateral sinus (*6*) are only incompletely separated in this case by a vertical bony ridge. 10 = the projection of the posterior ethmoidal cell onto the lateral wall of the sphenoidal sinus (described by Onodi). The outline of the middle turbinate is indicated by *grey ghosting*.

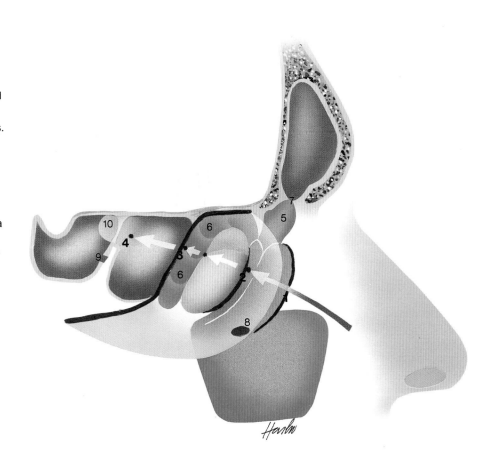

process with granulation tissue, occasionally marked crust formation or even osteitis. Such action may also endanger the ethmoidal vessels, requiring the use of packs, which also increase mucosal injury and lead to synechia formation. Care must be taken, however, that no recesses or spaces remain that could close off and become the site of renewed retention or a fresh nidus for disease.

DIFFICULTIES, TIPS, AND TRICKS

Local Anesthesia

When the inferior turbinate projects far medially, it may be difficult to reach and inject the posterior third of the uncinate process with a straight needle. Anesthesia in this area is extremely important since the ostium of the maxillary sinus lies behind the posteroinferior third of the uncinate process and work in this area is painful to the patient. A careful bending of the tip of the septal needle to the left or to the right (Fig. 7.25) allows the surgeon to inject this otherwise unreachable area.

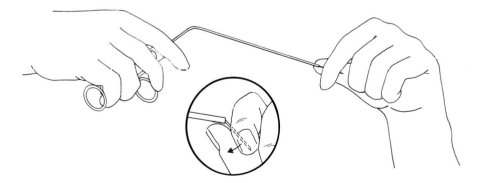

FIGURE 7.25 Bending the tip of the septum needle so that in difficult anatomic situations the laterally deviated parts of the uncinate process can be infiltrated. In most cases it is possible to infiltrate the most posterior extensions of the uncinate process past a laterally deviated middle turbinate or past a paradoxically bent middle turbinate.

Identification of the Site of Insertion of the Uncinate Process

Generally, the anterior insertion of the uncinate process roughly follows the projection of the free margin of the turbinate onto the lateral wall of the nose. There is frequently a small sulcus on the lateral wall of the nose at the insertion of the uncinate process. Posterior to this point, the uncinate process can be readily incised. By palpation with an instrument, the uncinate process can frequently be indented and observed to spring back medially. This "movable part" of the uncinate can then be resected at a flat angle.

The safest method, however, is to identify the uncinate process at its free posterior margin and, in case of doubt, to resect in strips from the back anteriorly with a curved blade or a reverse biting punch forceps. When attempting to identify the insertion of the uncinate process, the curved blade should never injure the mucosa at the insertion or the agger nasi. This only causes unnecessary bleeding, which can make the rest of the procedure most difficult and ultimately lead to granulation tissue and scar and synechia formation that may constrict the entrance of the middle meatus. When the agger nasi is extensively pneumatized, the bony lamella of the uncinate process may extend into the bony, medial wall of the agger nasi.

Identification of the Correct Point for Perforation of the Ground Lamella

When the ground (basal) lamella must be perforated on the way to the posterior ethmoid, the safest place to do so can be found in the following way.

After the ethmoidal bulla has been resected, the posterior third of the middle meatus is identified through the endoscope. Its root is formed by the here almost horizontally running ground lamella. This roof is followed from the back to the front, and the point at which the ground lamella changes its orientation from horizontal to almost vertical and at which point it bends sharply superiorly behind the (previously removed) ethmoidal bulla is identified. Three to four millimeters superior from this turn, the perforation is made *as far medially as possible* in order to reach the superior meatus and the posterior ethmoid. In this way the danger of getting too close to or perforating the roof of the ethmoid can be avoided even in cases where the lateral sinus extends far posteriorly or invaginates the ground lamella posteriorly and superiorly.

To create this perforation, the instrument, usually a small Blakesley forceps, is pushed through the bony lamella, with the jaws closed. Once through the lamella the jaws are opened and the opening is identified as a lumen and then enlarged. The lumen must always be clearly identified before a cutting or biting instrument is used.

Identification of the Sphenoid Sinus

After passing through the anterior and posterior ethmoid, the anterior wall of the sphenoid sinus is encountered *much more medially and inferiorly* than originally anticipated. To enter the anterior wall of the sphenoid sinus, the same technique as described in the previous section for the ground lamella is used. A J-curette (angled spoon) is suitable for this purpose, although it should always be used with its angled end pointing *downward* (see Fig. 7.17).

Even with minimal pneumatization, most of the posterior ethmoidal air cells lateral to the sphenoid sinus, the anterior wall of the sphenoid sinus is no longer in a frontal plane, but runs at an acute angle from anteromedial to posterolateral. If the anterior wall of the sphenoid sinus cannot be definitely identified, it is possible to find its natural ostium medial to all of the turbinates through the sphenoethmoidal recess and to enlarge the sphenoid sinus ostium inferiorly. This procedure requires the placement of anesthetic pledgets into the sphenoethmoid recess. We use this approach in those cases of isolated sphenoid sinus disease that require surgical management.

We *do not*, in the framework of the Messerklinger technique, perform *direct sphenoid sinus endoscopy* through a modified maxillary sinus trocar as described by Draf. When it is necessary to take a diagnostic biopsy from the sphenoid sinus, we use the technique described above, i.e., across the sphenoethmoidal recess, through the enlarged sphenoid sinus ostium under direct endoscopic vision.

There are some cases in which despite all attempts at identifying the anatomic landmarks, careful review of the CT scans, and even use of a C-arm image intensifier that there is still some doubt as to whether one is in the sphenoid sinus or in the last, most posterior, extensively pneumatized ethmoid cell. An additional complicating factor in these cases may be the presence of a bony thickening of the anterior wall of the sphenoid sinus. In such cases we have found the following approach helpful.

A long septal needle is attached to a saline-filled three-ring syringe. With this needle we perforate the presumptive sphenoidal sinus as far medially and inferiorly as possible. We then aspirate carefully. Usually a cellular space can be identified behind the bony wall, which can then be opened safely. The aspiration is done to prevent injury to blood vessels, an aberrant internal carotid artery being the greatest potential danger. We have never yet had such an injury in any of our patients, but we assume that a needle puncture of the carotid artery could be controlled without difficulty. In those extremely rare cases where we have had to use this technique to identify the sphenoid sinus, we have always had small pellets of "Tabotamp" at hand and ready for use.

In these trial punctures of the sphenoid sinus, it is important that the needle be firmly attached to the syringe and that the plunger of the syringe be completely airtight, otherwise, when air enters the syringe on aspiration, an erroneous conclusion could be drawn.

Identification of the Frontal Recess

When difficulties are encountered in visualizing the ostium of the frontal sinus "around the corner" anterosuperiorly from below the insertion of the middle turbinate, it is helpful to ask the patient to extend the head, i.e., to raise the chin. This small change in position frequently markedly improves the visibility of the frontal recess. When working in the frontal recess we prefer the Blakesley-Weil instruments. They have fenestrated jaws that allow a view of the structures behind them. This is particularly helpful when the tip of the endoscope must be very close to the jaws of the instrument. The otherwise satisfactory Takahashi forceps lack this advantage (see Fig. 7.17 C and D).

When we are unable to identify the ostium of the frontal sinus because of extensive scarring from previous operations or because landmarks such as the middle turbinate had been removed, it is possible to perform a Beck's procedure (frontal trephination) and to view the floor of the frontal sinus in this way. At the same time an angled Blakesley forceps is introduced into the frontal recess intranasally. When the tip of this instrument produces a bulge in the floor of the sinus, this point can usually be used safely to perforate the scar tissue plate. Normally, the periphery of the frontal sinus ostium is manipulated as little as posssible with the Messerklinger technique. Therefore, massive scar tissue, bony obstruction, or stenoses of the ostium of the frontal sinus are not indications for use of the Messerklinger technique.

If the frontal recess is involved by massive polyposis and there are no anatomic landmarks, it is sometimes helpful to introduce anesthetic and decongestant pledgets repeatedly, following the polypectomy. After a few minutes, endoscopic examination may identify small trickles of secretions and thus lead the surgeon directly to the ostium of the frontal sinus.

The cone of light projected by the 30 degree lens may also be useful on the way to finding the frontal sinus. Holding the endoscope in the chosen position and inspecting the area of the frontal sinus from the outside, the surgeon can often see that the light transilluminates the frontal sinus, even though the endonasal route has not yet been clearly identified. The 30 degree angle between the shaft of the endoscope and the direction of the light beam may then provide a guide in identifying the proper route to the frontal sinus ostium.

Identification of the Maxillary Sinus Ostium

If the ostium cannot be seen after resection of the uncinate process, it is probably because of edematous mucous membrane or, more commonly, to posteroinferior remnants of the uncinate process. These uncinate remnants should be identified and removed. Pressure against the fontanelles may make bubbles appear through the natural ostium and thereby reveal its location. When palpating for the ostium of the maxillary sinus, it is best to palpate along the bony insertion of the *inferior turbinate*. This prevents an accidental perforation of the orbit.

Similarly to the frontal sinus, it is possible to locate the ostium from the inner side of the lumen through the sinus. By maxillary sinus endoscopy through the canine fossa, the ostium can be inspected while a bent spoon is used to palpate from the middle meatus. This further minimizes the danger of creating the perforation in the wrong place.

Occasionally the maxillary sinus mucosa may be separated and pushed forward from the medial wall or from the roof of the sinus by the palpating spoon or other instrument. This situation is difficult to recognize. The lumen that becomes visible actually corresponds to the space between the displaced mucosa and the bone while, in fact, the sinus has not yet been entered (Fig. 7.26). Once this mistake has been recognized, it is frequently difficult to grasp the displaced mucosa, as these attempts usually just displace it further laterally. In this event, opening of the sinus is best accomplished with a bent Blakesley suction forceps with which the mucosa can both be held (suction) and opened. Only now should the newly created window be enlarged.

Another option is to close the nostril with gentle pressure over the endoscope and the instrument and ask the patient to inhale. The negative pressure created by inhalation may cause the mucosa to bulge medially making it easier to grasp.

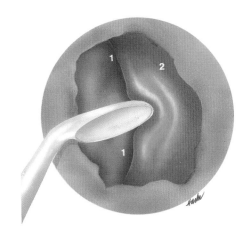

FIGURE 7.26   The situation after an *alleged* opening of the ostium of a left maxillary sinus. The medial bony wall of the maxillary sinus is fenestrated and the surgeon assumes that he or she is looking into the lumen of the maxillary sinus (1). In fact, the spoon is elevating the mucosa (2) of the maxillary sinus laterally and anteriorly, in toto, and thus denuding the posterior wall and, occasionally, even the roof of the maxillary sinus (1). In reality then, one is looking into a space between the maxillary sinus mucosa and the posterior wall of the maxillary sinus.

Injury to the Orbits

Surgeons who perform endonasal procedures under general anesthesia emphasize the need that the patient's eyes be visible to the surgeon and/or to the scrub nurse at all times. This may make it possible to recognize injury to the orbit by movement of the eyeball or the appearance of an intraorbital hematoma.

In most cases, encroachment of the orbit can be recognized by the identification of orbital fat, which can be distinguished from diseased mucosa by the fat's yellow color (Fig. 7.27). A less direct sign may be the presence of small fatty "eyes" (readily recognized through the endoscope) on the blood droplets in the ethmoid. Even a prolapse of orbital fat usually does not cause significant complications. If the periorbital tissues are only split, an attempt may be made to replace the fat carefully with a blunt instrument. *Under no circumstances should the fat be pulled out or resected.* At the end of the procedure the prolapsed fat can be "splinted" with a small Merocel sponge that stays in place for 1 to 3 days. The patient should be instructed not to blow the nose (to avoid orbital emphysema) and antibiotics are prescribed.

Injury to the orbit occurs most commonly at the time of the initial incision to open the infundibulum (resection of the uncinate process), on removing the ethmoidal bulla, and during the search for and enlargement of the ostium of the maxillary sinus. Pain is an important warning sign. Injury to the periorbital area is felt by the patient as pain *in* the eye. This warning sign is, of course, absent under general anesthesia.

The nurse should place all tissue removed from the nose during the procedure into a small container filled with normal saline or Ringer's solution. The nurse should be instructed to advise the surgeon immediately if any of the tissue floats in the solution. Such tissue should be inspected immediately. It could be a small portion of mucous membrane with a small air bubble caught in it. Pushing the tissue a few times with an instrument and turning it over should release the air and the tissue should then sink to the bottom. The only tissues that might float naturally are fat (orbital) and brain.

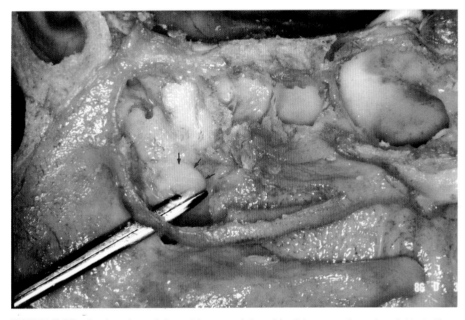

FIGURE 7.27 Perforation of the orbit and protrusion of orbital fat (*arrows*). The lesion in the lamina papyracea is located in the characteristic site. The orbit can be injured in this area when the sickle knife is carried too far laterally against the lamina papyracea during resection of the uncinate process.

Pain

It is always surprising to us how little local anesthesic is required to reach the sphenoid sinus, even when the injections are limited to the mucous membrane of the uncinate process and the insertion of the middle turbinate. In addition to the use of an appropriate analgesic and sedative premedication, the most important factors in providing freedom from pain are the correct application and adequate contact time of the anesthetic pledgets. There are some points, however, where even a well anesthetized patient may feel pain. These include the roof of the ethmoid, particularly in the area of the ethmoidal vessels and nerves, the medial wall of the orbit, the area around the ostium of the maxillary sinus, and (quite particularly) the posterior end of the middle turbinate.

The area of the anterior ethmoidal nerve is highly sensitive. This nerve occasionally accompanies the artery (either anterior or posterior to the artery) and it may divide into two or more branches. If the patient, previously free of pain, begins to complain of pain after the ethmoidal bulla has been removed, this is a clue to the surgeon to make sure about the anatomic relationships. The ethmoid roof is significantly more sensitive to pain than any of the adjacent areas.

When a patient who is uncomfortable throughout the entire procedure is asked where it hurts, the answer is frequently: ''Just where you are working,'' in other words a very diffuse localization. If, however, the periorbital area is touched or injured, the response is immediately ''I feel pain in the eye.'' Pain provides the most important warning sign and helps to avoid the more serious complications. This advantage is lost under general anesthesia.

The area around the ostium of the maxillary sinus, particularly the inferior and posterior margins, can be pain sensitive. This can be remedied by injecting local anesthetic below the mucosa of the most posterior extensions of the uncinate process. The mucosa over the posterior fontanelle can also be injected if topical anesthesia is not sufficient. The posterior end of the middle turbinate can also be especially pain sensitive. Frequently only 2 to 3 millimeters above this area, the vessels and nerves from the sphenopalatine foramen emerge and advance into the mucosa of the turbinates and the lateral wall of the nose. One of the few situations in which the Messerklinger technique is used in this area is in the the opening and resection of a concha bullosa if the pneumatization extends to the posterior end of the middle turbinate and if the lateral lamella of the concha bullosa must be resected as far as this point. There is a danger of direct injury to the vessels and nerves in this area. Additional injection of local anesthetic may be helpful even after the concha has already been opened. Removal of the most posterior fragments of the lateral lamella of the turbinate is better tolerated when the removal is performed by sharp dissection (scissors or a modified conchotome) rather than pulling, tugging, and twisting with a Blakesley forceps.

The application of local anesthesia may be particularly difficult in those patients who have undergone previous surgery for diffuse, polypoid rhinosinopathy with extensive scar formation from which new polyps originate. The best solution in these patients is to repeatedly apply the anesthetic and vasoconstrictor pledgets and operate in a "ping-pong" fashion. The anesthetic pledgets are placed in one side while the surgeon operates on the other side and then sides are switched. In repeat operations it is helpful to inject the scarred stalk of the new polyps with a small amount of local anesthetic and then resect them with sharp dissection.

Another source of pain may occur when the suction tip is introduced into an ethmoid cell or into a sinus through a small opening that fits tightly around the instrument. When suction is applied, the sudden negative pressure in the closed space may produce a sudden sharp pain. It is therefore important to ensure that air can enter the space around the suction tip in order to avoid the creation of an area of negative pressure.

The problems created by intraoperative bleeding are discussed in Chapter 13.

Chapter 8

PREOPERATIVE PREPARATIONS

As with any operation performed under local anesthesia, for which the patient's understanding and cooperation are important, the purpose and nature of the endoscopic nasal procedure must be explained in a manner comprehensible to the patient. The indications and purpose of the procedure have usually been discussed earlier, at the time of the diagnostic endoscopy. Tomograms or CT scans are helpful in showing the relationship between the diseased ethmoid and other paranasal sinuses and for pointing out the potential technical difficulties and risks inherent because of the topographic proximity of the neighboring structures. These relationships can be best demonstrated to the patient on coronal CT images.

It usually comforts the patient to know the steps and sequence that will be taken, and the approximate length of the procedure, since they will be a conscious participant.

Apart from obtaining an informed consent, we inform the patient that after premedication has been administered, he or she will become very drowsy, but not asleep, and consequently will be aware of most of the events taking place.

Patients are informed that although they will be aware that their nose is being operated upon, they will not feel pain. It is inevitable that there will be some blood loss, but the loss of blood is almost invariably small and should not affect them in any way. Patients should always be sufficiently awake to tell the surgeon if they wish to expectorate. Patients should always indicate promptly if they do not feel well, become nauseated, or feel faint. In this way patients are motivated to be participants in the procedure, rather than helpless objects.

Before the procedure, we show the patient the cotton pledgets and explain their purpose and how long they remain in the nose. We tell the patient that the pledgets feel cool on introduction and that they may initially generate a feeling of slight pressure. The patient is told that the subsequent injection of a local anesthetic may also generate a feeling of pressure or tension and that if a few drops of anesthetic reach the pharynx, they can be swallowed safely. We also warn about the sensation of pressure in the nostrils that may be produced by the instruments. It is particularly important to allay the patient's anxiety about the cracking and sometimes snapping noises and sensations that inevitably occur when the cellular septa and other bony structures of the ethmoid are removed.

In this way the fear of the procedure can be largely eliminated in most patients and their full cooperation obtained.

Once the premedication has been administered, the patient should not be distracted by unnecessary questions or extraneous noises.

With the exception of children, almost all our procedures are performed under topical and infiltration anesthesia in the premedicated, sedated patient. *General anesthesia should be reserved only for the exceptional case.* Whenever possible, we try to convince the patient of the advantages of local anesthesia. It is our conviction, supported by our clinical experience, that the Messerklinger technique should *not be performed under general anesthesia.*

PREMEDICATION FOR LOCAL ANESTHESIA

A number of premedications are available for procedures that are to be performed under topical and local anesthesia. The choice is determined by the preferences of the surgeon and the anesthesiologist combined with the individual requirements of the patient. The premedication administered should provide sedation, analgesia, and anxiolysis.

The surgical requirements that must be met by the anesthesiologist ordering the premedication are that the patient remain in contact, respond, and be able to follow simple commands, e.g., swallow, spit, and turn the head toward the surgeon. Furthermore, the swallowing and cough reflexes must be preserved. If the sedation is too profound and the surgeon loses "contact" with the patient, more problems are generated than resolved.

Our most commonly used and most satisfactory premedication consists of meperidine (pethidine hydrochloride) as a neuroleptic analgesic and promethazine both for sedation and as an antiemetic. Our standard dose for a healthy, 50-year-old adult weighing 70 kg is 100 mg meperidine and 50 mg promethazine, given intramuscularly 30–45 minutes preoperatively.

We do not use atropine for premedication because the resultant dryness of the mouth is extremely unpleasant for the patient and the decrease in secretions is of little, if any, benefit for the surgical procedure in the nose.

The amount of premedication recommended increases with the weight and decreases with the age of the patient. Arteriosclerosis can affect the circulatory compensatory mechanisms and in a patient with cerebrovascular disease a fall in blood pressure may lead to a disturbance in cerebral perfusion. In older people particularly, this may produce an increasing restlessness that is most undesirable during the endoscopic surgical procedure. Preexisting hypertension does not usually require any change in the dose of meperidine and promethazine.

Great caution is indicated in cases with cerebral pathology, particularly those accompanied by convulsions or increased intracranial pressure, e.g., idiopathic or posttraumatic epilepsy, post shunt procedures, or patients who have a history of unexplained bouts of dizziness or visual disturbances. Proven increased intracranial pressure is a contraindication for meperidine and epilepsy is a contraindication for promethazine. Meperidine should also be avoided in patients with liver disease or respiratory problems in whom respiratory depression must be avoided. Meperidine when combined with a phenothiazine, can cause significant hypotension, and should never be used in patients who are receiving MAO inhibitors. An ambulatory patient must be warned about the longer lasting central depressant effects of premedication (e.g., driving, walking on the streets).

Promethazine should not be used in patients with sulfite sensitive asthma since it contains sulfite. Promethazine may also potentiate the effects of antihypertensive drugs.

Another useful premedication combines droperidol (2.5 mg) and fentanyl (0.05 mg). This neuroleptic analgesic combination demands careful monitoring of the patient because of the respiratory depressant effects of fentanyl. A decrease in dosage reduces the respiratory and circulatory depressant effects, but also causes an undesirable decrease in the amount of analgesia. We only use this combination in exceptional cases.

Another method of achieving sedation is the addition of a small amount of flunitrazepam orally to the intravenous premedication. Flunitrazepam (1–2 mg) is administered with a sip of water 30 to 60 minutes preoperatively. The attention and reaction potential of the patient can be adversely affected for up to 24 hours by this drug. In older patients, flunitrazepam may produce extrapyramidal motor activity, which is the exact opposite of the desired effect.

The patient is brought to the operating room 10 minutes before the start of surgery and the pledgets are placed into the nasal cavity.

Respiration and circulation are monitored, an intravenous infusion having been started even before the premedication was given. If possible, the IV should be on the left side so that it remains accessible without disturbing the surgeon.

POSITIONING THE PATIENT

The head of the supine patient is slightly extended and turned to face the surgeon sitting on the right (Fig. 8.1). The surgeon's legs fit under the table approximately at the level of the patient's neck. In elderly patients it is sometimes necessary to support the head when decreased mobility of the cervical spine no longer permits a completely flat supine position. We do not like the semirecumbent position (with the head and trunk slightly elevated) since this position makes it more difficult for the surgeon to assume a fully relaxed posture and also makes it much more difficult for the surgeon to visualize the frontal recess. The frontal recess can usually be more easily examined by slightly hyperextending the patient's head. Close to the surgeon (on the left), is a small table (Fig. 8.2A) that holds the endoscope and its handle, a storage vessel half-filled with saline and lined with absorbent cotton (Fig. 8.2B), antifog solution, the cotton pledgets, and

A
B

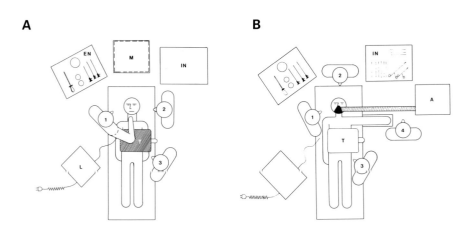

FIGURE 8.1 *A,* This schematic representation shows the position of the patient for functional endoscopic sinus surgery under topical and local infiltration anesthesia. 1 = surgeon; 2 = scrub nurse; 3 = assistant; L = light source; EN = movable table with endoscope and accessories; M = video monitor, alternate location for light source; IN = movable instrument table; and T = Mayo stand to hold suction tips and other equipment and serve as an armrest for the surgeon. *B,* This illustration shows the position of the patient and the arrangement of equipment for an endoscopic sinus surgical procedure to be performed under general anesthesia. 1 = surgeon; 2 = scrub nurse; 3 = assistant; 4 = anesthesiologist; T = Mayo stand for instruments and armrest; IN = movable instrument table; and A = anesthesia machine and its connections.

epinephrine and Pontocaine for topical anesthesia (Fig. 8.2C). The surgeon changes and cleans the endoscopes and applies the antifog solution to the lens. Arm rests on the chair are advantageous to prevent fatigue. The left elbow may also rest on the endoscope table. A Mayo stand on which the right elbow may rest is placed over the patient's chest (as for micro-laryngoscopy). The scrub nurse sits or stands at the patient's left, across from the surgeon. Another assistant (to handle the suction tip) stands at the level of the knees of the patient, either on the left or right side. The handing and changing of instruments must be performed smoothly so that the surgeon's eyes need not leave the endoscope. A frequent change from the eyepiece to room light is distracting. It should be noted that in this set-up, no instrument is ever passed across the face of the patient. This prevents injury if an instrument is accidentally dropped.

FIGURE 8.2 *A*, The set-up of the endoscopy table. 1 = endoscopes (the 2.7-mm endoscope is used only in diagnostic endoscopy); 2 = spray attachment for Pontocaine-vasoconstrictor mixture; 3 = glass jar with cotton pledgets and metal cup for mixing Pontocaine and epinephrine; 4 = bottles with 2% Pontocaine and 1:1,000 epinephrine; 5 = antifog solution; 6 = decongestant nose drops; and 7 = glass cup with cotton lining for cleaning the endoscope and applying the antifog solution. *B*, The storage receptacle for the endoscopes used during the procedure. The container is filled with lukewarm saline and the bottom lined with cotton to protect the lenses. This prevents the accumulation and drying of blood, mucus, and debris on the endoscope lens. *C*, The Pontocaine and epinephrine solution with cotton pledgets. The cotton pledgets measure approximately 12 × 12 × 3 mm when dry.

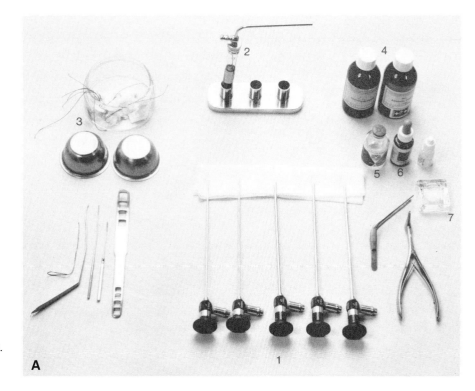

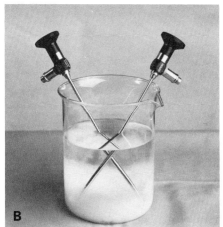

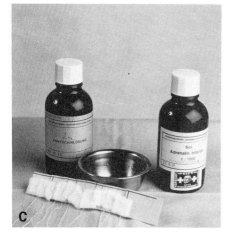

Endoscopic ethmoid surgery is not a particularly sterile procedure: the inside of the nose cannot be sterilized. After cleansing the patient's face, a drape with a hole is placed over the face, leaving the mouth and nose free. The hole is wide enough to permit access to the eyes, if necessary.

The patient is covered with a sterile sheet. The nurse removes the required instruments from a sterile container just before the procedure and lays them out on the instrument table (Fig. 8.3). The endoscopes are sterilized in a glutaraldehyde solution, dried, and covered with a sterile towel on the endoscope table.

It is especially important that the tomograms are displayed in the operating room so that the surgeon can see them by simply raising his eyes from the patient. Even after the most thorough preoperative study of the tomograms, there are frequently situations where another review provides great reassurance to the surgeon. This is even more important if several patients are scheduled one after the other and provides additional safety for both patient and surgeon.

The light source and television screen for trainees and observers are located at the head of the table (see Fig. 8.1). When photography or videotaping is planned, the light source is placed behind the surgeon to allow the cable to run in a straight line. This is particularly important for gel- or fluid-filled cables, which suffer considerable loss of light through internal reflection if the cables are bent or looped (see Chapter 14).

Some light sources are very noisy because of their built-in cooling fans. The patient should be cautioned about this noise, which is generated directly alongside his or her head.

FIGURE 8.3 The standard instruments for endoscopic procedures. At the bottom left: a 2 ml 3-ring syringe with a septum needle for local anesthesia. A detailed description of the instruments can be found in the Appendix.

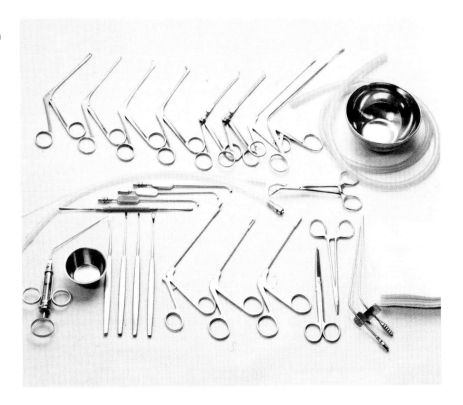

TOPICAL AND INFILTRATION ANESTHESIA

For topical anesthesia and vasoconstriction of the mucous membranes, we use a mixture of 2 percent Pontocaine (4 to 5 parts) and 1:1,000 epinephrine (1 part). This mixture is prepared in a small metal cup (Fig. 8.4) into which we place a number of small, 1 × 1 cm, cotton pledgets each having a ligature tail. These cotton pledgets are more convenient to use than standard neurosurgical sponges, since they are more absorbent and can be more easily molded. They are also easier to introduce into the recesses and corners of the common and middle meatus. It is particularly important that the pledgets be *completely wrung out* prior to their introduction into the nose and after they have been soaked in the Pontocaine-epinephrine solution (Figs. 8.5 and 8.6). The pledget must *not be dripping wet* when applied to the mucosa. This gives us the best guarantee that only a minimal amount of Pontocaine and epinephrine comes into contact with the mucosa. With careful attention to this principle, we have used this technique in several thousand cases without a single serious complication or side effects from either the Pontocaine or the epinephrine. In older patients with hypertension, coronary artery disease, or cardiac arrhythmias, the surgeon should consult with an internist and the anesthesiologist to determine if Pontocaine and epinephrine can safely be used.

The pledgets are introduced with bayonet forceps. Ideally, they should be advanced right up to the entrance of the middle meatus, although this is not always possible due to the presence of pathology. Regardless of the extent of the proposed procedure, an attempt should be made in each case to fill *the entire nasal cavity* with the pledgets. We usually push the first pledget to the end of the middle turbinate, both below and medial to it. We then place pledgets into the spheno-ethmoidal areas and fill the space anteriorly from this point between the septum and the middle turbinate, after having placed several pledgets into the middle meatus itself. It is important that the pledgets come into direct contact with the mucosa at the attachment of the middle turbinate along the lateral wall of the nose and the mucosa over the uncinate process as well as in the area of the agger nasi. The anterior third of the nose is then loosely packed with pledgets all the way to the vestibule.

Under no circumstances should the mucous membrane be injured during placement of the pledgets. If rough handling causes even minimal bleeding, e.g., in the area of the septum or the lateral wall anterior to the middle turbinate, this can become a very real nuisance for the rest of the procedure and transform an ordinarily simple procedure into a troublesome and difficult operation. The pledgets

FIGURE 8.4   Mixing Pontocaine (4–5 parts) and epinephrine (1 part) in a small metal cup. Usually about 2 ml of this mixture are prepared, so that there is some extra left in case of later need.

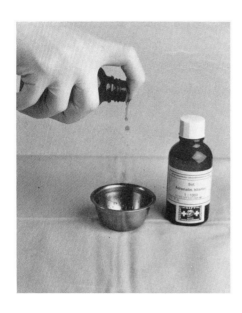

FIGURE 8.5   The pledgets soaked in the solution are well wrung out before they are introduced into the nose. Under no circumstances should they be dripping wet. This precaution prevents the excessive use of Pontocaine and epinephrine.

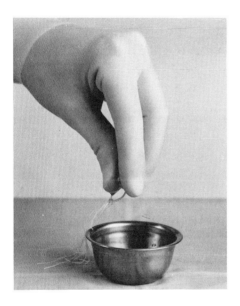

FIGURE 8.6   The pledgets soaked in Pontocaine and epinephrine and well wrung out, are spread out and opened up. They are then introduced, one at a time, into the nose.

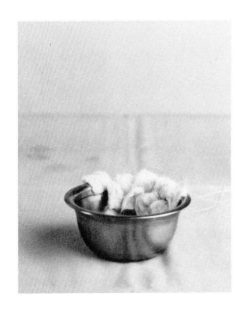

must be placed very carefully and without any force, blood stains on the pledgets on removal indicate that these guidelines were not followed.

Cocaine may be used as a topical anesthetic instead of Pontocaine and epinephrine. We have no personal experience with cocaine. David W. Kennedy has reported good results with cocaine flakes that he puts into place with a nasal applicator. The advantage of cocaine flakes over a cocaine solution is that the flakes remain in place longer. The excellent anesthesia provided by Pontocaine, combined with the good vasoconstriction produced by epinephrine and the total absence of side effects, when used with the technique described above, has in our view obviated the need for any other topical anesthetic.

The pledgets are left in place for at least 10 minutes and then removed first from the operative side. Removal is accomplished by carefully pulling on the suture attached to the pledget. The Pontocaine-epinephrine mixture in the small cup is preserved throughout the procedure for use in case the need for additional anesthesia occurs during the procedure.

For infiltration anesthesia we use 1 percent lidocaine with 1:200,000 epinephrine. The injection is made under endoscopic guidance with a three-ring syringe and a special septal needle (see Fig. 8.3). In Figure 8.7, the typical injection sites under the mucosa of the uncinate process are shown. The technique of infiltration is the same as in septoplasty. The needle is introduced under the mucosa and the solution is injected until the mucosa is slightly elevated from its base. This is readily indicated by the mucosa blanching. Since in most cases the procedure begins with an incision into the ethmoidal infundibulum, 1 to 1.5 ml lidocaine are injected at 3 to 4 injection points maximally. The most important points are in the area of the insertion of the middle turbinate, since the terminal branches of the anterior ethmoidal artery and nerve, proceeding from above, pass on to the middle turbinate and the agger nasi. It is also important to locally anesthetize the attachment of the uncinate process to the inferior turbinate because if the ostium of the maxillary sinus must be enlarged, the area of the fontanelles may be exposed to considerable pressure by the instruments.

As few injection sites as possible should be used to minimize oozing from puncture sites. Great care must be exercised when introducing the needle not to injure any of the more anterior areas of the mucous membranes. The mucosa may be very thin over the nasal septum and also over the uncinate process and thus it may be difficult to introduce the needle under the mucous membrane and elevate it with the injected solution. If the bone in the area of the uncinate process is very thin or absent, the needle may inadvertently be advanced into the infundibulum with the injected solution entering

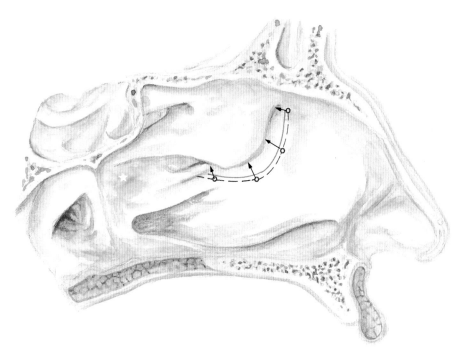

FIGURE 8.7 This semischematic representation shows the injection sites for local anesthesia along the anterior insertion of the uncinate process. The anterior outline of the uncinate process is marked with a *red line*. The number of injection sites should be kept to a minimum and the injections should always be made 2 to 3 mm from the insertion of the uncinate process, under the mucous membrane (*o*, along the *broken line; arrows* indicate direction of infiltration). A *star* marks the area of the palatine foramen, where an additional injection may be made, if needed. *Note*: the middle turbinate is very short and small in this illustration (this corresponds to the skull cross-section used in Chapter 7). As a result, the uncinate process appears to extend far beyond the turbinate anteriorly and inferiorly. In the majority of cases, the insertion of the uncinate process runs parallel to the projection of the outline of the head of the turbinate onto the lateral wall of the nose (see Chapter 7). (Drawn by M. Schröckenfuchs, M.D.)

the nasopharynx. The patient must be advised about this possibility and informed that small amounts of the anesthetic solution can be swallowed without any problem.

Only rarely are more than 1 to 1.5 ml of lidocaine required for each side. Under no circumstances should so much solution be injected under the mucous membrane of the uncinate that it balloons up and obscures the view into the middle meatus and distorts the contours of the uncinate itself. If this happens, it can be very difficult to find the proper place for the incision through the uncinate process. Occasionally it is helpful to bend the tip of the needle laterally to the right or left, particularly when the posteroinferior end of a far lateral uncinate must be reached across a medially protruding inferior turbinate. After injection of the local anesthetic, it is advisable to wait 1 to 2 minutes before commencing the operation. During this period, the points of injection may be gently compressed with the tip of the aspirator to prevent even minimal oozing.

If the procedure includes resection of a concha bullosa, injections are performed in a similar fashion under the mucosa of the head of the middle turbinate and along its free margin toward the rear. If the entire middle turbinate is pneumatized, resection of the lateral lamella of the turbinate may present increased hazards and the surgeon must remember that he may come perilously close to the sphenopalatine foramen and the vessels and nerves that emerge from it. It is, therefore, particularly important to provide thorough anesthesia in the area of the end of the turbinate.

It is a source of constant amazement to us that in most cases it is possible to work in the area of the sphenoid without any additional anesthesia if the mucosa of the uncinate process was infiltrated really well.

If the patient reports pain during the operation, we use Pontocaine-epinephrine soaked pledgets to repack the surgical field loosely. This is most likely to occur when there is scarring from a previous procedure or in the presence of an acute inflammatory process.

The most pain-sensitive areas are the posterior end of the middle turbinate close to the sphenopalatine foramen and the inferior edge of the ostium of the maxillary sinus. Pain in the area of the roof of the ethmoid suggests the proximity of the anterior ethmoid nerve and constitutes an important warning signal.

We have no experience with the transorbital block of the anterior and posterior ethmoidal nerves and we perform sphenopalatine block only rarely.

ADVANTAGES OF LOCAL ANESTHESIA

The advantages of local anesthesia are obvious. In most cases local anesthesia provides excellent hemostasis and thus excellent visibility during the surgical procedure. This is practically never the case under general anesthesia. Local anesthesia makes it easier to distinguish healthy mucosa from diseased mucosa, to recognize anatomic narrowings as such, and to remove sections carefully with the least radical procedure. This results in more rapid wound healing and less stress on the patient. With few exceptions, packing is not required in patients operated upon under local anesthesia.

The risks of local anesthesia are less than those of general anesthesia and even older and cardiac risk patients can usually be operated on, without any problems. As already indicated, intraoperative pain has an important *warning function* that contributes greatly to the avoidance of injury to the roof of the ethmoid, the orbit, and the optic nerve. Another important feature is that local anesthesia forces the surgeon to exert the greatest care and to proceed as atraumatically as possible. Even the well sedated patient will not tolerate roughness under local anesthesia. The postoperative recovery time is clearly shorter after local anesthesia. Even after a total sphenoethmoidectomy, most patients can be up and about after 2 to 3 hours, take nourishment, and breathe through the nose.

ENDOSCOPIC PROCEDURES UNDER GENERAL ANESTHESIA

General anesthesia should be reserved only for the exceptional case. Children obviously require general anesthesia, and we are extremely conservative in the indications for endoscopic sinus surgery in children (see Chapter 6).

We may consider general anesthesia in adults when there is extensive scarring following previous surgery, if surgical revision of scarred and compartmentalized maxillary sinuses becomes necessary, or if osteitic changes or scars preclude local anesthesia for an approach to the frontal sinus. The incidence of general anesthesia use in our patient population is less than 5 percent of all procedures. Even hypotensive anesthesia does not provide as bloodless a field as local anesthesia. Posthypotensive rebound hypertension makes packing necessary more frequently.

If general anesthesia must be used, the nose is prepared in the same way as for local anesthesia, except that phenylephrine is used instead of epinephrine as an additive to Pontocaine. When halothane is used for general anesthesia, topical and submucous application of epinephrine may cause cardiac arrhythmias in some patients. Therefore, if epinephrine or lidocaine with epinephrine is used, as we would recommend, some other anesthetic gas should be used.

Even in the hands of an experienced surgeon, the amount of blood lost under general anesthesia can be 5 to 12 times as much as under local anesthesia (150 to 360 ml versus less than 35 ml). In more than 6,000 cases of local anesthestic surgery, blood transfusion was required because of massive blood loss in one case only (see Chapter 13).

Chapter 9

SINUS PROBLEMS AND ENDOSCOPIC SOLUTIONS

In this chapter, the surgical techniques used for the treatment of different disease processes are illustrated with appropriate examples. Because of the difficulty of operating and taking pictures at the same time and the absorption of light produced by even a few drops of blood, in some cases not all of the surgical steps can be documented. Since the results of intraoperative photographs can only be evaluated after the film is developed, it is unavoidable that some stages are irretrievably lost as the result of errors of lighting or other technical problems. For this reason, we have included some illustrations that are not perfect photographic documentation. We have however, made every effort to select the pictures so that the individual pictures can be appreciated even when they are taken out of sequence. In some particularly dynamic processes, such as the opening of a mucocele and the rapid flow of its contents, or in massive polyposis with bleeding, useful documentation is frequently impossible. A diffuse polyposis that practically fills the entire nasal lumen, makes flash photography impossible since there is no space for the light to diffuse. The surgical procedure in these cases is better documented by videotaping.*

Where in a sequence illustrations from a different case were included for the purpose of clarification, it is clearly indicated.

---

* Videotapes showing the surgical procedure in mucoceles, all paranasal sinuses, diffuse polyposis and choanal polyps, as well as in other indications, have been made by the author of this book and are available from the American Academy of Otolaryngology, Head and Neck Surgery, or from the A&G Company, Reifensteinweg 2, D-8701 Sommerhausen, Germany.

POLYPOID RHINOSINUSITIS

This 45-year-old patient suffered for several years from recurrent, bilateral purulent infections of the frontal and maxillary sinuses. Medical therapy was beneficial in the acute stages, but it never resulted in a complete disappearance of the patient's symptoms. A type I allergy could not be demonstrated and topical steroid therapy had no major effect. The numerous sinus X-ray films that the patient brought with him on his first visit all showed various degrees of density and fluid levels in both the frontal and the maxillary sinuses. Tomography of the paranasal sinuses, performed on the basis of the endoscopic findings, showed characteristic, severe disease in the anterior and posterior ethmoids and secondary mucosal swelling and retained secretions in the frontal and maxillary sinuses. The sphenoid sinus was affected to a lesser degree.

Figure 9.1 shows the initial endoscopic findings on the left side after removal of the Pontocaine-epinephrine pledgets, i.e., after maximal decongestion. The findings on the right side were almost identical.

In Figure 9.2, the injection of approximately 1.5 ml of 1 percent lidocaine with 1:200,000 epinephrine under the mucosa of the uncinate process with a septum needle in 3 to 4 different sites is demonstrated. The blanching of the mucosa, due to ischemia, can be clearly seen. The mucosa is raised from the underlying bone by the local anesthetic.

Even when obvious polyps are present, we always try to go past these polyps to identify and inject the uncinate process. To achieve this, it may be useful to push large anterior polyps posteriorly or to

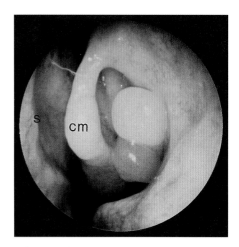

FIGURE 9.1 Initial endoscopic findings after decongestion in a patient with recurrent sinus infections. cm = middle turbinate.

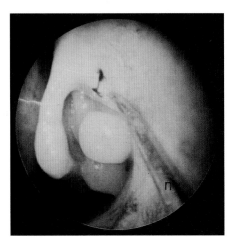

FIGURE 9.2 Submucosal injection of lidocaine at the uncinate process. n = septum needle.

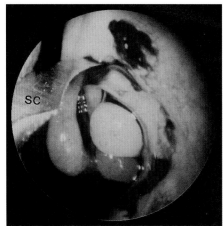

FIGURE 9.3 Incision of the uncinate process with the sickle knife. sc = sickle knife.

displace them superiorly. If it is possible to resect the uncinate process, the most anterior polyps are usually removed at the same time. This produces less hemorrhage than when the anterior polyps are removed first and the uncinate process is resected afterward. The anterior polyps are removed only in extreme situations, or when as the result of previous surgery, the anatomic conditions are likely to be confusing. In such cases a small amount of local anesthetic is injected into the stalk or the presumptive insertion of the polyp. This is also one of the few situations, where a laser (Neodymium-Yag or KTP 532) may be useful, since the laser permits an almost bloodless approach. Particularly when bony septa must be removed, however, we see no advantage in using a laser, which in fact only makes the procedure more expensive, complicated, and prolonged.

After injecting local anesthetic under the mucosa of the uncinate process, we wait for 1 minute. During this time we exert gentle pressure on the injection sites with the suction tip, to avoid even minimal oozing. This is followed by the incision of the uncinate process with the sickle shaped knife (Fig. 9.3). The curved blade is pushed through the uncinate process and immediately upon the tip entering the ethmoidal infundibulum, the handle of the knife is held almost parallel to the lateral nasal wall in order to avoid entering the orbit (Fig. 9.4). The uncinate process is then incised inferiorly (Fig. 9.5) and somewhat luxated medially. At this time additional polyps can be seen, deep in the infundibulum. The uncinate process is then carefully twisted off, first at its superior and then at its inferior insertion. The small tear in the mucosa up to the middle turbinate, as shown in Figure 9.6, can usually be avoided.

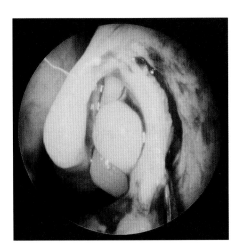

FIGURE 9.4 The handle of the sickle knife is held almost parallel to the lateral nasal wall to avoid entering the orbit.

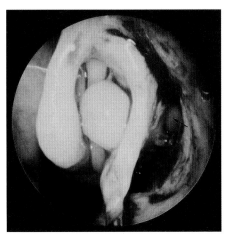

FIGURE 9.5 Inferior incision of the uncinate process with medial luxation. *Arrow* indicates additional polyps coming into view deeply in the ethmoidal infundibulum.

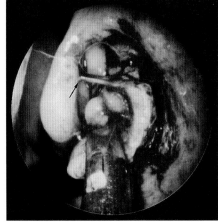

FIGURE 9.6 Removal of the uncinate process. The small tear in the mucosa of the middle turbinate (*arrow*) can usually be avoided.

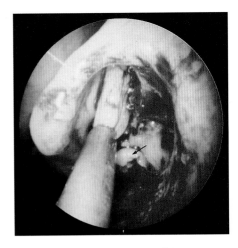

FIGURE 9.7 After removal of the uncinate process and its attached polyps, a large polyp arising from the anterior and medial face of the bulla can be seen being pulled anteriorly by the aspirator. A smaller polyp that occluded the ostium of the maxillary sinus like a valve can also be seen (*arrow*).

In Figure 9.7, the uncinate process was removed except for small superior and inferior remnants. The polyps that were seen between it and the middle turbinate were also removed at the same time. On looking at the anterior surface of the ethmoidal bulla, one sees that the large polyp aspirated into the suction tip, and that had been visible in the depth of the middle meatus, originated in the cleft between the middle turbinate and the ethmoidal bulla and not from an air cell. In the depth, behind the inferior remnant of the uncinate process, another, smaller polyp can be seen that occludes the ostium of the maxillary sinus like a valve. Next, the superior remnants of the uncinate process are resected and polyps from the frontal process are removed with a curved Blakesley-Weil forceps (Figs. 9.8 to 9.10). The frontal recess is not yet entered for any distance and only the polyps that originated from the superior uncinate remnants are removed.

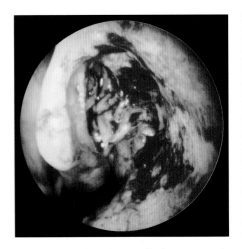

FIGURE 9.8 Appearance, before removal, of polyps in the frontal recess.

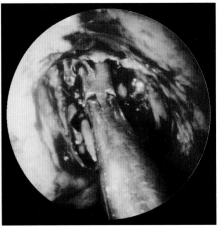

FIGURE 9.9 Upbiting Blakesley-Weil forceps grasping the polyp.

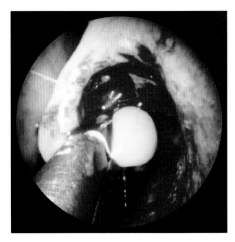

FIGURE 9.10 Removal of the polyp from the frontal recess.

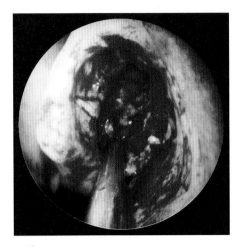

FIGURE 9.11 The ground lamella of the middle turbinate is visible after removal of the ethmoidal bulla.

In Figure 9.11, the ethmoidal bulla has been removed entirely and one can see the ground lamella of the middle turbinate, curving slightly posteriorly and superiorly, as the posterior border of the lateral sinus. Directly above the suction tip, a lighter area can be seen that is shown better in Figure 9.12. Here the bone of the ground lamella has already been removed and polypoid mucosa of the posterior ethmoid bulges through the bony defect anteriorly. After removal of the polypoid mucous membrane and preservation of the normal mucosa, the anterior wall of the sphenoid sinus is carefully pushed inward and one can see into a cavity lined by unremarkable mucosa. The course of the optic nerve and the bulge produced by the internal carotid artery can be seen (Figs. 9.13 and 9.14).

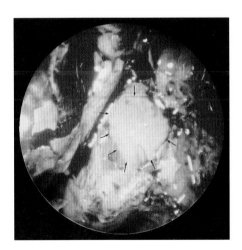

FIGURE 9.12 Polypoid mucosa (*arrows*) bulging through the defect formed after perforation of the ground lamella.

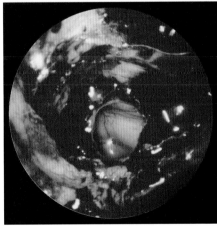

FIGURE 9.13 View into the sphenoid sinus after an opening has been made in the anterior wall.

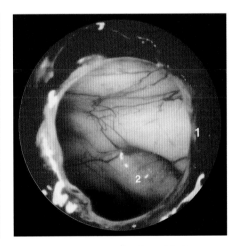

FIGURE 9.14 Normal sphenoid sinus mucosa, the course of the optic nerve (*1*) and the course of the internal carotid artery (*2*) are visible through the opening seen in Figure 9.13.

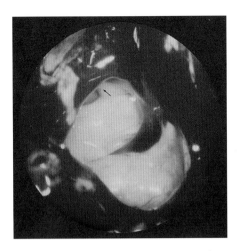

FIGURE 9.15 The course of the anterior ethmoid artery (*arrow*) across the roof of the ethmoid is seen here.

In Figure 9.14, the opening into the sphenoid sinus has not been enlarged, but the endoscope moved closer to gain a better view into the cavity. There is no additional resection of the anterior wall of the sphenoid sinus.

We then switch from the 0 degree lens to the 30 degree endoscope and inspect the base of the skull and the roof of the ethmoid. After removal of additional small polyps and bone remnants from the bulla lamella, the remainder of the mucosa on the roof of the ethmoid was unremarkable. The channel of the anterior ethmoidal artery can just be seen (Fig. 9.15).

The path to the frontal sinus is still not free, and only after further removal of polypoid mucous membrane and remnants of the uncinate process, is there an unobstructed view of the ostium of the frontal sinus (Fig. 9.16). In this instance, the frontal sinus ostium was located far medially, between the middle turbinate and the insertion of the uncinate process. On approaching the frontal sinus ostium with the 70 degree endoscope, a good view was obtained into the relatively small

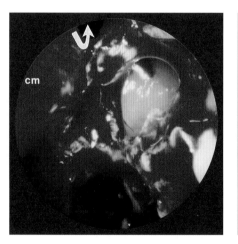

FIGURE 9.16 The ostium of the frontal sinus (*curved arrow*) after removal of all of the polypoidal mucosa and the remnants of the uncinate process. cm = middle turbinate.

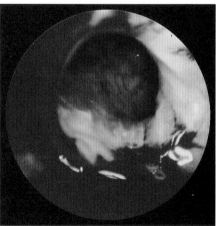

FIGURE 9.17 A view into the frontal sinus with the 70 degree endoscope showing edematous mucosa.

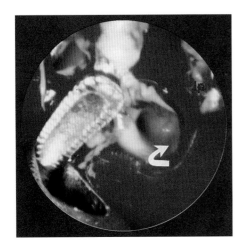

FIGURE 9.18 Removal of the inferior remnant of the uncinate allows access to the ostium of the maxillary sinus (*curved arrow*).

frontal sinus. Its mucosa showed some edematous changes (Fig. 9.17). The mucosa in the sinus and in the area of the ostium must not be touched.

Removal of the most inferior remnants of the uncinate process also removed a small polyp that was attached to them and permitted an unrestricted view of the ostium of the maxillary sinus (Fig. 9.18). With a reverse cutting rongeur, the ostium was enlarged at the expense of the anterior fontanelle, until a good view into the maxillary sinus was obtained (Figs. 9.19 and 9.20). With a curved aspirator, some retained secretions were removed from the floor of the sinus. No other manipulation was undertaken, except for the incision of a small retention cyst.

If there are polyps *medial* to the middle turbinate, for example originating between the middle turbinate and the septum, this is the time to remove them. Such a finding is shown in Figure 9.21. These polyps originated on a broad base from the septum on the right side (of a different patient).

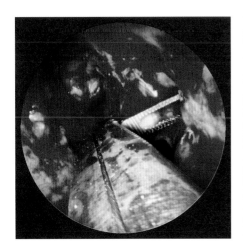

FIGURE 9.19 The ostium is enlarged with the reverse cutting rongeurs at the expense of the anterior fontanelle.

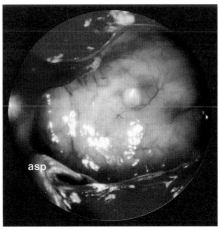

FIGURE 9.20 After enlargement of the natural ostium, a good view of the maxillary sinus is obtained, demonstrating a tiny retention cyst. Some secretions are removed with an aspirator. asp = aspirator.

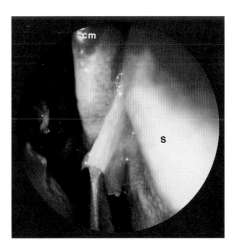

FIGURE 9.21 Polyps may also be located medial to the middle turbinate. cm = middle turbinate and s = nasal septum.

Figures 9.22 to 9.25 are also a different patient. They show the localization and opening of a maxillary sinus ostium in the middle meatus on the left side as seen from within the maxillary sinus. For this purpose, the trocar used in the earlier maxillary sinus endoscopy was left in place, and the individual steps were documented photographically through a 30 degree endoscope.

Figure 9.22 shows the head of a bent spoon extending through the ostium into the maxillary sinus. The middle meatus was already treated surgically and the ostium of the maxillary sinus was located with the spoon. The light bulge in the foreground is the lacrimal eminence behind which the nasolacrimal duct is hidden. By pulling the spoon in the maxillary sinus ostium gently in an anteroinferior direction, the opening was enlarged at the expense of the anterior fontanelle. A ring curette (Fig. 9.23) and a reverse cutting rongeur (Fig. 9.24) were also used. The resulting ostium was approximately 10 × 6 mm in size. This allows the introduction of a curved suction tip (Fig. 9.25) and other special instruments, should additional manipulations become necessary.

Even in extensive polyposis, the surgical procedure can be largely limited (conservative). Only the grossest pathology should be removed and constricted areas enlarged. We do not resect the middle turbinate, even in cases of severe polyposis. We remove the polyps that originate on the middle turbinate and occasionally some parts of the middle turbinate are inadvertently removed. This is most likely if the turbinate is markedly compressed and thinned out by pressure from the polyps and if there is also some decalcification of the bony lamellae. In such cases it is futile to worry about the preservation of such a thinned structure.

It is only rarely necessary to use supplemental local anesthesia on the way to the sphenoid. When needed, the local anesthetic is injected into the stalk or into the body of the polyps. Pledgets with Pontocaine and epinephrine can also be used. They should be left in place for at least 1 minute. These pledgets also provide additional hemostasis.

Nasal polyps can be cystic and/or extremely gelatinous. In these cases a clear liquid may seem to be mixed with the blood droplets in the surgical area. This makes the novice insecure, since it suggests a CSF leak. In contrast to a CSF leak, however, this type of clear liquid flow stops after a few seconds or at the latest when the corresponding polyp or cyst has been removed.

Difficulties may be encountered during surgery for recurrent nasal polyps. In addition to the difficult topographic anatomic conditions caused by the absence of important landmarks, the combination of polyps and scar tissue may be extremely coarse. If these are attached to the lamina papyracea or the roof of the ethmoid, the greatest caution is required. Under no circumstances must these polyp-scar combinations be handled roughly in the vicinity of the skull base. Sometimes it is impossible to tell whether these scars are adherent to the dura. Two of the three CSF fistulas that occurred in our institution were seen in patients who had undergone several previous procedures for recurrent polyposis. We consider it entirely proper in such cases, for reasons of safety, to leave such fibrotic plaques alone, even with a few coarse polyps attached and the patient must be informed accordingly.

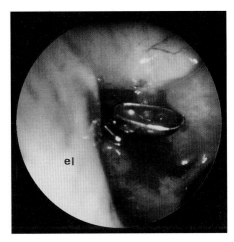

FIGURE 9.22   Enlarging a maxillary sinus ostium on the left as seen from within the sinus, using a 30 degree endoscope through a sinuscopy canula (see also Figs. 9.23 to 9.25). Location of the position of the ostium with the bent spoon. el = lacrimal eminence.

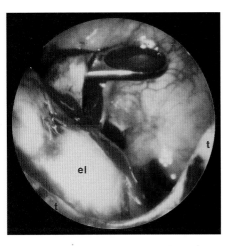

FIGURE 9.23   The ostium is enlarged with a ring curette. el = lacrimal eminence and t = trocar canula.

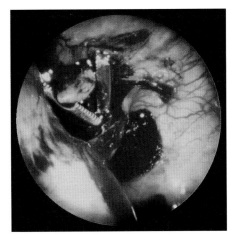

FIGURE 9.24   The ostium is enlarged with a reverse cutting rongeur.

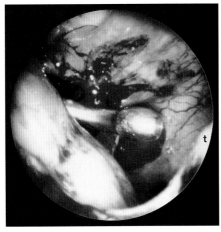

FIGURE 9.25   The enlarged ostium will now allow the passage of suction tips and other instruments if necessary. t = trocar canula.

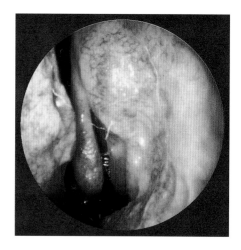

FIGURE 9.26 The appearance of the middle meatus in a patient with recurrent sinusitis.

ETHMOID DISEASE IN SINUBRONCHIAL SYNDROME

Figure 9.26 shows the endoscopic appearance of typical severe infundibular disease. The patient had suffered for years from recurrent sinusitis. During the acute phases, her asthma symptoms were always exacerbated. Following resection of the uncinate process (Fig. 9.27), a large ethmoidal bulla that almost completely filled the middle meatus was seen. It lay in intimate contact with the mucosa on the lateral surface of the middle turbinate. In the anterior surface of the bulla was a slit-like opening from which copious secretions were suctioned (Fig. 9.28). These secretions were extremely viscous. In some instances the mucus thread could be pulled out for a distance of 10 cm without breaking (Fig. 9.29). Such tenacious mucus is found frequently in diseased sinuses, particularly in patients with asthma.

In Figure 9.30, the ethmoidal bulla has been removed and through a perforation in the ground lamella, there is an unobstructed view into

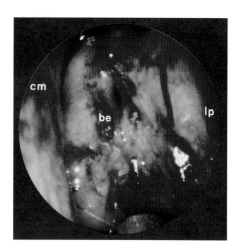

FIGURE 9.27 Removal of the uncinate reveals a large ethmoidal bulla filling the middle meatus. cm = middle turbinate; lp = lamina papyracea; and be = ethmoidal bulla.

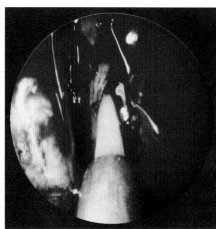

FIGURE 9.28 Thick mucus is aspirated from an opening in the bulla.

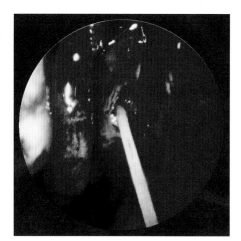

FIGURE 9.29 The mucus is often extremely viscous, especially in asthmatic patients.

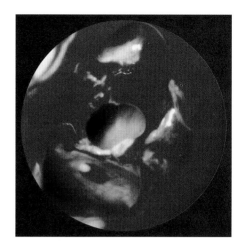

FIGURE 9.30 The ethmoidal bulla is removed and the posterior ethmoidal cells entered through the ground lamella. Normal mucosa is seen in the posterior ethmoidal cell.

the unremarkable posterior ethmoid. No additional steps were required. Figure 9.31 shows the ostium of the maxillary sinus in its normal position. After resection of the uncinate process, the ostium showed no appreciable stenosis and was therefore not further enlarged. Macroscopically, the mucous membrane of the maxillary sinus appeared normal.

In Figure 9.32, an unrestricted view is presented into the frontal sinus, through the frontal ostium. There was a somewhat edematous swollen mucosa, which was not removed, over the lamina papyracea.

Figure 9.33 shows good healing several days postoperatively. The slight traces of blood are due to the removal of crusted secretions. In the depths, the recovering mucosa of the surgically repaired ethmoid can be seen clearly. The ostium of the maxillary sinus is patent.

Since the surgical intervention (3 years to date), the patient is much improved. Even her pulmonary complaints are much decreased and she no longer requires steroids for the management of her asthma.

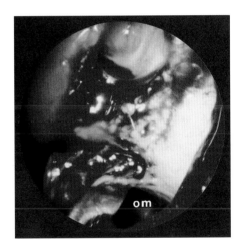

FIGURE 9.31 In this patient, the maxillary sinus ostium is normal and is therefore not enlarged. om = maxillary ostium.

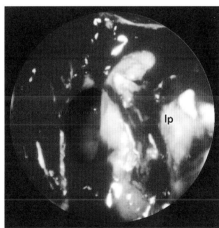

FIGURE 9.32 The frontal sinus is seen through its ostium. The mucosa over the lamina papyracea is somewhat edematous. lp = lamina papyracea.

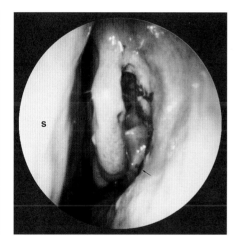

FIGURE 9.33 The appearance several days post surgery shows that the mucosa has returned to normal. The *arrow* indicates the maxillary sinus ostium. s = nasal septum.

ANTROCHOANAL POLYPS

As already indicated in Chapter 5, choanal polyps are a classical indication for endoscopic surgery with a good prognosis and low rate of recurrence.

In our experience, antrochoanal polyps usually have two components. One that is cystic, which frequently completely fills the maxillary sinus, the other a solid polypoid part, which extends into the middle meatus and the nasopharynx. This arrangement was found in more than 80 percent of the choanal polyps in our surgical series. The point of origin in the maxillary sinus was almost always from the posterior wall in the vicinity of the maxilloethmoidal angle. A second point of attachment was found in more than 50 percent of the cases, where the stalk of the polyp emerged from the maxillary sinus, i.e., at the posterior, inferior part of the exit ostium. In about 70 percent of our patients, the choanal polyp left the maxillary sinus through an accessory ostium in the posterior fontanelle. In only 29 percent did the polyp exit the maxillary sinus through the natural ostium. Even in these latter cases, we could never be certain that the pressure exerted by the stalk of the polyp did not cause a preexisting accessory ostium to merge into the natural ostium.

The first step in the surgical removal of an antrochoanal polyp is an endoscopic examination of the maxillary sinus through the canine fossa. The introduction of the maxillary sinus trocar usually breaks open the cystic portion of the polyp and allows the suction removal of its contents. Any remaining cyst can be punctured with a sharpened polyethylene catheter, as described in Chapter 5, and their wall can be removed through the trocar sheath. This procedure has already been described in detail and is not discussed further in connection with the present case.

If the stalk of the polyp exits from the maxillary sinus through an accessory ostium in the posterior fontanelle, it may not be necessary to remove the uncinate process in order to resect the polyp.

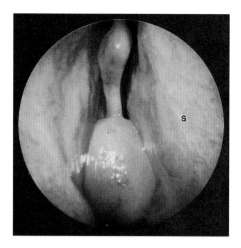

FIGURE 9.34 The endoscopic appearance of a patient with an antrochoanal polyp. s = nasal septum.

In the present case (Fig. 9.34), it could not be determined with any certainty whether the stalk of the polyp emerged through the natural or through an accessory ostium. For this reason the uncinate process was incised in the usual manner (Fig. 9.35) and we first gained the impression that the polyp emerged into the middle meatus through the natural ostium of the maxillary sinus. In Figure 9.36, the natural ostium has already become somewhat enlarged at the expense of the anterior fontanelle. As shown in Figure 9.37, it became obvious, after pushing the polyp back in the direction of the choana, that the polyp extended into the nose through an accessory ostium in the posterior fontanelle and not through the natural ostium. The bulk of the polyp was removed and in Figure 9.38 we can see a small part of the stalk still attached to the inferior circumference of the accessory ostium in the posterior fontanelle. The remnant of the stalk is held by the suction tip.

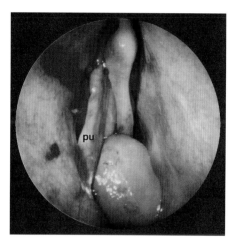

FIGURE 9.35 The uncinate process is incised in the usual way. pu = uncinate process.

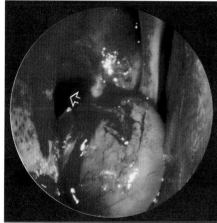

FIGURE 9.36 The natural ostium (open arrow) is found to have been enlarged by the polyp at the expense of the anterior fontanelle.

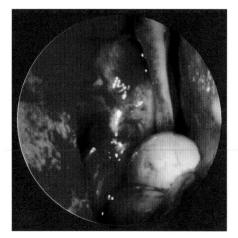

FIGURE 9.37 Deflection of the polyp posteriorly allows the stalk to be seen, arising from an accessory ostium in the posterior fontanelle.

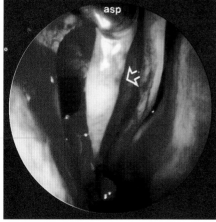

FIGURE 9.38 After removal of the bulk of the polyp, a remnant of the stalk (open arrow) can be seen at the inferior margin of the accessory ostium. asp = suction tip.

In Figure 9.39, the rest of the attachment of the polyp has been removed from the rim of the accessory ostium and one can clearly see the bony and mucosal division between the two ostia. The accessory ostium in the posterior fontanelle can be seen. A good view can be obtained through the anteriorly enlarged natural ostium into the maxillary sinus.

Figure 9.40 shows how the dividing bony ridge can be resected with a reverse cutting rongeur and the accessory ostium enlarged into the natural one.

Figure 9.41 shows the resulting enlarged ostium through which the trocar sheath, still in the sinus, can be seen. In this way the results of the procedure can be assessed from both sides. Figure 9.42 is a final look through the trocar sheath into the sinus cavity, at the enlarged ostium, and at the place from which the polyp had been removed. One can see the free margin of the middle turbinate, reduced in thickness by the pressure from the polyp, and the septum. The site of attachment of the cystic part of the polyp in the maxilloethmoidal angle is also visible, as are the additional points of attachment at the posterior inferior margin of the accessory ostium.

Figure 9.43 shows the solid portion of the polyp.

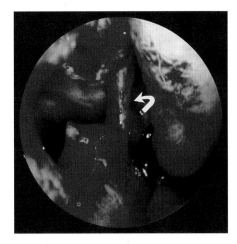

FIGURE 9.39   After removal of all of the stalk, the dividing ridge of bone between the two ostia can be seen. The *curved arrow* indicates the accessory ostium.

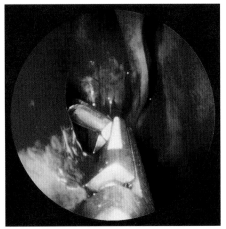

FIGURE 9.40   The ridge of bone seen in Figure 9.39 is excised with a reverse cutting rongeur, combining the two ostia into one.

FIGURE 9.41 The resulting large ostium allows a good view into the sinus. Note the trocar canula still in the maxillary sinus.

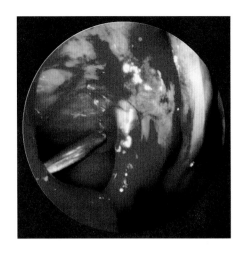

FIGURE 9.42 The enlarged ostium is well seen through the trocar canula, along with the site of attachment of the cystic part of the polyp in the maxilloethmoidal angle. The point of attachment at the margin of the accessory ostium is shown by the *white arrows*. s = nasal septum.

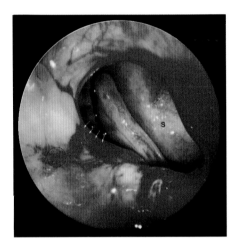

FIGURE 9.43 The solid part of the antrochoanal polyp.

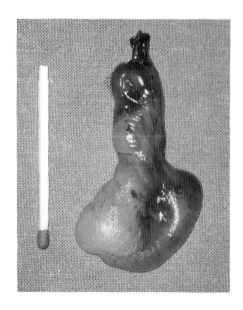

349

CONCHA BULLOSA

If a concha bullosa contributes to the disease of the ethmoid or if it is itself diseased, the first step is the resection of its lateral lamella. The medial lamella, which serves as the attachment of the turbinate to the roof of the ethmoid and, via the ground lamella, to the lamina papyracea, is left alone in order to create the most physiologic conditions possible. If it is not certain that the lateral nasal wall will also require surgical intervention, such as resection of the uncinate process and removal of the ethmoidal bulla, then only the mucosa over the concha bullosa is infiltrated with local anesthetic. This avoids oozing from the puncture sites over the uncinate process and allows for better evaluation of the anterior ethmoidal clefts after the removal of the lateral lamella of the concha bullosa.

Figure 9.44 shows a concha bullosa on the left side after removal of the Pontocaine-epinephrine pledgets. The uncinate process is medially bent and is evidently in contact with the lateral lamella of the concha bullosa. Depending upon the extent of pneumatization of the middle turbinate, it may be necessary to extend the procedure as far as the posterior end of the turbinate. It is therefore important to insert the Pontocaine-epinephrine pledgets posteriorly as far as this point.

Figure 9.45 shows the infiltration of the local anesthetic. It is administered at 3 to 4 places in the insertion, the frontal surface, and along the inferior free margin of the turbinate. If the mucosa is thin and the bony plate of the turbinate is also thin, it frequently happens that the needle breaks through into the turbinate cell. Great care must be taken that the local anesthetic is deposited between the mucous membrane and the bony surface. The mucosa at the most anterior portion of the insertion of the turbinate is injected from the agger nasi (Fig. 9.46).

FIGURE 9.44   The endoscopic appearance of a left concha bullosa after decongestion.

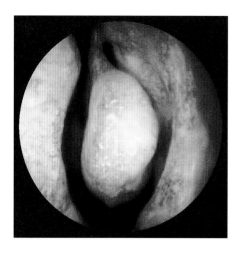

FIGURE 9.45   Infiltration of local anesthetic for surgery on the concha bullosa.

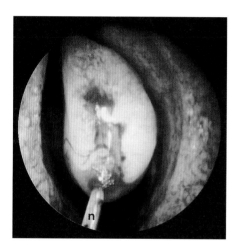

FIGURE 9.46   Infiltration at the agger nasi anteriorly.

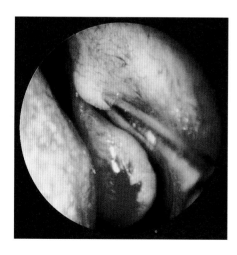

The turbinate cell is now entered with a curved blade in the area of the most pronounced pneumatization (Fig. 9.47). This area may be located far posterior in some cases. It is usually obvious when the tip of the blade "drops into the turbinate cell." The incision is carried downward along the free inferior margin with a sawing motion. After this, the cutting edge of the blade is turned superiorly and the incision is extended up to the insertion of the middle turbinate. If the insertion of the middle turbinate is delicate, great care must be taken not to break off the turbinate during these perforating maneuvers. This is particularly likely to happen when the bony shell of the turbinate cell is thick and hard. In such cases it is advisable to open the turbinate cell with straight scissors or with a Struyken conchotome, since this avoids direct pressure on the insertion of the turbinate. Figure 9.48 shows how the incision is carried along the free inferior margin with the scissors until just before the end of the pneumatized space. In the displacement of the lateral lamella superiorly, care must be taken to keep the upper jaw of the scissors lateral to the insertion of the turbinate. The two leaves of the turbinate can usually be easily spread with the scissors and a good view can be gained into the interior of the turbinate cell and whatever mucosal pathology may be present. Frequently, the cell can be entered with the endoscope and the ostium of the cell, that is the point of origin of the pneumatization, can be identified.

Figure 9.49 shows how the lateral lamella of the concha bullosa can be grasped with a delicate straight Blakesley forceps and sheared off with a careful rotatory maneuver and removed. This removal is not always possible in toto, if the middle turbinate is extensively pneumatized. In such cases the lateral lamella must be removed, piece by piece with the scissors and the straight Blakesley forceps.

Figure 9.50 shows in a different case, an inspissated, friable old empyema in a right concha bullosa, just after it had been opened, but before removal of the lateral lamella.

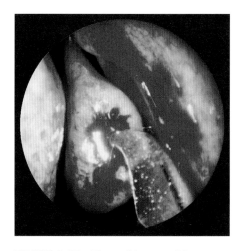

FIGURE 9.47   The turbinate cell is
entered with the sickle knife at the area
of most pronounced pneumatization.

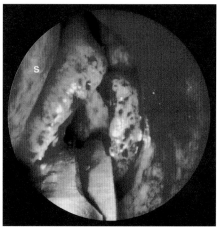

FIGURE 9.48   The incision is carried
along the inferior margin with scissors.

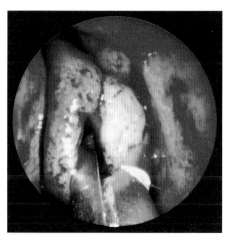

FIGURE 9.49   The lateral lamina of the
concha is then removed with the
Blakesley-Weil forceps.

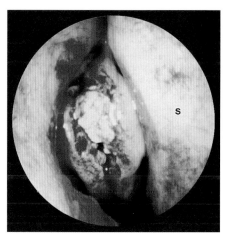

FIGURE 9.50   An inspissated empyema
of a right concha bullosa is shown just
after opening into the cell. s = nasal
septum.

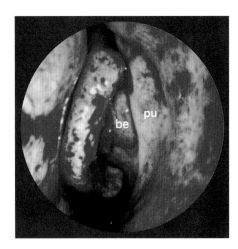

FIGURE 9.51 Following removal of most of the lateral lamella, a good view of the middle meatus can be obtained. be = ethmoidal bulla and pu = uncinate process.

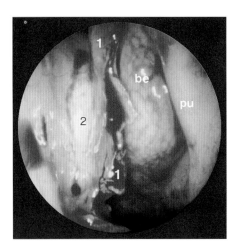

FIGURE 9.52 The middle meatus after resection of the lateral half of a concha bullosa shows remnants of the lateral lamella (1) and the posterior wall of the turbinate cell (2).

In Figure 9.51, most of the lateral lamella has been removed. An unimpeded view and access has been gained to the middle meatus. Posteriorly and inferiorly, there are small remnants of the lateral lamella. These only need to be removed if they are bulky or if they interfere with ventilation. The closer one gets to the posterior end of the middle turbinate, the greater the danger of hemorrhage and pain. At this point, the sphenopalatine foramen and the vessels and nerves exiting through it are immediately adjacent.

Depending on the pathology present, the procedure may be limited to a resection of the lateral lamella of the concha bullosa. The advantage of an endoscopic procedure is that an intraoperative staging is always possible. It can be decided on the spot, whether the edematous mucosa is in the hiatus semilunaris or over the bulla and whether the infundibulum is narrow and requires additional surgical intervention in this area. Should this be the case, an additional 1 ml of local anesthetic solution should be injected under the mucosa of the uncinate process, prior to continuing the operation. Before proceeding, it is important to ascertain that the lateral lamella of the concha bullosa had been removed completely and that only the medial leaf remains.

Figure 9.52 shows the key sites of the middle meatus through a 30 degree lens. Remnants of the lateral lamella of the turbinate can be seen clearly. They are anterior to the ethmoidal bulla and in contact with it. The posterior wall of the turbinate cell blocks the view

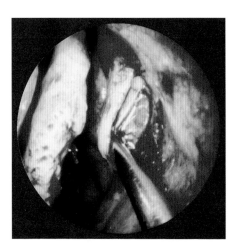

FIGURE 9.53 The uncinate process being incised with the sickle knife, and diseased mucosa of the ethmoidal infundibulum is exposed.

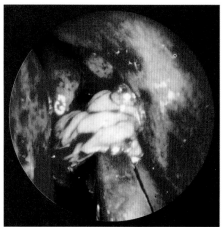

FIGURE 9.54 The uncinate process is removed.

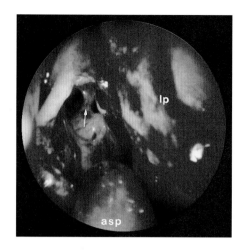

FIGURE 9.55 With a 30 degree endoscope, a good view is obtained of the frontal recess. The *arrow* indicates a mucosal bridge across the frontal sinus ostium. asp = suction tip and lp = lamina papyracea.

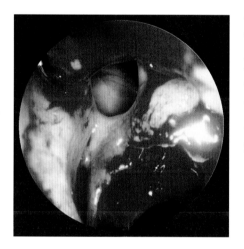

FIGURE 9.56 A view of a normal frontal sinus after the bridge (Fig. 9.55) has been resected.

between the ethmoidal bulla and the posterior vertical portion of the middle turbinate. Between it and the anterior surface of the ethmoidal bulla, there are some blood-tinged secretions in the hiatus semilunaris.

Figure 9.53 shows the incision of the uncinate process. After it has been reflected, copious polypoid mucosa can be seen in the ethmoidal infundibulum. This is removed (Fig. 9.54) yielding an unimpeded view, with a 30 degree lens, superiorly into the frontal recess (Fig. 9.55). There are two openings in the frontal sinus that are separated from each other by a narrow sagittal tissue bridge. Removal of this bridge permits a good look into the otherwise unremarkable frontal sinus (Fig. 9.56 and 9.57).

One week after surgery, there is already good healing and only moderate crusting. The path to the maxillary sinus is clear (Fig. 9.58).

If, in addition to the excision of a concha bullosa, the lateral nasal wall must also be treated, then this automatically leads to the creation of opposing wound surfaces. If the middle meatus is constricted or if there has been an unintentional injury to the head of the middle turbinate, we recommend that a small Merocel sponge moistened with beclomethasone be placed in the middle meatus for 1 or 2 days to prevent adhesions. Such cases must be monitored and followed closely to recognize the formation of adhesions and to treat them in a timely fashion. These adhesions may appear only after a few weeks and always extend from the insertion of the middle turbinate inferiorly.

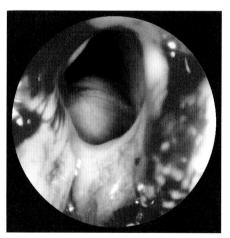

FIGURE 9.57 A view of a normal frontal sinus, close-up view.

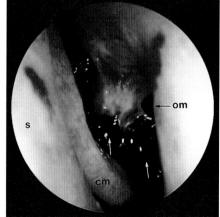

FIGURE 9.58 One week post surgery, healing is progressing well, with only moderate crusting (*arrows*). s = nasal septum and om = maxillary sinus ostium.

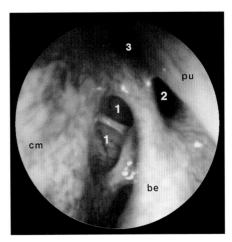

FIGURE 9.59 A view into the frontal recess with a 30 degree endoscope in a patient with recurrent frontal sinusitis. Three openings are visible; a blind pouch between the bulla and the middle turbinate (*1*), and two other openings that could extend to the frontal sinus (*2* and *3*). cm = middle turbinate; be = ethmoidal bulla; and pu = uncinate process.

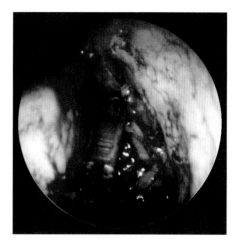

FIGURE 9.60 A view of the anterior surface of the bulla after removal of the uncinate process.

ISOLATED DISEASE OF THE FRONTAL SINUS

Isolated, recurrent disease of the frontal sinus is almost always due to the extension of disease in the frontal recess. In many cases it can be treated without performing a total ethmoidectomy. The procedure is the same in principle as in acute frontal sinusitis that is resistant to medical therapy and to focused endoscopic, topical management. The external approach to the frontal sinus is used only in the case of life-threatening complications of frontal sinusitis, e.g., osteomyelitis (Pott's puffy tumor) or following previous surgery that has left the frontal recess and the ostium of the frontal sinus coarsely scarred or ossified. Trephination of the frontal sinus (Beck procedure) or obliteration procedures have not been performed in our institution in 15 years.

As shown in Chapter 7, endoscopic exploration of the frontal recess may present the greatest challenge a surgeon is likely to encounter.

Figure 9.59 shows a view into the left frontal recess of a patient who had suffered recurrent frontal sinusitis with empyemas and headache for several years. Medical therapy improved the symptoms during the acute attacks and prevented complications, but never succeeded in completely eliminating the headaches. During a relatively symptom-free interval, endoscopic revision of the frontal recess was performed.

The view is into the frontal recess and the 30 degree endoscope is already lateral to the middle turbinate. On the right, inferiorly the uncinate process can be seen extending superiorly toward the skull base. It is not possible to tell endoscopically whether it turns further laterally and forms a recessus terminalis or whether it extends to the skull base. The ethmoidal bulla also extends a projection of its lamella superiorly toward the base of the skull. This projection extends medially and fuses with the middle turbinate and also extends laterally and reaches the lamina papyracea. These structures form three recesses or openings: a blind pouch subdivided by a small bony bridge between the bulla lamella and the middle turbinate; an opening that can be inspected for only a few millimeters with the endoscope (possibly an anterior opening to the lateral sinus, but it may also open further anteriorly into the frontal sinus); and another opening that can also be inspected for only a few millimeters (possibly a blind pouch extending to the base of the skull, the entrance to an agger nasi cell, or the path to the frontal sinus). A definitive diagnosis can be made only by additional dissection.

In Figure 9.60, the uncinate process has been removed and the anterior surface of the ethmoidal bulla can be seen. It is not touched, but is dissected further superiorly with curved forceps, under the insertion of the middle turbinate.

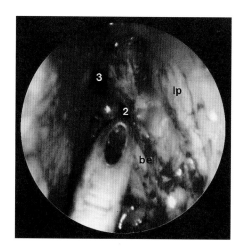

FIGURE 9.61 The transverse bony septum representing a remnant of bulla lamella is removed with forceps. lp = lamina papyracea; be = ethmoidal bulla; and 2 and 3 = openings as in Figure 9.59.

Figure 9.61 shows this situation in a close-up view. One can clearly see the anterior surface of the ethmoidal bulla and its insertion on the lamina papyracea. The forceps removes the transverse bony septum that represents a remnant of the bulla lamella, split and turned into the frontal plane.

In Figure 9.62 it becomes apparent that both openings lead to a common space, the frontal recess that is almost completely filled by a mucosal polyp. It is removed and now a completely unrestricted view to the ostium of the frontal sinus is obtained (Figs. 9.63 and 9.64). Nothing was done to the ostium of the frontal sinus. The mucosa inside the frontal sinus is unremarkable.

Within a few days the patient recovered completely and has remained free of any frontal sinusitis symptoms for the past 4 years.

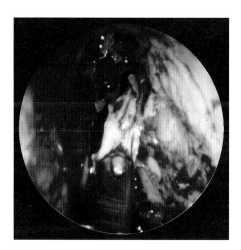

FIGURE 9.62 The openings lead to the frontal recess, which is found to be blocked by a polyp. This is removed with forceps as shown.

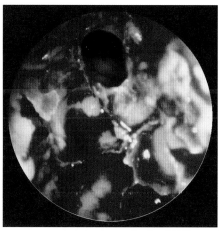

FIGURE 9.63 The frontal recess is clear to the frontal sinus ostium following removal of the polyp.

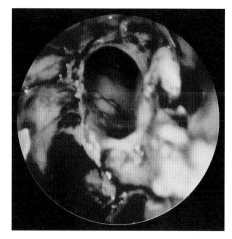

FIGURE 9.64 The frontal sinus ostium and mucosa are normal and are not touched.

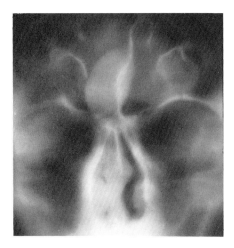

FIGURE 9.65   A CT scan of a patient complaining of headaches, showing a large frontal sinus cyst.

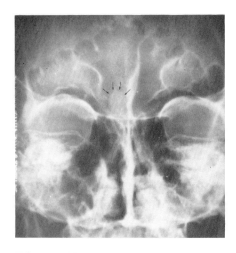

FIGURE 9.66   Following endoscopic surgery for concha bullosa and frontal recess disease, the cyst shrank to the size of a pea in 10 days (*arrows*).

FRONTAL SINUS CYST

It is not always possible to reach pathologic tissues originating from the floor of the frontal sinus or from other areas of the frontal sinus directly. In the present case there was a large cyst in the frontal sinus that caused characteristic headaches (Fig. 9.65). The underlying cause was identified as a diseased frontal recess and a marked concha bullosa of the middle turbinate. Surgically, there were no difficulties in correcting the problems in the concha bullosa, the frontal recess, and in the ostium of the frontal sinus (the technique was described in the previous section). Because of the bulging frontal ridge and the frontal extension of the frontal sinus, it was not possible to reach into the sinus with an instrument and remove the cyst.

Since the patient was much improved after repair of the frontal recess and volunteered information concerning the obvious reduction in symptoms, it was decided to wait and not to approach the removal of the cyst from externally. Within 10 days the cyst shrank to the size of a pea (Fig. 9.66) and after 14 more days it had disappeared completely (Figs. 9.67 and 9.68). In this case, there has been no recurrence after several years.

If in this case the cyst had not regressed spontaneously, and the complaints had persisted, an external approach or a radical endonasal procedure could have been performed at any time.

We believe that this example beautifully illustrates that many secondary manifestations regress spontaneously when the basic problem (in this case a concha bullosa and diseased frontal recess) has been removed. A primary approach to the frontal sinus from the front, appeared to us to be far less physiologic.

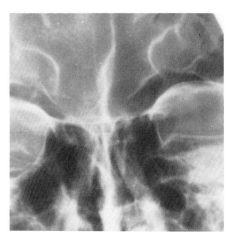

FIGURE 9.67   Radiographs performed 24 days post surgery show complete disappearance of the cyst.

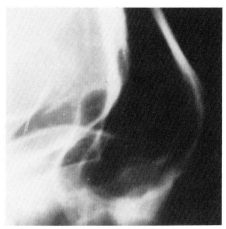

FIGURE 9.68   Lateral view of the situation in Figure 9.67.

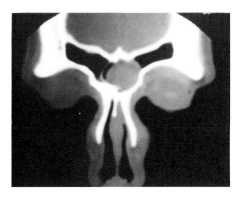

FIGURE 9.69 This patient had frontal headaches, and from the coronal CT scan appeared to have a frontal sinus cyst along with absence of the interfrontal septum.

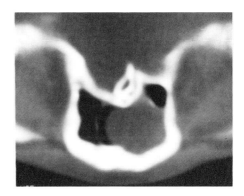

FIGURE 9.70 An axial CT scan had similar findings.

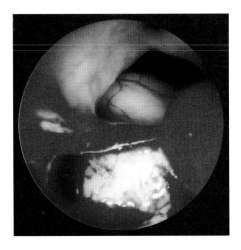

FIGURE 9.71 At operation a meningoencephalocele was found arising from the posterior wall of the frontal sinus. For details, see text.

MENINGOENCEPHALOCELE

In this patient who had been suffering from frontal headaches for several months, a frontal sinus cyst was diagnosed. The CT of the paranasal sinuses seemed to confirm this diagnosis. It was noteworthy that the cyst had either destroyed the frontal sinus septum, or that this patient had a congenital absence of this septum (Figs. 9.69 and 9.70, coronal and axial CT). Other than the headaches and some respiratory obstruction, this patient was symptom-free. There were no neurologic signs or any other indications of the presence of a CSF fistula.

During the endoscopic procedure, the path to the frontal recess was difficult because of the constricted conditions. When the ostium of the frontal sinus was finally visualized (it was unusually large), a good view of the frontal sinus could be obtained. There was a pulsating, semicircular, whitish-yellow structure bulging from the posterior wall. It was covered by a translucent "skin," containing a fine vascular network (Fig. 9.71). This was a meningoencephalocele.

The repair was done at a later date, transethmoidally and under general anesthesia.

The potential danger of such pathology lies in the fact that a meningoencephalocele can be easily mistaken for a polyp or a cyst, particularly if there are any in the area. It is also surprising how few symptoms a meningoencephalocele may produce. When questioned specifically, our patient recalled that he had minor trauma from a fall 8 years previously, but had never attributed any problems to the fall and has never had a skull X-ray film done. He never had meningitis or any symptoms that would have suggested a CSF fistula.

There are cysts at the base of the skull and, particularly, in the area of the frontal sinus that on opening give the surgeon the strong impression of having perforated the dura. On opening such a cystic structure there may be a pulsating flow of a watery clear fluid that may contain a few flecks of a more solid whitish material. We had two such cases and one more was related to us by a colleague (Dr. Kennedy) where clear liquid emerged for 5 to 8 minutes, but where the most careful search failed to reveal any injury to the base of the skull or any defect in the dura. After all the mucosa was removed from the area, the flow of secretions stopped. These are evidently a special form of secreting mucous membrane cyst. In none of the three cases were there any postoperative complications.

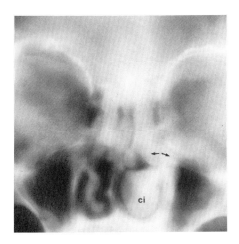

FIGURE 9.72   This coronal CT scan shows "hyperplasia" of the left inferior turbinate. There is also thickened mucosa over the ethmoidal bulla and obstruction of the infundibulum (*arrows*). ci = inferior turbinate.

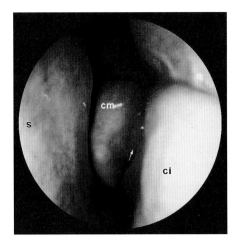

FIGURE 9.73   An endoscopic view of the patient in Figure 9.72 with thickened mucosa over the inferior turbinate shows a reduction in the thickening beyond the anterior end of the turbinate. There is also typical middle meatal disease with polyps (*arrow*). ci = inferior turbinate and cm = middle turbinate.

HYPERPLASTIC INFERIOR TURBINATE

During the past several decades, a number of techniques have been described in the literature for the extirpation or "plastic" reduction, or partial submucous resection of the "hyperplastic inferior turbinate." In a number of institutions the enlarged inferior turbinate was routinely resected, either totally or partially, in cases of allergic rhinitis or "obstructed nasal breathing."

We have found little reason in our clinical experience for a surgical approach to the hyperplastic inferior turbinate. In the few cases where this procedure was indicated, we limited our resection to the posterior hyperplastic end and only if there was documented osseous hypertrophy and corresponding respiratory obstruction. In the vast majority of the other cases where the inferior turbinate was significantly enlarged, we could show inflammatory disease in other parts of the nose. Once these areas were healed, the hyperplastic mucosa of the inferior turbinate returned to normal. In these cases, there was apparently a reactive hyperemia and hyperplasia of the mucosa of the inferior turbinate. The mechanism for this reactivity is not clearly understood.

The evaluation of a "hyperplastic inferior turbinate" is largely one of technique. When inspecting the nose with the naked eye and the speculum, the first thing one sees is the head of the inferior turbinate. A moderate enlargement or swelling of this structure can be interpreted as being of great clinical significance. Since we examine all patients with nasal complaints endoscopically, we pay less and less attention to an "enlarged" inferior turbinate. The author has performed no partial or total resection of the inferior turbinate for "hyperplasia" for the past 15 years. Even in a patient population that is alleged to suffer from "hyperplastic inferior turbinates" (from the Arabic countries) we have yet to find an indication for such a procedure.

We are aware of the fact, however, that there may be regional or racial differences in this disease entity.

Figure 9.72 shows the tomographic findings in a case with a left hyperplastic inferior turbinate. A typical ethmoid involvement can also be seen clearly, with thickening of the mucosa over the ethmoidal bulla and with obstruction of the ethmoidal infundibulum. In evaluating such changes in the turbinate, one must always consider that the nasal cycle with its increase in nasal perfusion, may also affect the radiographic findings.

Figure 9.73 shows the endoscopic view of an inferior turbinate with a thickened mucosa. The thickening is found to be not nearly as massive, once the endoscope is passed beyond the head of the middle turbinate. We now see a typical diseased infundibulum with polyps

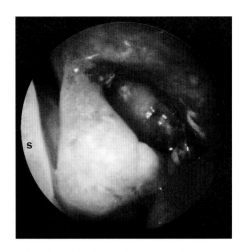

FIGURE 9.74 Polypoid mucosa becomes visible on the surface of the ethmoidal bulla after resection of the uncinate process.

emerging from the area of contact between the middle turbinate and the uncinate process.

Figure 9.74 shows the edematous polypoid mucosa on the anterior surface of the ethmoidal bulla that became visible after resection of the uncinate process. The bulla is so large that it completely fills the entire turbinate sinus. Both the bulla and the lateral sinus were markedly involved. Figure 9.75 shows the polypoid inflammatory gelatinous mucosa being removed from the lateral sinus.

Good healing can be seen already 1 week after the endoscopic procedure (Fig. 9.76). The mucosa is already completely normal over the roof of the ethmoid. There are still some crusts adhering to the ground lamella. At the same time, the inferior turbinate has "shrunk" almost to its normal size without ever having been touched (Fig. 9.77). Subsequently, healing was complete and the inferior turbinate was never large enough to interfere with respiration. We have had the same experience in almost all of our cases of hyperplastic inferior turbinates.

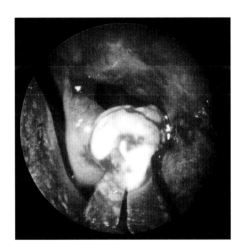

FIGURE 9.75 Polypoidal mucosa being removed with forceps from the lateral sinus.

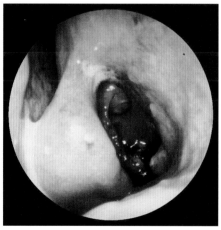

FIGURE 9.76 The appearance 1 week postoperatively shows good healing already progressing.

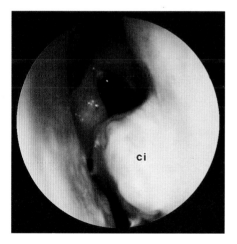

FIGURE 9.77 The inferior turbinate has also shrunk almost to normal size. ci = inferior turbinate.

COMPLICATIONS OF ACUTE SINUSITIS

In 82 percent of our pediatric patients who have initial acute sinusitis with incipient orbital complications, the inflammatory changes can be managed successfully with medical therapy and target-oriented local management (see Chapter 6). In children who again develop orbital complications during recurrent sinusitis, only 15 percent require no surgery. In adults who have orbital complications, history reveals chronic sinusitis in almost all cases. In all of these, we perform endoscopic repair after the acute phase has been reversed by medical therapy. The contraindications for endoscopic intervention in these cases have been discussed in Chapter 6. A rule of thumb for the indications for endoscopic surgery is a lack of clear improvement or worsening of the general condition after 24 hours of intensive intravenous antibiotic therapy and corresponding local decongestant measures (see Chapter 5). Incipient endocranial complications (epidural or subdural abscess, meningitis, intracranial abscess formation, or severe visual disturbances) are contraindications for a primary endoscopic procedure.

In children, the intervention is performed under general anesthesia. For this reason and also because the acute inflammation leads to more extensive bleeding, in addition to the frequently confusing anatomic situation, this procedure requires great skill on the part of the surgeon. With skill and experience it is usually possible to manage the case without external incision and drainage and thus interference with the patient is considerably less. With this technique, we have successfully managed not only sinusitis with periorbital cellulitis, but also cases with marked periorbital abscesses and even intraorbital abscesses.

We always advise the patient, or the parents, preoperatively, that increased bleeding may force us to resort to a transethmoidal approach during the same sitting. This became necessary in only one case in our institution during the past few years. During an operation for acute frontal sinusitis in a patient with cystic fibrosis with a mucocele of the ethmoid, it was possible to open the mucocele endonasally, but we were unable to reach and safely remove the rubbery masses of secretions from the lateral parts of the frontal sinus. For this reason we had to open the frontal sinus from the front during the same procedure.

If the procedure is done under general anesthesia, we always use additional decongestant pledgets with Pontocaine-epinephrine and inject lidocaine under the mucosa of the uncinate process in order to improve hemostasis.

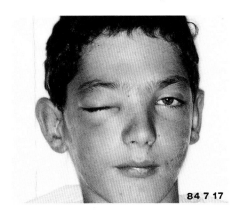

FIGURE 9.78 This 11-year-old boy developed right orbital swelling with restriction of movement of the eye during treatment of acute sinusitis with oral antibiotics.

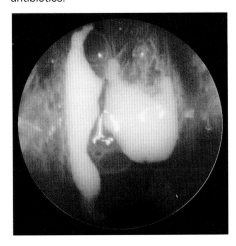

FIGURE 9.79 The endoscopic findings were of massive acutely inflamed polyps protruding from the middle meatus, along with streams of pus.

Figure 9.78 shows an 11-year-old boy with acute sinusitis who was treated at home by the general practitioner with oral antibiotics for a week. Two days prior to admission, he developed swelling of the right upper eyelid and on admission, both eyelids were swollen, external movements of the eye were limited, and the eye was protruding.

Figure 9.79 shows the endoscopic findings. The massive inflammatory swelling of the mucosa in the middle meatus can be clearly seen. Polyps protrude into the meatus and there are streams of pus along the polyps. With high-dose intravenous antibiotics and target-oriented decongestant inserts, conditions had *not* clinically improved within 24 hours. A CT of the paranasal sinuses showed a typical pansinusitis on the right with a separation of the periorbita from the lamina papyracea.

Figure 9.80 shows the operative field after resection of the uncinate process. The bony structure of the bulla can barely be seen. The remaining bony septa were soft and appeared to be eroded. Acute inflammatory and partly gelatinous polyps were removed from the entire anterior and posterior ethmoid and there was copious pus between the polypoid masses (Fig. 9.81). The entire ethmoid was carefully cleared all the way to the anterior wall of the sphenoid. The frontal recess was cleaned and the ostium of the maxillary sinus enlarged. The maxillary sinus also contained some purulent secretions that were removed by suction. After identifying the lamina papyracea, this was opened carefully in a circumscribed area. No free pus was encountered. The orbit itself was not opened in this case and the incision of the periorbita, as performed for intraorbital abscesses was omitted.

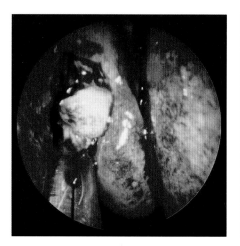

FIGURE 9.80 Following removal of the uncinate, the bony bulla and ethmoidal septa appeared eroded.

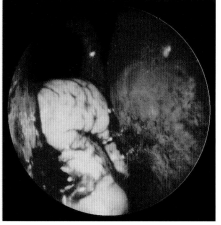

FIGURE 9.81 Inflammatory and gelatinous polyps were seen surrounded by copious pus.

Figure 9.82 shows the middle meatus at the end of the procedure. A Merocel sponge, moistened with beclomethasone, was placed into the middle meatus and left there for 24 hours.

Intravenous antibiotic therapy was continued and by the next morning, the general condition of the youngster was definitely improved (Fig. 9.83). The right eye could be opened, the eyeball's upward mobility was no longer restricted, and there was no diplopia. In the right nares, the ventilated Merocel sponge can be seen. It was removed later that same day.

Figure 9.84 shows the patient 36 hours after the surgery. The mobility of the eye has returned to normal and the patient was discharged home shortly afterwards.

At a routine postoperative visit 8 weeks later, the mucous membranes in the ethmoid were entirely normal. The open communication into the frontal sinus could be seen anterosuperiorly (Fig. 9.85).

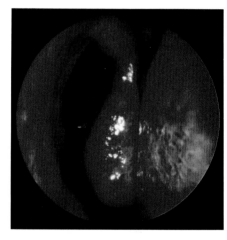

FIGURE 9.82   The appearance of the middle meatus at the end of the procedure.

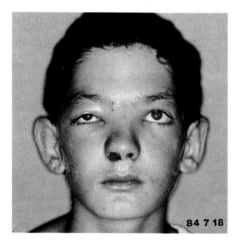

FIGURE 9.83   Within 24 hours there was improvement in the swelling and mobility of the eye.

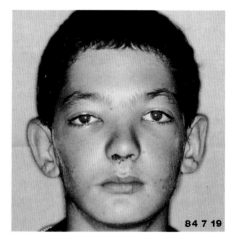

FIGURE 9.84   At 36 hours post surgery the mobility of the eye was normal.

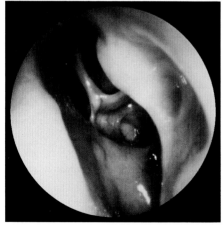

FIGURE 9.85   At follow-up 8 weeks later, the ethmoidal mucosa was normal with free communication with the frontal sinus.

MUCOCELES

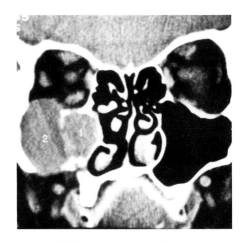

FIGURE 9.86 This coronal CT scan shows a two-chambered mucocele, which developed following a Caldwell-Luc operation. The lateral mucocele had eroded the floor of the orbit and extended posteriorly to the angle of the mandible. 1 and 2 = two chambers of the mucocele.

In general, mucoceles are an ideal indication for endoscopic surgery. This is particularly true for mucoceles of the maxillary sinus that are typical late complications of a Caldwell-Luc procedure or of radical operations. They can be diagnosed and treated without undue difficulty. In a mucocele of the maxillary sinus, we fenestrate the middle meatus at the site where the natural ostium would be under normal circumstances. The secretions are removed and the ostium is enlarged (up to a diameter of 1 × 1 cm, if possible) but the mucosa is usually not removed from the mucocele cavity. Healing is almost always rapid and complete.

Even complex mucoceles can be managed endoscopically. The two-chambered mucocele, shown in Figure 9.86, developed in a right maxillary sinus 27 years after a Caldwell-Luc procedure. In this instance the first mucocele was opened and drained from the middle meatus. Subsequently, the anterior wall of the second mucocele was opened by a bi-meatal approach through the enlarged ostium and through a trocar introduced through the anterior wall of the maxillary sinus. This resulted in a wide passage into the middle meatus, through the first mucocele and through the window. The mucosa was not removed. The bony floor of the orbit was extensive and stable enough to prevent a descent of the bulb and there was no postoperative diplopia.

This case was unusual, since there was a complete septation between the two mucoceles and also since the lateral mucocele had eroded not only into the orbit, but also far posteriorly to the angle of the mandible. It was the discomfort during swallowing and chewing that brought the patient to the physician.

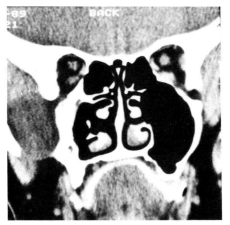

FIGURE 9.87 The operative bony defect in the facial wall of the maxillary sinus can be clearly seen.

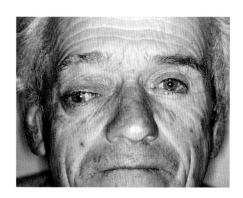

FIGURE 9.88 A case of an extensive mucocele of the right frontal sinus and anterior ethmoid.

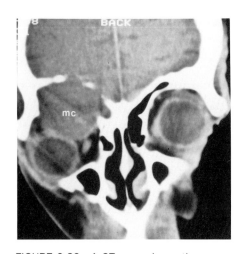

FIGURE 9.89 A CT scan shows the enormous size of the mucocele and displacement of the globe.

Figures 9.88 and 9.89 show the findings in an extensive mucocele of the frontal sinus and of the anterior ethmoid. Endoscopic management was not successful. Because of a large number of inflammatory episodes, the bone in the area of the frontal recess was so sclerotic that it could not be opened with the endoscopic instruments. More caudally and somewhat posteriorly, where the bone was thinner, one immediately got into orbital fat that was displaced medially and caudally by the enormous pressure exerted by the mucocele. The endoscopic procedure had to be discontinued and surgical repair had to be done from the outside. Note the major displacement of the eyeball inferiorly and laterally by the mucocele.

Figure 9.90 shows that mucoceles usually have a typical, unmistakable appearance. We see a large mucocele of the anterior ethmoid and the maxillary sinus. The bulging mucocele has pushed the middle turbinate inferiorly, against the septum. Precisely because the endoscopic appearance of the mucocele is supposed to be unmistakable, we show here a similar endoscopic finding on the left side (Fig. 9.91). There was a leiomyosarcoma hidden behind it. Even in apparently obvious findings, appropriate radiologic diagnostics must be performed in order to avoid unpleasant intraoperative surprises.

Figure 9.92 shows a maxillary sinus mucocele bulging into the inferior meatus. The inferior turbinate had been partially resected, many years previously, during a radical maxillary sinus procedure.

Figure 9.93 was photographed several weeks after opening a large maxillary sinus mucocele via the middle meatus. We can see a perfectly unremarkable maxillary sinus on the left. The course of the infraorbital nerve can be seen in the roof of the sinus and we can even see a few fibers extending anterocaudally into the facial wall of the maxillary sinus.

The endoscopic potential in mucoceles of all paranasal sinuses has been demonstrated on a videotape (see footnote on first page of Chapter 9).

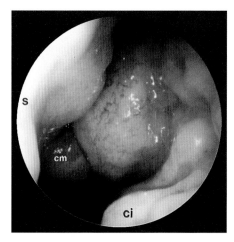

FIGURE 9.90 An endoscopic view of a large mucocele of the right ethmoid and maxillary sinus shows how the middle turbinate is pushed against the nasal septum. ci = inferior turbinate; cm = middle turbinate; and s = septum.

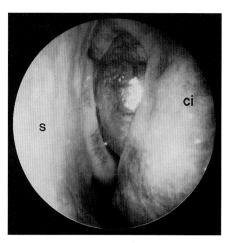

FIGURE 9.91 These endoscopic findings in another patient's left side were similar to those in Figure 9.90, but this bulge was due to a leiomyosarcoma.

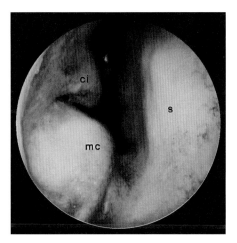

FIGURE 9.92 An endoscopic view of a maxillary sinus mucocele bulging into the inferior meatus on the right. s = nasal septum; ci = inferior turbinate; and mc = maxillary sinus mucocele.

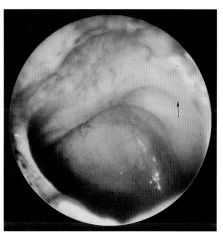

FIGURE 9.93 The result several weeks after opening a left-sided maxillary sinus mucocele via the middle meatus, shows normal mucosa, and an easily visible inferior orbital nerve with some fibers extending down the anterior wall of the sinus (arrow).

Chapter 10

POSTOPERATIVE CARE

As discussed in Chapter 7, we do not routinely insert packing into the middle meatus or the nose, since at the end of the procedure there is usually little if any bleeding. At the end of the procedure, the surgical area is examined with the endoscope and the larger clots removed. Because of the adhesive forces generated between these clots and the mucosal lining, their removal may start some capillary oozing. If an area of capillary oozing is identified (something that occurs most commonly when the surgery was performed for an acute inflammatory problem), we place a small piece of Oxycel mesh, 100 percent regenerated oxidized cellulose (Johnson & Johnson), over the bleeding site. The Oxycel mesh can be easily draped over the bleeding surface and it immediately adheres to the raw surface and in most instances controls the bleeding. The Oxycel is usually absorbed within a few days.

Finally, the nasopharynx is carefully inspected, and any clots that may have accumulated in this area are removed. We routinely place a cotton pledget into the nasal vestibules to prevent blood-tinged secretions from running down the patient's face during the first few postoperative hours.

In those cases where opposing wound surfaces were created, or where the spaces are extremely narrow, we usually place strips of compressed Merocel sponge into the middle meatus, which are then expanded by moistening them with a beclomethasone solution (e.g., Beconase aqueous solution). The strips of Merocel sponge are transfixed with a suture and the end of the suture is taped to the patient's cheek. These sponges are kept in place for no more than 1 or 2 days, and during this time they are moistened with the beclomethasone solution several times each day.

It is important to inform the patient that the presence of some blood-tinged secretions in the nasopharynx is perfectly normal during the first few postoperative hours. These secretions should be expectorated and not swallowed. This makes it easier for the recovery room nurse to monitor blood loss and to recognize the appearance of a fresh hemorrhage. The patient is also requested not to blow his or her nose at all during the first 24 hours. These instructions must be strictly followed, especially if maxillary sinus endoscopy was performed through the canine fossa or if the lamina papyracea has been injured during the procedure. If the patient wishes to clear the nasal passages, sniffing inwardly as frequently as necessary is recommended.

Depending on the type and amount of premedication administered, the patient may take nourishment 1 to 2 hours postoperatively. During the first few days, extensive physical activity, e.g., lifting heavy weights, and all activities that could elevate blood pressure and increase perfusion of the surgical site must be avoided. The patient should be informed that even after the topical and local anesthesia wears off, there should be little pain. For the first few hours, or even 1 to 2 days there will probably be a reactive swelling of the nasal mucous membranes, and consequently, the nasal passages may be more obstructed than preoperatively.

POSTOPERATIVE DRUG THERAPY

In the past, we instilled antibiotic and corticosteroid ointments into the middle meatus. However, in recent years we have ceased this practice (see Local Postoperative Care). The instillation of ointments has no advantages as far as wound healing or the prevention of synechiae and crusts is concerned. Within minutes or hours after instillation, the ointment is transported into the nasopharynx where it affects the patient with its unpleasant taste. In some cases with recurrent problems, we found remnants of the ointment in obstructed sections of the ethmoid, although there was no evidence that it was the ointment that was responsible for the recurrence of disease. The occasional observation of fungal growth on top of such encapsulated ointment has further induced us to abandon this practice.

We are aware of several cases where the ointment was introduced into the orbit where it produced serious complications (persistent diplopia). In addition to the inadvertent direct instillation of the ointment into the orbit through an unrecognized perforation of the lamina papyracea, it is also possible for the ointment to penetrate into the orbit through the site of a minor prolapse of orbital fat that was missed intraoperatively. Such cases have also contributed to our discontinuing the use of ointments in the surgical field.

In most cases, we prescribe an oral antibiotic, usually penicillin or a cephalosporin, for a variable period of time, but usually no less than 1 week. While in many cases there is no pressing need for antibiotic coverage, our rationale for using antibiotics follows. Postoperatively, there is a large wound surface with open mucosal areas measuring several square centimeters. There is always the danger of infection from the outside and the administration of antibiotics can be regarded as a prophylactic measure. There is no doubt about the propriety of giving antibiotics if (intraoperatively) pus-filled cells were opened or the disease process was an infectious or inflammatory one (or the complication of such a disease process).

We give *no* antibiotics in mycotic infections of the paranasal sinuses, except when there is a concurrent, massive bacterial superinfection. This is frequently seen in the maxillary sinus, in the presence of fungus balls.

Corticoids are not used routinely and neither are antihistamines. The latter are used only if the patient has a clear history of an allergic component. Corticoids are used only for the management of coincidental disease, e.g., asthma, when we are dealing with an inflammatory problem with polyp formation, or in some cases of diffuse polypoid rhinosinusitis. In the latter two circumstances we also administer antihistamines. In diffuse polypoid rhinosinusitis, the administration of steroids is a rather desperate attempt to reduce the high recurrence rate if possible and to promote wound healing.

An aqueous solution of beclomethasone nose drops has proven to be a useful local agent, which we administer 4 to 5 times on the first postoperative day. The patient is requested to have the head maximally extended or to assume the "Mecca" position, recommended by Lund, Drake-Lee, and Mackay. In the latter position, the drops are introduced deeply into the nose with the head maximally flexed and the kneeling patient is instructed to sniff. Less sporting, but just as effective is to place the nose drops with the patient sitting in a chair with the head bent downward (Fig. 10.1).

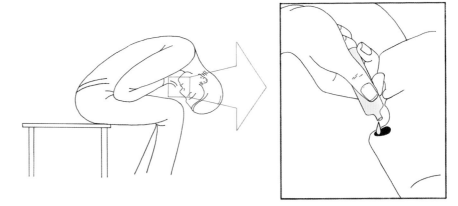

FIGURE 10.1 The recommended position for the instillation of nose drops.

With both of these methods there is a reasonable chance that the nose drops actually reach the ethmoid area and not just run along the base of the nose to the pharynx. In marked polypoid disease we recommend steroid nose drops for a period of at least 10 days, although this may vary widely.

Some patients tend to form thick crusts in the operated area. The instillation of oily nose drops will soften these crusts and makes their removal easier. If maxillary sinus endoscopy through the canine fossa produces mucosal swelling, the administration of an anti-inflammatory drug for a few days usually is of benefit.

LOCAL POSTOPERATIVE CARE

Careful local postoperative care is an important component of our therapeutic concept, although it must be emphasized that the majority of the operative cavities require no extensive care. In some instances, however, the ultimate success of the surgical procedure depends largely on the postoperative care given.

On the first postoperative day, clots, secretions, and crusts should be removed carefully from the surgical site by suction. This must be done by the operating surgeon, since the surgeon who actually performed the surgery is the only one who knows the precise extent of the procedure and the areas where special caution is necessary. When suctioning on the first day, it is important that the suction tip be introduced under the middle turbinate and that secretions not just be removed from the nasal vestibule and the floor of the nose. This removal of the secretions prevents the formation of scabs and fibrin bridges that may contribute to the later formation of synechiae. These procedures must be performed carefully to avoid new trauma. In many cases, this first suctioning can be performed without anesthesia and with the naked eye. In some cases, especially when the passages were very narrow, the endoscope must be used and the suctioning must be performed under direct vision. Depending on the sensitivity of the patient, a local anesthetic spray or pledgets may be required.

When Merocel sponges are removed, a liquid solution such as beclomethasone should be dripped onto the sponge about an hour before removal to make it more pliable. This reduces the risk of mucosal injury by the irregular surface of the Merocel sponge.

When necessary, it may be possible to remove clots or tenacious secretions from the maxillary and/or frontal sinuses with a curved aspirator. In order to avoid fresh injury to the ostium, we prefer not to perform this before the third postoperative day.

Nasal irrigation with saline or Ringer's solution are *not* routinely done during the first few postoperative days.

The suctioning is performed again on the second and third postoperative days and the patient is instructed to return 1 week later for another check (Figs. 10.2 to 10.5). At this time, inspection with the endoscope is essential as it is usually possible to identify developing problems (synechiae, ostial stenosis, disturbances of wound healing, etc.) or most commonly to observe an uncomplicated recovery. At this time the dates for further visits can be discussed. If there are no problems, we usually see the patient in 4 to 6 weeks and decide then on the date of future visits. In problem cases, individual schedules must be developed.

FIGURE 10.2 *A*, A view into the right side of a nose 3 days after endoscopic ethmoid surgery for mycotic sinusitis. The entrance into the middle meatus is covered with crusts. *B*, After removal of the crusts, some granulation tissue is found immediately below the insertion of the middle turbinate. The ethmoid cavity behind it is already healing nicely. g = granulation tissue. *C*, After suctioning the wound secretions, a good view of the ostium of the maxillary sinus can be obtained. On the floor of the maxillary sinus, there are still some inspissated secretions, mixed with old coagulum. Note that in spite of the wound surfaces, the mucociliary transport already functions over a considerable area (the *arrows* indicate the paths of the secretions from the ostium of the maxillary sinus and from the frontal recess). *D*, A view into the maxillary sinus after aspiration of the wound secretions. The mucosa is still edematous and swollen, but healing well. Note that the posterior rim of the ostium of the maxillary sinus was *not* traumatized, but that the ostium was enlarged anteriorly at the expense of the fontanelles. The more firmly adherent fibrin deposits have not been removed yet. *E*, The view at an endoscopic check-up 6 weeks after surgery. Note the patent passage into the frontal sinus through the enlarged frontal recess (*large arrow*). The posterior wall of the recess and its normal mucosa can be readily seen. The *thin arrows* point to a small anterior ethmoidal artery in the area of the lateral sinus. The mucosa has returned to normal in all areas. ru = remnants of the uncinate process and rbe = remnants of the ethmoidal bulla.

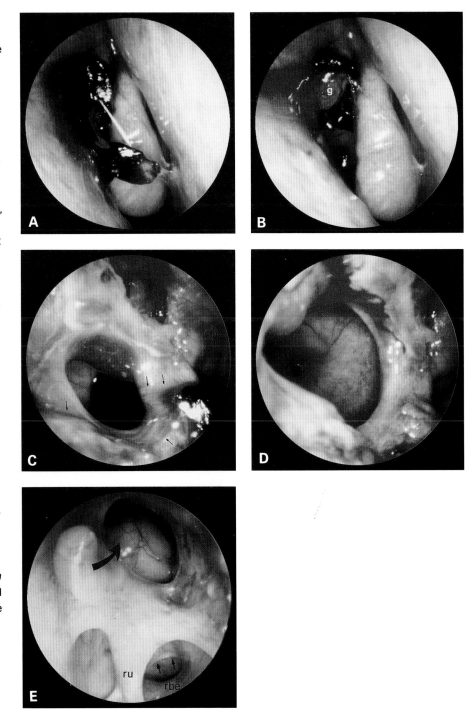

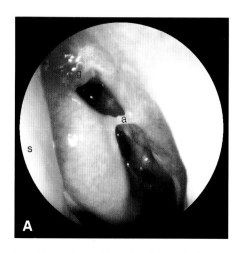

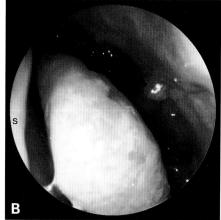

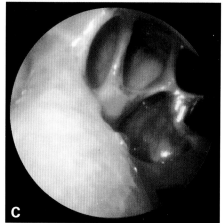

FIGURE 10.3 *A*, The view into a left middle meatus 8 days after surgery for severe polypoid disease. The mucosa is still somewhat thickened and loosened over the lamina papyracea, but already shows good recovery. Only at the insertion of the middle turbinate can some polypoid granulation tissue be seen. g = polypoid granulation tissue; a = a small adhesion between the head of the middle turbinate and the lateral nasal wall, obviously due to some intraoperative injury to the head of the middle turbinate; s = septum. *B*, The appearance post removal of the granulations and transsection of the adhesion. s = septum. *C*, A further 10 days later, the mucosa in the ethmoid is unremarkable.

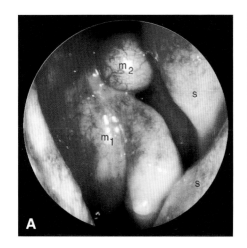

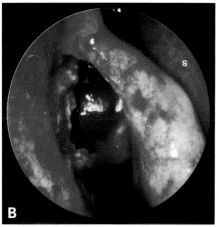

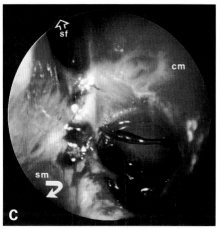

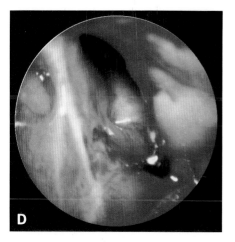

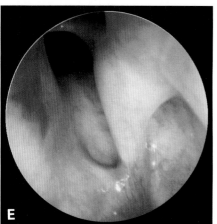

FIGURE 10.4 *A*, The preoperative appearance in a right nasal cavity, following a polypectomy several years previously. There are two mucoceles (m_1 and m_2) present. The middle turbinate is displaced medially in the area of the infundibulum, by the larger mucocele (m_1). m = mucocele and s = septum. *B*, The appearance immediately after the end of the endoscopic procedure. Both mucoceles have been opened and their walls largely removed. s = septum. *C*, The endoscopic appearance 1 week postoperatively. After removal of some crusts, there is an unimpeded view, through the frontal recess, to the frontal sinus (*open arrow*) and to the maxillary sinus (*curved arrow*). In the cavity produced by mucocele m_1, the mucosa was not disturbed during the operation. It contained some crusts that were subsequently removed. The mucosa over the lateral surface of the middle turbinate still shows some inflammatory thickening. sf = to frontal sinus; sm = to maxillary sinus; and cm = concha media. *D*, One month after surgery, the conditions at the roof of the ethmoid are essentially normal. A look through the ostium of the frontal sinus into the sinus shows well visible, normal mucosa on the walls of the frontal sinus. There is a small secretion crust on the roof of the ethmoid, just posterior to the ostium of the frontal sinus. The slight hemorrhage was caused by the endoscope and the suction tip. *E*, One year later, the conditions are normal. The ostium of the frontal sinus and the cavity of the mucocele have shown no tendency to shrink.

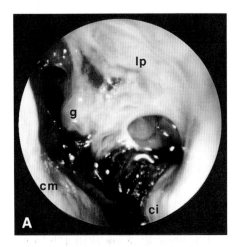

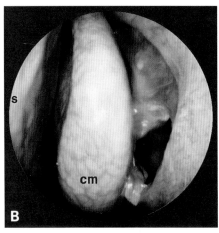

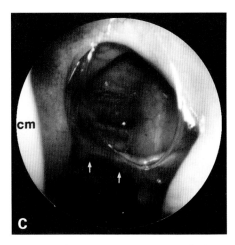

FIGURE 10.5 *A*, A view into a left middle meatus 1 week after endoscopic surgery for polypoid disease of the anterior ethmoid. Over the lamina papyracea, the mucosa is still edematous and thickened by inflammation. In some areas, small granulations may be seen. These were carefully removed. Crusts extending from the maxillary sinus into the middle meatus were also removed. lp = lamina papyracea; g = granulation; cm = concha media; and ci = concha inferior. *B*, Three days later, the mucosa over the lamina papyracea is much improved and the mucosa of the maxillary sinus is almost normal. On the posterior aspect of the enlarged ostium of the maxillary sinus, there are some fibrinous wound secretions, which were removed by suction. s = septum and cm = concha media. *C*, Seven weeks postoperatively, the mucosa of the entire ethmoid is normal. (View with a 30 degree lens at the roof of the ethmoid.) The *arrows* indicate the course of the anterior ethmoidal artery. The thin layer of secretion that can be seen is due to the spray that was used for topical anesthesia. cm = concha media.

As mentioned earlier, the patient must be advised that the healing phase, particularly the reepithelialization will take at least 2 to 3 weeks, but it may take as much as 6 weeks, and in exceptional cases, even longer. During this time it is quite normal for some secretions to appear, and for crusts to be expelled during sneezing or while blowing the nose. In severe polyposis, it may take several weeks before the pathology in the maxillary and/or frontal sinuses completely reverts to normal (Fig. 10.6). For this reason, it makes no sense to have a repeat X-ray study in less than 6 to 8 weeks. Since the operative field can usually be seen well with the nasal endoscopes, we do not use postoperative X-ray examinations routinely, but reserve these for problem cases and complications.

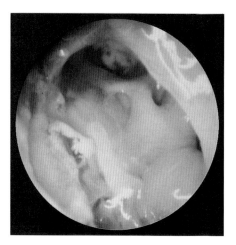

FIGURE 10.6 In this patient, the mucosa shows no healing tendency 2 months after an endoscopic procedure for severe polypoid ethmoidal disease. The patient complained continuously about mucopurulent secretions, which reached the pharynx and about a feeling of fullness. The poor healing tendency was probably due to an underlying osteitis. After 10 days of therapy with ciprofloxacin IV and a combination of cortisone and antihistamine, b.i.d. orally, the symptoms rapidly regressed and the mucosa returned to normal.

POSTOPERATIVE PROBLEMS AND COMPLICATIONS

Some patients respond during the first few postoperative hours or days with a marked reactive mucosal engorgement, so that nasal breathing is initially more obstructed than it was preoperatively. The patient must be told in advance that this is not a complication, and that it should be considered an entirely normal event. Even a minor crust can, on occasion, give rise to significant symptoms. As a precursor to epithelialization, these scabs or crusts consist of inspissated secretions and fibrin deposits. They can solidify and, on occasion, they may fill the entire surgical area like a cast. They must be removed with the greatest care, in order not to cause additional injury or renewed bleeding. Even a tiny 1- or 2-mm crust, if located at the entrance to the middle meatus, and particularly if it is situated in a transverse direction, may give the patient the impression of complete respiratory obstruction. They may feel this sensation of complete respiratory obstruction even though objectively, there is practically no interference with the air stream. It is always astonishing, how the removal of such a tiny crust leads to a subjective improvement in nasal respiration even though rhinometric measurements fail to demonstrate any significant change in flow. This is one of the reasons why we abandoned rhinometry as an adjunct in the evaluation of surgical success.

Occasionally, patients feel pain when the aspirator is introduced to the ethmoid. If this happens, a local anesthetic solution should be applied to the surgical area prior to further manipulation.

It is particularly important, when the passages are very narrow, that the suction tip be advanced between the middle turbinate and the lateral wall of the nose to break up and remove fibrin bridges and to prevent the mucous membrane edges from narrowing the ostia of the sinuses. If this should produce some bleeding, it can usually be easily controlled by the application of Oxycel.

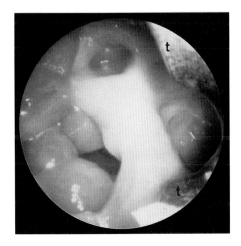

FIGURE 10.7 A view into a right middle meatus 3 weeks after endoscopic surgery for diffuse polypoid rhinosinopathy. The mucosa shows the typical diffuse hyperplastic thickening that produces polyps, particularly in the area of the ostium of the maxillary sinus. The large maxillary sinus ostium is the result of a previous operation, at which time a transmaxillary ethmoidectomy and radical maxillary sinus operation were performed. In spite of intensive antibiotic and steroid therapy, orally and topically, there was no appreciable improvement.

In cases of diffuse polypoid rhinosinusitis, we can see granular and/or polypoid changes recurring in the mucous membranes within a few postoperative days. Occasionally, glassy polyps reappear in the ethmoidal sinus on the first or second postoperative day and these should be removed promptly. It is often painful and frustrating to see that in spite of intensive and expensive local management, removal of crusts and secretions, and the application of steroids, the diffuse mucosal changes characteristic of this disease regress only extremely slowly and, in some cases, may even get worse during therapy (Fig. 10.7).

We must distinguish the persistently granulating changes, hypersecretion, and disturbances of wound healing that occur in those cases where an osteitis of an underlying bony structure exists.

Clinically, this is characterized by a finely granular, weepy mucosal surface with frequently smeary, purulent secretions and occasionally, small glassy inflammatory polyps in this area. These cases usually require prolonged and careful local management and the administration of a specific high-dose long-term IV antibiotic regimen. These are the cases where a combination therapy of antibiotics and steroids is frequently successful.

Using the Messerklinger technique, the enlarged ostium of the maxillary sinus in the middle meatus shows surprisingly little inclination toward stenosis (see Chapter 13). In order to traumatize the ostium as little as possible postoperatively, we do not irrigate the maxillary sinus routinely, and only suction retained secretions when they spontaneously liquefy after the third or fourth postoperative day. If the maxillary sinus has been diseased for months or even years, it may take many days or weeks before ciliary activity returns to normal and before mucus having a normal consistency is produced.

Serious Complications During Aftercare

In Chapters 5 and 11 we report cases in which the instillation of antimycotic ointment into the middle meatus or into the maxillary sinus was followed by extremely painful and persistent granulomatous infiltrates into the soft tissues of the cheek. Apparently the antibiotic ointments reached the soft tissues through the openings in the canine fossa, which were created by the insertion of the maxillary sinus trocar. In those cases where maxillary sinus endoscopy is performed as part of the surgical procedure, we instill antimycotic preparations, if at all, only after the fifth or sixth postoperative day by which time it can be assumed with reasonable certainty, that the trocar openings have completely closed.

When foreign substances like cotton pledgets or Merocel sponges are "forgotten" in the operative field, they may lead to serious complaints. All pledgets or sponges introduced into the nose must be marked with a long suture that assures their recognition and removal. When a sponge is left intentionally for some time, the thread attached to it should be taped to the patient's cheek to prevent the sponge from advancing into the pharynx and to alert the aftercare team to its presence.

DISCHARGE INSTRUCTIONS TO THE PATIENT

For at least 1 week postoperatively, the patient should "take it easy," avoid engaging in vigorous sports, and generally avoid all activities that may lead to sudden hypertension (e.g., bending, lifting heavy loads, sauna, excessive alcohol intake, sun bathing, etc.). The patient must be made aware of the various phases of wound healing, and he or she should understand that reepitelialization may take several weeks and that the presence of secretions and crust formation are normal during this period. The patient's expectations must be kept within reason and they must be made to understand that the operation will not immunize them against future upper respiratory infections. They may well develop colds with nasal and paranasal sinus symptoms and even sinusitis, which would then need to be treated appropriately. The incidence and severity of such infections should, however, be appreciably less than preoperatively. They should also be of shorter duration and, most importantly, should not become chronic.

Chapter 11

SPECIAL PROBLEMS

WHEN FENESTRATION AND CALDWELL-LUC FAIL

We have seen many patients who had previously undergone
fenestration procedures or Caldwell-Luc operations performed for the
control of paranasal sinus problems and continued to suffer from the
same symptoms without any appreciable improvement. Since the
history and symptoms were almost identical in most of these patients,
we conducted a more detailed study of 200 similar cases. The patients'
histories were reviewed, the operative reports from the previous
surgical procedures examined, and the radiographic and endoscopic
findings analyzed. The results of this study confirmed the extraordinarily important role that the ethmoidal sinus plays in the
pathophysiology of paranasal sinus disease. We can conceive of no
better (involuntary) example to demonstrate the dependence of the
frontal and maxillary sinuses on their relationship with the
prechambers of the anterior ethmoid.

Symptoms

All of the patients in this study had previously undergone fenestration
or Caldwell-Luc procedures and some had undergone multiple
operations. When there were multiple operations, one or two
fenestration procedures were usually followed by a radical maxillary
sinus operation. The previous operations were performed from 3
months to 10 years prior to the study period.

This study was performed in collaboration with D.W. Kennedy and S.J. Zinreich et al at
the Johns Hopkins University, Baltimore, MD and published in HNO 1987; 35:93–105.

All patients either continued to suffer postoperatively from the same symptoms for which they had undergone the original surgical procedure or else the original symptoms recurred promptly. The patients continued to complain of nasal obstruction; headache; pressure between and behind the eyes; increase in pathologic secretions; postnasal discharge; tearing; and recurrent, acute rhinosinusitis.

In order to get the most information from this study, we did not include in our assessment those specific, postoperative problems that may be attributed directly to a radical maxillary sinus operation, e.g., the well-known neuralgias, or paresthesias due to scarring, injury, or irritation of the infraorbital nerve. Patients with allergies were excluded as were those who had diffuse, polypoid rhinosinopathy and ASA intolerance, since this group of patients has a high incidence of recurrence, regardless of surgical technique used.

All patients had a diagnostic endoscopy, and the maxillary sinus was inspected through the fenestration, if this was patent. If the fenestra was not patent and it was appropriate to examine the maxillary sinus, maxillary sinus endoscopy was performed through the canine fossa. All patients underwent a repeat tomographic examination.

Endoscopic Findings

It is known that inferior meatal fenestrations tend to stenose or even close completely. This is not necessarily an undesirable event, especially if the fenestration has accomplished its purpose while it was patent and led to a complete resolution of the maxillary sinusitis. The patients in this study however, represented a uniformly negative outcome group, i.e., in each and every case, the surgical procedure(s) failed to accomplish their goal of an improvement in the patient's symptoms. We were therefore not surprised that on endoscopic examination we found a great degree of variation in the status of the inferior meatal antrostomy, which varied from a widely patent window in the inferior meatus to marked stenosis or even total obliteration (Figs. 11.1 to 11.4). It became obvious to us that there was no direct relationship between the severity of the patients' symptoms and the size and patency of the fenestration (see below).

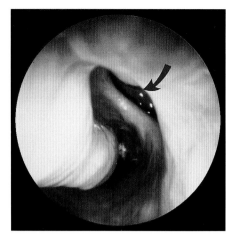

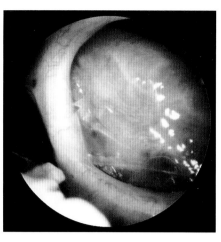

FIGURE 11.1   The wide window of the inferior meatal antrostomy (*arrow*) is clearly
seen in this view into a left inferior
meatus.

FIGURE 11.2   In this view through the
window into the maxillary sinus with a 30
degree lens, edematous polypoid mucosa
can be seen bulging forward from the
posterior wall and maxilloethmoidal angle
of the maxillary sinus. Note the copious,
tenaceous secretions.

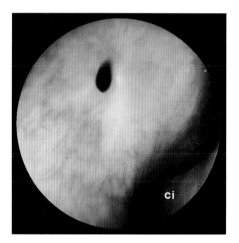

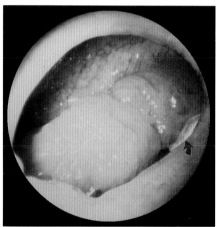

FIGURE 11.3   In this view into a right
inferior meatus, the inferior meatal
window has stenosed to a diameter of
1.5 mm. The corresponding middle
meatus is shown in Figs. 11.15 and
11.16. ci = inferior turbinate.

FIGURE 11.4   This right inferior meatus
has a large patent window. Polypoid
strands of diseased mucous membrane
and granulation tissue can be seen on
the floor and posterior wall of the maxillary sinus. The changes extended to the
maxilloethmoidal angle and to the natural
ostium. The arrow points to the viscous,
purulent secretions in the maxillary sinus.

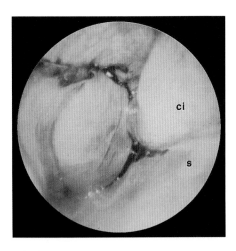

FIGURE 11.5   This large window in a right inferior meatus is completely blocked by a cyst bulging out from the maxillary sinus. ci = inferior turbinate; s = septum.

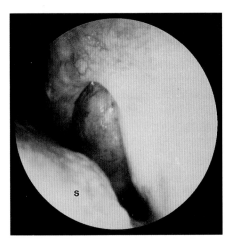

FIGURE 11.6   The inferior turbinate has been partially resected in this left inferior meatus. A large polyp can be seen bulging into the inferior meatus from the maxillary sinus. s. = septum.

As far as the extent of the pathology within the maxillary sinus was concerned, the spectrum of involvement ranged from minimal mucous membrane changes to the most massive alterations. Even here, there was still only a very indirect correlation between the extent of the pathology and the patient's symptoms. Even more surprising to us was the discovery that the amount of disease in the maxillary sinus was not directly related to the patency of the inferior meatal window.

We found marked maxillary sinus mucous membrane changes in about half of our patients (n = 116) examined in this study. These changes included edematous, inflammatory mucous membranes; polyps; cysts; granulation tissue; highly viscous secretions; and even pus, so that there was practically no normal mucosa left. In two-thirds of these patients with marked mucous membrane changes (n = 75), the window into the inferior meatus was patent, while one-third of the patients had significant stenosis or complete obliteration of the window. Occasionally an otherwise patent window was obstructed by a polyp or a cyst protruding from the sinus (Figs. 11.5 to 11.7).

Twenty-five patients had only minimal macroscopic mucous membrane changes at the time of the study, although in most of these patients there was some mucosal swelling in the area of the natural ostium, which partially or completely occluded the ostium. This group also contained patients with patent maxillary sinus windows or windows that were partially or completely obstructed.

Twelve percent of the patients had completely unremarkable maxillary sinus mucosa, with only slight narrowing of the natural ostium and no pathology discernible within the sinus. In one-half of these patients, windows into the inferior meatus were patent (Fig. 11.8), whereas in the other half, the windows were either stenotic or completely occluded.

In four patients, no free maxillary sinus lumen could be found by endoscopy. As seen in the radiographs (Figure 11.9) this was due not so much to scar formation but to a total postoperative collapse of the bony walls of the maxillary sinus.

In each of these groups there were patients with a wide range of complaints. There was no statistical relationship between any group characteristics and the time elapsed since the previous procedure. There was also no relationship between the maxillary sinus pathology (endoscopic or radiographic) and the patient's symptomatology: minimal radiographic and/or endoscopic findings did not necessarily mean that the patient had only minimal or no symptoms.

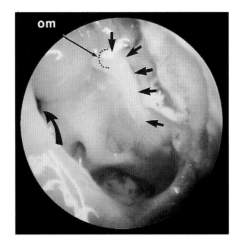

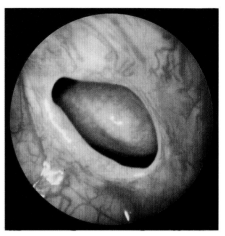

FIGURE 11.7   This is a view through the canine fossa into a left maxillary sinus 3 years after a Caldwell-Luc procedure. The entire mucous membrane shows inflammatory, edematous changes. The window into the inferior meatus is somewhat narrowed, but still patent (*bent arrow*). The viscous, purulent secretions in the maxillary sinus are transported primarily (*row of arrows*) in the direction of the natural ostium (*stippled*), even though the ostium is mostly blocked. om = maxillary ostium.

FIGURE 11.8   This is a view into a left maxillary sinus through the canine fossa 6 months after a fenestration procedure. The free margin of the inferior turbinate can be seen medially through the inferior meatal window. The mucous membrane of the maxillary sinus shows increased vascular markings in the area of the ostium, but is otherwise unremarkable.

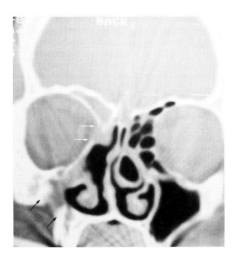

FIGURE 11.9   This is the coronal CT scan of a patient who had undergone a fenestration procedure and a subsequent de Lima operation on the right side. There is no longer any maxillary sinus lumen as the maxillary sinus has collapsed. Note the "curled" and osteitic bony margins in the area of the previous transantral window (*black arrows*). The middle turbinate had been resected and the frontal recess is largely obliterated by scar tissue. Copious retained secretions were present in the frontal recess and in the frontal sinus (not shown in this section). Note the bony defect in the lamina papyracea, which has been filled in by scar tissue (*white arrows*). On the left side a large concha bullosa is in close contact with the ethmoidal bulla. A small Haller's cell narrows the infundibulum from above.

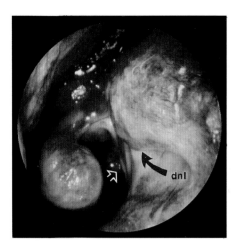

FIGURE 11.10 This is a left inferior meatus after a fenestration procedure. The middle turbinate has been partially resected, posterior to the ostium of the nasolacrimal duct (*curved black arrow*). Behind this, the patent window into the maxillary sinus can be seen (*open white arrow*). Fleshy polyps can be seen protruding from the middle meatus. dnl = nasolacrimal duct.

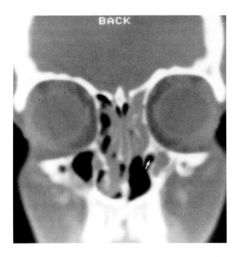

FIGURE 11.11 This is the tomogram of the patient shown in Figure 11.10. The absence of the inferior turbinate is apparent. The plane of the section cuts precisely through the opening of the nasolacrimal duct (*arrow*). Note the obvious bilateral, anterior ethmoidal sinus disease.

This observation clearly demonstrates the lack of usefulness of standard plain X-ray films in evaluating the postoperative paranasal sinus. A normal finding does not exclude pathology, nor does the finding of massive pathology allow the surgeon to conclude that there are correspondingly severe symptoms. If the radiologist knew that the patient had previous maxillary sinus surgery, the X-ray report not uncommonly stated: "Opacities in the maxillary sinus as a consequence of radical sinus surgery, consistent with fibrosis." The endoscopic findings showed that no reliance could be placed on the radiologist's conclusion that the shadows on the survey film in fact actually represented "fibrosis." In only 4 of 200 patients was the maxillary sinus lumen actually absent, and indeed, complete obliteration of the sinus cavity by fibrosis appears to be a rare occurrence.

It is noteworthy how often significant changes in the mucosa of the maxillary sinus occurred, even though the inferior meatal windows were patent. A look through these windows into the maxillary sinus revealed granulation tissue, cysts, diffusely swollen mucous membranes, and a variable amount of secretions (see Figs. 11.2, 11.4, 11.7, and 11.8).

We observed repeatedly in this group of patients that the inferior turbinate had been partially or completely resected. In many cases the turbinate had been removed as far as the ostium of the nasolacrimal duct (Figs. 11.9 to 11.11). Apparently, this was supposed to have made access to the inferior meatus and creation of the window easier.

In some cases we found the window to the inferior meatus occluded by cysts. After these were punctured and collapsed, we occasionally discovered that these cysts did not originate from the wall of the maxillary sinus but apparently arose from the ethmoid and progressed through the ostium of the sinus and into the maxillary sinus itself (Fig. 11.12).

A more or less pronounced pathology in the middle meatus was a universal finding in these patients. This was particularly true in the group that had practically no maxillary sinus left.

Thus, the patient whose left inferior meatus is shown in Figure 11.13 had windows placed on two previous occasions and had also undergone two radical sinus procedures within a 2-year period. A slight, scarred recess in the inferior meatus is all that was left of the maxillary sinus. The persisting symptoms were explained on the basis of the findings in the middle meatus (Fig. 11.14) where there was evidence of a very diseased ethmoid.

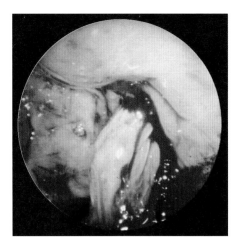

FIGURE 11.12   A view into a right maxillary sinus after a large cyst had been punctured and collapsed. It is now evident that the cyst originated in the infundibulum and the ethmoid, projecting through the natural ostium into the maxillary sinus.

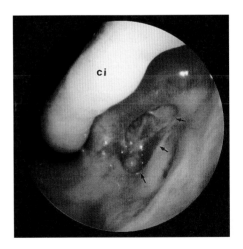

FIGURE 11.13   A left inferior meatus after two Caldwell-Luc procedures. The inferior turbinate has been partially resected. All that remains of the maxillary sinus is a shallow depression (*arrows*). ci = inferior turbinate.

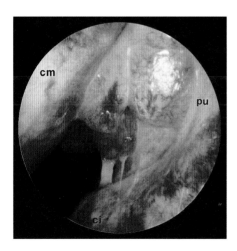

FIGURE 11.14   The view into the middle meatus of the same patient. Massive, polypoid ethmoid disease and tenaceous secretions are clearly visible. cm = middle turbinate and pu = uncinate process.

In another case, where the window had stenosed down to a 2-mm opening, a bizarre pathology was encountered in the middle meatus (Fig. 11.15). An attempt had evidently been made to remove the anterior ethmoid through a transmaxillary approach or fragments of the ethmoid had been displaced into the middle meatus by maxillary packs ultimately occluding it with scar tissue. On endoscopic repair (Fig. 11.16), severely diseased ethmoidal air cells were encountered, which had been worsened by the distorted anatomic situation combined with extensive scar formation.

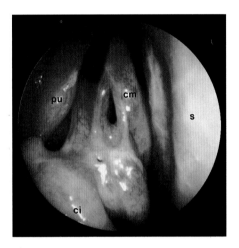

FIGURE 11.15 Bizarre anatomy of a right middle meatus after a Caldwell-Luc procedure and an apparent attempt to eradicate the ethmoid through the maxilla. The uncinate process is shifted anteriorly, the middle turbinate is fractured medially. Parts of the anterior ethmoid are shifted anteriorly and medially and fused extensively with both the middle and inferior turbinates. pu = uncinate process; cm = middle turbinate; ci = inferior turbinate; and s = septum nasi.

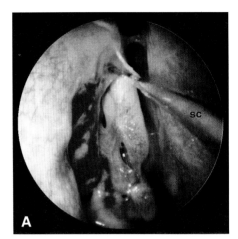

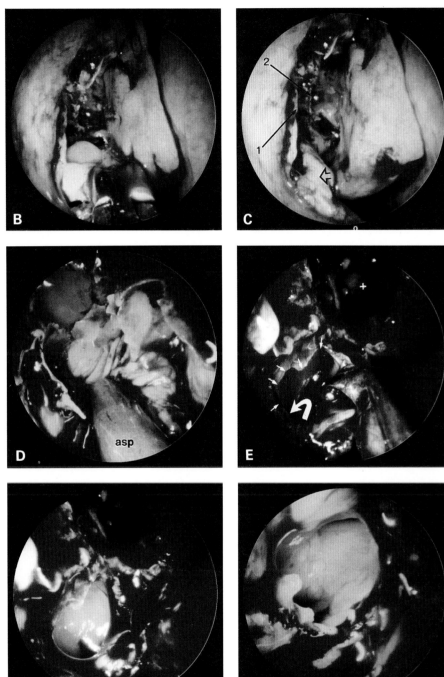

FIGURE 11.16   This sequence of photographs shows the endoscopic surgical procedure performed on the patient shown in Figure 11.15. *A,* After injecting the local anesthetic, the uncinate process is circumferentially incised. sc = sickle shaped knife. *B,* Removal of the uncinate process and its attached polyps. *C,* The view into the anterior ethmoid after removal of the uncinate process and its attached polyps. Numerous polyps can be seen emerging from the region of the maxillary sinus ostium (*open arrow*). 1 = margin of resection of the uncinate process and 2 = margin of resection of the ethmoidal bulla. *D,* After removal of the ethmoidal bulla, the diseased mucous membrane of the lateral sinus can also be removed. asp = tip of the aspirator. *E,* The ostium of the maxillary sinus is explored and carefully enlarged with the bent spoon (*arrows*). The perforation through the basal lamella can be seen in the depths. The posterior ethmoid was inspected through this perforation (+). Since the mucous membrane there did not show any appreciable changes, no further surgery was performed. *F,* The appearance after the enlargement of the maxillary sinus ostium with the bent spoon. It was possible to obtain a good view of the somewhat edematous mucosa covering the posterior wall of the maxillary sinus. *G,* The appearance of the ostium after it had been enlarged with the backbiting forceps.

Radiologic Findings

While the hallmark of the endoscopic findings in these patients was extraordinarily variable, in contrast, the tomographic findings can be described as constant. Regardless of the size or patency of the window in the inferior meatus, there was always pronounced disease in the key sites of the ethmoid with a variable degree of secondary pathology in the associated maxillary or frontal sinuses. In reviewing some of the

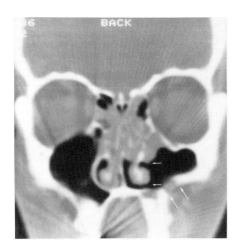

FIGURE 11.17 This is the CT scan of a patient who had persistent complaints following a left Caldwell-Luc procedure. Note the bony defects in the anterior wall of the maxillary sinus (*long arrow*). The untreated disease in the ethmoid sinuses is clearly visible. Note that the nasoantral window is patent (*shorter arrow*).

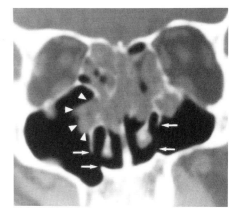

FIGURE 11.18 Note in this scan of a patient with bilateral patent inferior meatal antrostomy windows (*arrows*) the massive disease of the ethmoid with protrusion of polypoid mucosa through the infundibulum into the maxillary sinus (*arrowheads*). Courtesy of SJ Zinreich, M.D.

tomograms, one gets the impression that the affected mucous membrane literally protrudes into the maxillary sinus from the ethmoid (Figs. 11.17 and 11.18). In other tomograms, it was again apparent that relatively minor, circumscribed disease in the key sites can trigger or sustain considerable responses in the maxillary and frontal sinuses (Fig. 11.19 and 11.20). It was not the extent of the pathologic findings that was of overwhelming importance, but their location.

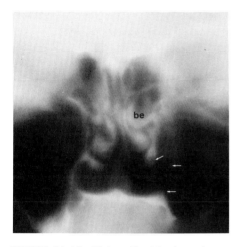

FIGURE 11.19 This patient had previously undergone bilateral inferior meatal fenestration procedures. On the right side, the inferior meatal window has closed while on the left it remained patent (*arrows*). The inferior turbinate has been partially resected bilaterally. The patient's persistent symptoms are due to untreated disease in the middle meatus. The ethmoidal bulla almost completely fills the turbinate sinuses, particularly on the left side. be = bulla ethmoidalis.

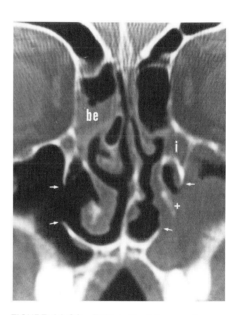

FIGURE 11.20 This patient has undergone bilateral Caldwell-Luc procedures. The windows into the inferior meatus are patent bilaterally (*arrows*). On the left, the inferior turbinate has bent across the window (+). Note the bilateral infundibular disease. On the right side the ethmoidal bulla is also involved. The ethmoidal bulla is in extensive and close contact with the middle turbinates bilaterally. be = bulla ethmoidalis and i = ethmoidal infundibulum. Courtesy of SJ Zinreich, M.D.

Secretion Transport

We were also able to repeatedly observe the phenomenon of secretion transport, as described in Chapter 2. In general, the bulk of the secretions consistently tried to avoid the fenestration window into the inferior meatus, regardless of the size of the window and instead progressed toward the natural ostium of the maxillary sinus. In some patients, however, we did observe a transport of secretions through the fenestration window. Normally these were associated with those "secretion pathways" that had their natural course toward the center of the window. All of the other secretion pathways went around the window and joined the secretions going toward the natural ostium (see Chapter 2).

When the secretions were plentiful and the mucus transportation system was easily observed, the amount of the secretions that passed into the inferior meatus through the fenestration window represented only a negligible fraction of the total secretions.

Naturally, secretions can *pour* through the window into the inferior meatus. If there is an excess of secretions, these may flow or slide by gravity and following the suction created by the inspired air into the inferior meatus through the window. This could be well seen when there was extensive infection in the maxillary sinus. As shown in Figures 11.21 and 11.22, purulent secretions are transported primarily to the natural ostium of the maxillary sinus, even though it is constricted by inflammation. Since these secretions cannot pass through the ostium, they accumulate around the natural ostium to slip back to the floor of the maxillary sinus, from whence some of them slide out through the artificial window into the inferior meatus. The secretions adhering to the mucosa, or those freshly produced, are again transported toward the ostium. We also observed that during the Valsalva maneuver, pus can be squeezed back into the maxillary sinus from the infundibulum.

In those cases where unusually large windows permitted a good view into the maxillary sinus, we attempted to study the movement of the secretions. We first placed a drop of blood on the floor of the sinus and then observed the transportation of secretions as described above. The majority of the secretions bypassed the window and were carried in the direction of the natural ostium. Even when the drop of blood was placed directly on the edge of the artificial window, the direction of transport was *into* the maxillary sinus and in the direction of the natural ostium. The amount of secretions carried to the outside remained small by comparison. When the windows were extremely large, we could observe the entry of secretions *into* the maxillary sinus, as described above (Figs. 11.23 and 11.24). Clear or turbid

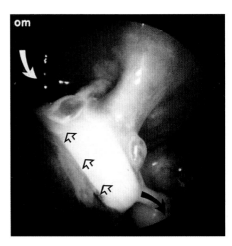

FIGURE 11.21 The transportation of pathologic secretions in the direction (*open arrows*) of the natural ostium (*curved white arrow*) in a right maxillary sinus following a fenestration procedure. Only a portion of the purulent secretions slide into the inferior meatus, through the antrostomy window (*black arrow*).

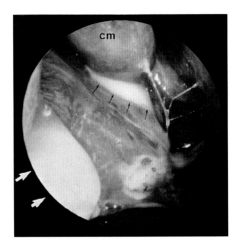

FIGURE 11.22 A view into the inferior meatus and nasal cavity on the right side of the same patient. The inferior turbinate is almost completely absent. Purulent secretions are seen sliding through the window into the inferior meatus (*double arrow*). The pathway of pus from the middle meatus to the nasopharynx is clearly visible (*small black arrows*). cm = middle turbinate.

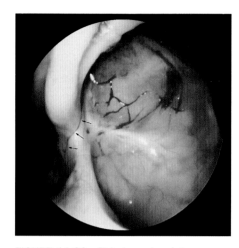

FIGURE 11.23 This is a view into an inferior meatus which has an extremely wide antrostomy window. Blood introduced into the maxillary sinus is carried primarily to the natural ostium. Only a small amount of the blood leaves the maxillary sinus through the artificial antrostomy window (*small black arrows*).

viscous secretions passed through the window into the maxillary sinus and were carried in the direction of the natural ostium.

Only when an *excessive amount* of blood was injected, did it flow out through the artificial window (Fig. 11.25). In about 12 percent of the cases in which the maxillary sinus was examined endoscopically, there was either no transportation of secretions or only unsatisfactory secretion transport. The markers either did not move at all during the observation period or the secretion pathway bypassed the natural ostium and accumulated in the maxilloethmoidal recess or on the floor of the maxillary sinus. We could not tell whether all of these observed behavior patterns were due to artifacts (e.g., the heat of the endoscope light) or the result of structural damage to the mucous membranes or perhaps to dyskinesia of the cilia. Individual mucosal biopsies showed some of the ciliary changes described in Chapter 5. It is obvious, however, that single biopsies are not necessarily representative, particularly in electronmicroscopic studies.

Following endoscopic therapy, there were no more secondary failures in the group with transportation abnormalities than in the remainder of the patients. This result suggests that in most cases the observed dysfunctions were reversible.

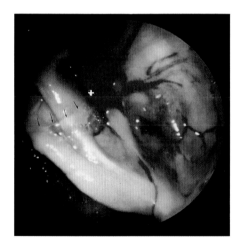

FIGURE 11.24 This is a view with a 90 degree lens into the maxillary sinus shown in Figure 11.23. The principal direction of the transportation of the bloodstained secretions to the natural ostium (+) is easily visible. The *small black arrows* point to a tenacious ribbon of secretions that is carried *into* the maxillary sinus through the artificial window and then up to the natural ostium. The upper edge of the maxillary sinus window can be seen running from 9 o'clock to 5 o'clock.

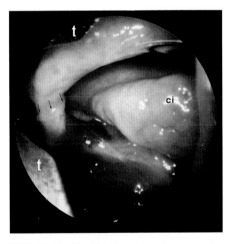

FIGURE 11.25 This is a view through the canine fossa into a right maxillary sinus. When excess blood is introduced, it *flows* through the artificial window into the inferior meatus. Note, that despite the presence of the wide window, the mucosa on the floor of the maxillary sinus is inflamed and discolored. The *thin black arrows* point to a viscous ribbon of secretions that is being transported into the maxillary sinus from the inferior meatus. ci = concha inferior.

Conclusions

What conclusions can be drawn from these findings? The first conclusion is that when fenestration or Caldwell-Luc procedures do not provide the expected results and when the symptoms that led to the procedure persist or promptly recur, there is a high probability that the underlying process is disease of one of the key sites of the ethmoid. These patients should undergo a diagnostic endoscopy and paranasal sinus tomography.

In those cases where the operative report of the previous procedure was available, another curious fact became apparent. Those procedures described as radical Caldwell-Luc or de Lima procedures frequently *did not* fulfill the postulates of these authors. In most cases the maxillary sinus was opened from the vestibulum oris in the canine fossa. Either the entire mucosa was removed or only the most severely affected parts. A window was then created in the inferior meatus, packing was inserted, and the facial wall of the maxillary sinus was again closed, even though Caldwell-Luc, de Lima, and Boenninghaus, Sr., all stated in their publications that the affected parts of the ethmoid should be included in the procedure. According to these authors the "middle and posterior" ethmoid had to be approached through the maxilla and the anterior ethmoid through the nose as part of the general procedure. Zinreich and Kennedy, in a similar study also found that the results of maxillary sinus operations were statistically significantly better when there was some kind of ethmoid procedure performed at the same time.

When approaching the anterior ethmoid by the transmaxillary route, the following considerations must be kept in mind. If the ethmoid is opened from the maxillary sinus and if there are Haller's cells developed at the floor of the orbit above the ostium of the maxillary sinus, these are usually entered first. The route of the procedure then leads toward the roof of the ethmoid and through the basal lamella into the posterior ethmoid. The most anterior portion of the ethmoid, however, primarily the frontal recess and the ethmoidal infundibulum are extremely difficult to approach from this direction, since the anatomic configuration mandates that the approach be "backwards and around a corner." Thus, pathologic changes in these fissures can be missed easily.

In some cases another observation could be made, but its clinical significance is not yet entirely clear. It is apparently a common practice to fracture the inferior turbinate medially and superiorly to facilitate the fenestration of the inferior meatus. If the fracture line of the inferior turbinate is lateral to the insertion of the uncinate process, the medial displacement of the inferior turbinate pushes the uncinate process laterally. This further narrows or occludes the infundibulum (Fig. 11.26) and hardly serves to improve the physiology of the maxillary sinus.

The complaints persisting after a Caldwell-Luc procedure or fenestration usually bear no relationship to the size and patency of the window in the inferior meatus or to the degree of persisting maxillary sinus pathology. There was no distinction in the frequency, intensity, or type of complaints between those patients with patent windows and those in whom the window was occluded. The time of symptom recurrence also gave no clear indication as to the patency of the window. The symptoms did, however, correlate well with pathology in the ethmoid. The correlation was considerably stronger with the location of the pathology than with its extent, and thus it was the site of the disease that correlated well with the patients' symptoms.

We do not say this to decrease or deny the importance of fenestration or Caldwell-Luc procedures in the management of chronic sinusitis in special cases. If, however, the patient's symptoms persist or recur postoperatively, then a more precise exploration of the middle meatus and the lateral wall of the nose must follow. Since we were able to identify and treat the underlying pathology in this region in most cases, it would seem that there are few indications for a radical surgical procedure as the first step in the surgical management of the maxillary or frontal sinus. Based on our more recent experience, we believe that most of those patients whom we previously treated with fenestration procedures in order to cure their maxillary sinusitis, could be successfully treated today without any surgical intervention. We can now achieve complete cures in most cases by a goal-oriented direct medical therapy of the key sites in the lateral wall of the nose (see Chapter 6).

We occasionally still perform fenestration procedures in those cases where highly viscous secretions are produced that can no longer be transported by the mucous membranes and that cannot pass through a wide window into the middle meatus. In these cases it may be advantageous to have a window through which the secretions can be removed by suction. This approach is satisfactory in some patients with diffuse polypoid rhinosinopathy, cystic fibrosis, and/or highly viscous secretions of unknown etiology. In these cases, the fenestration facilitates management, but it does not resolve the underlying problem.

Today we perform maxillary sinus operations (other than for invasive disease and neoplasms) for only two indications: in aspergillosis with abundant hard mycotic concretions that can not be removed through the middle meatus and in those patients who were subjected to previous surgery (see Chapter 6).

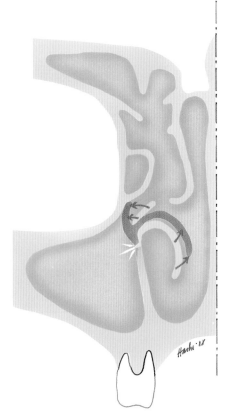

FIGURE 11.26 This is a schematic representation of the potential infundibular obstruction that can be caused by a lateral displacement of the uncinate process following out-fracture of the inferior turbinate. For details, see text.

Surgical Therapy

When a disease of the ethmoid is identified as the cause of persistent symptoms, therapy follows the principles of endoscopic surgery as discussed previously. The purpose is to promote the healing of diseased segments of the ethmoid and to reestablish ventilation and drainage through the physiologic pathways.

In those patients whose disease has been present for months or even years, additional problems may be encountered. There may be conditions in which the entire mucous membrane may, as the result of chronic purulent infection, have undergone inflammatory or granulomatous changes and massive exudation (see Fig. 11.22). In the coronal CT scan, there may be a thickening of the delicate bony structures and of the walls of the maxillary sinus. These indicate the presence of a periosteitis or osteitis of the respective structures. Every attempt should be made in these patients to improve their medical condition preoperatively by administering a carefully planned antibiotic regimen. In those cases where the infection is caused by hard to manage pathogens (e.g., *Pseudomonas*, *Proteus*, and some strains of *Staphylococcus*) we treat the patient for up to 2 or 3 weeks with high dose intravenous antibiotics. This therapy is maintained postoperatively for several days at which time the patient is switched to oral antibiotics. The addition of a steroid has proven beneficial in a few patients.

When there are marked polypoid or granulomatous changes in the maxillary sinus, we try to remove them. In many cases this can be accomplished through the window in the inferior meatus.

As previously discussed, the changes wrought by previous surgery can make endoscopic procedures very difficult. Postoperative scarring or synechia may have plastered the inferior or middle turbinate to the septum or against the lateral wall of the nose. The olfactory fissure may be largely obliterated by scars or granulation tissue and in the absence of anatomic landmarks, such as the middle turbinate (see Figs. 11.15 and 11.16), orientation may become very difficult. It is therefore critical to have a recent tomogram in previously operated patients. Under no circumstances should the clinical observations made *prior to the previous operation* be relied upon, and even a detailed operative report describing the last surgical procedure is also unsatisfactory in this regard. Primary attention must be directed toward tissue loss and scar formation in the area of the ethmoid and of the lamina papyracea.

There are three possible approaches that may be helpful in avoiding injury to the orbit during exploratory probing in cases where coarse scar tissue prevents identification of the natural ostium and the fontanelles in the middle meatus.

1. Palpation of the lateral wall of the nose immediately above the insertion of the inferior turbinate. This usually prevents advancing the probe too far superiorly (see Chapter 7).

2. If the inferior turbinate is absent, or if the ostium simply cannot be identified, an endoscope can be passed into the maxillary sinus through the canine fossa or through a persisting window in the inferior meatus and the palpating probe can be guided visually from within the maxillary sinus. The bulge created by the probe on the medial wall of the maxillary sinus can usually be seen very clearly and this area can then be perforated with safety.

3. If there is a patent window in the inferior meatus, a bent spoon can be introduced through this window and gently pushed medially and superiorly. The small bulges produced by this maneuver can be seen in the middle meatus. The spoon pressing from within the maxillary sinus allows the surgeon to identify the wall of the sinus accurately and permits the placement of an appropriate incision.

We are reluctant to perform maxillary sinus endoscopy, even in the presence of the appropriate indications in those patients who have developed an infraorbital nerve neuralgia following radical maxillary sinus surgery. If maxillary sinus endoscopy is essential in these patients, we prefer an approach through the inferior meatus in order not to further traumatize the canine fossa.

There have been some cases where there was a surprising improvement in the neuralgia following recovery from the ethmoid disease. This has occurred even in patients in whom we assumed the symptoms to be clearly because of an irritation of the infraorbital nerve and therefore not reversible. Because there are no signs that can be used to predict such an improvement, we always tell the patient that while they may count on an improvement in nasal breathing, secretions, and the sensation of pressure between, above, and behind the eyes, that the symptoms produced by irritation of the infraorbital nerve will in all likelihood persist.

In severe cases of infraorbital nerve neuralgia, we inform the patient about the option of surgical neurolysis of the infraorbital nerve, but we also indicate that even this procedure does not guarantee improvement and that no odds for success can be given.

As discussed in more detail in Chapter 13, there are unfortunately still a number of patients who cannot be helped with our present pharmacologic or surgical armamentaria. This group includes: most commonly those patients with ASA sensitive, diffuse polypoid rhinosinopathy, and for this reason this group has been excluded from the present study. ASA sensitive, diffuse polypoid rhinosinopathy cannot be cured by a "functional" microscopic or endoscopic surgery or even by extensive radical procedures, and consequently, in this group of patients, we feel justified in recommending a conservative approach. Since in these patients, even radical surgery will not guarantee a good result, the trauma, morbidity and specific postoperative problems will be significantly less after endoscopic surgery. Endoscopic surgery is the more sparing and sensible procedure, particularly in view of the great probability of the need for subsequent surgical procedures.

MYCOSES

In recent years, there has been a world-wide increase in the reported incidence of mycotic infections of the nose and paranasal sinuses. This increased incidence is probably the result of two factors: improved diagnostic methods, which enable more frequent recognition, and an increase in those factors that predispose to fungal infections. These include: diabetes, a decrease in the defense mechanisms of the body, radiation or chemotherapy for malignancy, immunosuppressive therapy, long-term antibiotic and steroid therapy, and immuno-deficiency diseases, such as AIDS. Many reports indicate, however, that mycotic infections of the paranasal sinuses occur most commonly in otherwise perfectly healthy individuals. This observation suggests the presence of some *local factor that favors the development of paranasal sinus mycosis.*

In addition to those minor cases in which fungal growth occurs only in crusted secretions or around indwelling feeding tubes, there are, more frequently, mycotic invasions of excoriated mucosal surfaces, e.g., malignancies during or after radiation. In cases of mycotic encrustations, therapy can usually be limited to symptomatic management. A careful removal of the crust with oily nose drops is usually sufficient. The mucosa underneath the mycotic crusts must be carefully examined, since even minimal changes may indicate a specific pathologic process, or even an underlying malignancy (e.g., malignant lymphoma, nasopharyngeal carcinoma, Wegener's granulomatosis, etc.) and *must not* be ignored (Figs. 11.27 to 11.30).

Mycotic invasion of the paranasal sinuses seems to be much more common than previously suspected. In the patient population of the ENT clinic at Graz University, almost 10 percent of all patients requiring surgical management for sinusitis had a mycotic etiology. There are about 35 new cases each year and the principal pathogen is *Aspergillus fumigatus* (Table 11.1, p. 425).

Even though the majority of ENT mycotic infections in our area are secondary saprophytic and noninvasive infections, there are also some

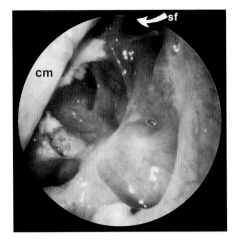

FIGURE 11.27 This is a view into a left middle meatus, 6 weeks after endoscopic ethmoid surgery. The mucosa is generally healthy, but there is obvious fungal growth on the crusted secretions. This patient was on long term therapy with a steroid aerosol. Culture revealed a mixed fungal infection with *A. fumigatus* and *Candida.* cm = middle turbinate and sf = frontal sinus.

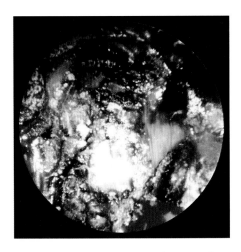

FIGURE 11.28 *Aspergillus niger* growing on top of a squamous cell carcinoma in a left maxillary sinus.

cases with severe complications and occasionally even a fatal outcome.

Orbital complications with destruction of bone and retrobulbar invasion, fungal meningitis with a potentially fatal outcome, osteomyelitis with complete destruction of the maxilla, involvement of the CNS with mycotic granuloma formation, and subarachnoid hemorrhages from mycotic aneurysms have been described.

Our knowledge concerning the dangers inherent in the toxins produced by fungi is limited. The aflatoxins produced by some species of *Aspergillus* are highly carcinogenic to the liver, even in minute quantities. They are also (as shown in animal studies) potentially teratogenic and mutagenic.

Penicillic acid produced by some species of *Penicillium* also has carcinogenic properties. Sterigmatocystine, produced by *Aspergillus versicolor* can produce carcinoma and liver tumors in experimental animals.

There is increasing evidence that some mycotoxins, such as gliotoxin, can be produced by all species of *Aspergillus* in man. These mycotoxins seem to be capable of producing both local reactions and systemic effects (including immunosuppression).

In our patients we have seen several cases of optic nerve neuritis, paralysis of the extrinsic eye muscles, and even total ophthalmoplegia in noninvasive paranasal sinus mycosis. We have no explanation for these occurrences, other than the possibility that these may be caused by mycotoxins.

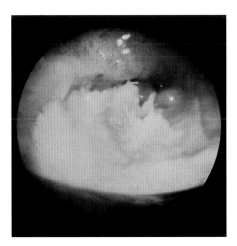

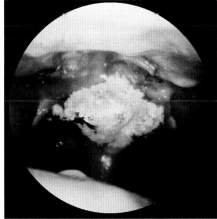

FIGURE 11.29 In a left maxillary sinus, a squamous cell carcinoma heavily super-infected by *Candida*. The tumor had already invaded the entire lateral wall of the nose.

FIGURE 11.30 *Candida* growing on top of a carcinoma in the nasopharynx. Courtesy of R Jakse, University ENT-Hospital, Graz.

After elimination of the mycosis, these symptoms disappeared without any additional therapy.

In view of the large number of fungi that are pathogenic in man, the number of species encountered as pathogens in the paranasal sinuses is relatively small. In Europe and North America the *Aspergillus* species predominate, particularly *A. fumigatus*.

The next most frequent groups are the mucormycoses and candida. Case reports of ear, nose, and throat infections caused by *Cladosporium, Alternaria, Penicillium,* and *Fusarium* are rare, and ENT diseases caused by *Petriellidium boydii* and *Paecilomyces* species are even less common.

Because of the importance and increasing frequency of *Aspergillus* mycoses in our area, this clinical entity is discussed in detail, especially since noninvasive mycotic infections can be diagnosed and treated endoscopically.

Aspergillosis of the Paranasal Sinuses

The first case of aspergillosis of the nose and paranasal sinuses was reported by Schubert in 1885. By 1972, Kecht had assembled from the world literature a total of 98 cases of aspergillosis of the ear, nose, and throat. The incidence of mycotic infections of the paranasal sinuses has increased over the past decade. At the ENT clinic of Graz University, between 1976 and 1989 more than 340 patients most of whom had severe mycotic infections of the nose and paranasal sinuses were treated. More than 90 percent of these mycotic infections were caused by *Aspergillus* (primarily *A. fumigatus*) (see Fig. 11.31).

This increasing incidence may be attributed to a variety of causes. In addition to better diagnostic capabilities and an increase in predisposing factors, e.g., long-term and repeated antibiotic therapy, local predisposing factors are also important. These local predisposing factors include: chronic recurrent sinusitis, increased exposure to spore-containing air, contact with contaminated food, domestic pets, potting soil, and some textiles. We also suspect that aberrant dental or root canal filling materials may have an etiologic or supporting role in mycotic infections of the paranasal sinuses.

Aspergillus fumigatus: Ecology and Physiology

Aspergillus fumigatus (Fresenius, 1863) is a mycelial fungus that is present as a saprophyte, primarily on decaying organic material. *Aspergillus fumigatus* is abundant in potting soil, and food is frequently contaminated with this fungus. The "mold" on old bread or marmalade is frequently *A. fumigatus* as is the mold found on damp walls.

Many species of *Aspergillus* are capable of decomposing organic substances in nature, especially those with a high osmotic pressure as found in substances that have a high sugar content. This may be the reason diabetic patients have a higher incidence of mycotic infections.

The hyphae of *Aspergillus* grow longitudinally in the apical zones of growth. The tubular hyphae that are formed by *A. fumigatus* have a characteristic 45 degree Y-shaped division. Chitin and cellulose in the cell wall of this fungus provide mechanical stability, and explain the resistance of this fungus to antibiotics. A genetically linked tendency for marked rhythmic growth periods produces a reproducible and characteristic colonization pattern in fungal cultures, which is used to identify the fungus.

Because of the centrifugal, and longitudinal growth pattern, cultures grown on a suitable laboratory culture medium are always more or less circular in shape. When growing on tissue with low resistance or within a sinus cavity, aspergillosis may assume a globular shape (fungus ball). In vivo, the structure of the fungal growth is affected by the surrounding anatomic configuration and by inflammatory or other host reactions. In mycotic infections of the sinuses, the tendency to form a fungus ball is common.

In 1973, Messerklinger and Eggeman coined the term "fungal concretions" to describe the dense, hard and frequently friable, fungal masses in the paranasal sinuses.

The mass of fungal hyphae is termed the mycelia. We must distinguish between vegetative and nonvegetative mycelia. The vegetative mycelia sit directly on the surface of the mucosa in mucous membrane mycosis and ingest nutrients from the surface of the mucous membrane. Special hyphae may protrude into the host tissues or into secretions (pus) and draw dissolved nutritional elements from them. Because *A. fumigatus* lacks keratolytic properties, it can not invade intact skin or mucous membranes, unless the surface has been damaged.

The nonvegetative mycelia of the fungus consist of numerous hyphae that are grouped in parallel bundles and are known as conidia. Particularly dense bundles can separate from the mycelium and survive for years under unfavorable environmental conditions, such as cold, dryness, and lack of nutrients. When the environment becomes more favorable, the fungus can develop active mycelia from these conidia.

The persistent nonvegetative mycelia may be hidden together with the active vegetative fungal masses behind the brown-black, variably firm crusts that the patient may sneeze out or that may be rinsed out of the maxillary sinus by irrigation.

Aspergillus fumigatus does not require light for growth, since it lacks chlorophyll, it does however, need a host to supply the elements necessary for the synthesis of its cellular components. *A. fumigatus* requires glucose, nitrogen, sulfur, phosphorus, potassium, calcium, and trace elements, e.g., magnesium, iron, and zinc as catalysts. The most favorable environment for fungal growth is mildly acidic.

These are precisely the conditions encountered by the fungus within the paranasal sinuses in chronic sinusitis. The presence of pathologic secretions in viral or bacterial superinfection in combination with the genetically determined growth rhythm of the fungus produces a periodic growth of peripherally oriented fungal hyphae. This gives the fungal mass the characteristic onion-like appearance on histologic sections (Fig. 11.31).

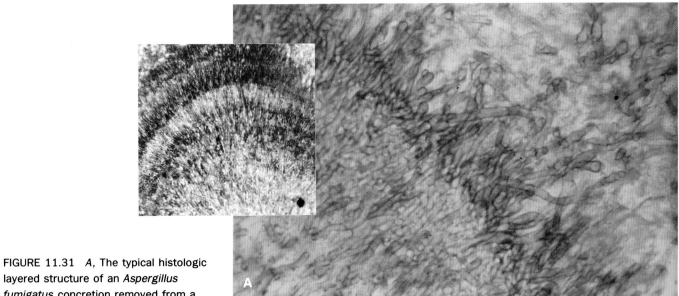

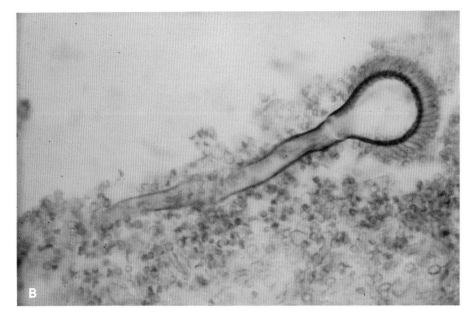

FIGURE 11.31 *A*, The typical histologic layered structure of an *Aspergillus fumigatus* concretion removed from a maxillary sinus (histologic section). Each "layer" corresponds to a period of growth. PAS-stain, magnification: 160 ×; insert: survey magnification: 25 ×. *B* and *C*, A higher power view of *A. fumigatus* showing the fruiting heads covered by multiple spores. H and E-stain, magnification: 400 ×. *D*, Necrotic and partially lysed fungal hyphae from the center of a maxillary sinus concretion. Note the clearly visible deposits of calcium. PAS-stain, magnification: 250 ×. *E*, Thickened, inflamed paranasal sinus mucous membrane with a mass of *Aspergillus* adherent to its surface. Note the interwoven and tangled mycelia. PAS-stain, magnification: 180 ×.

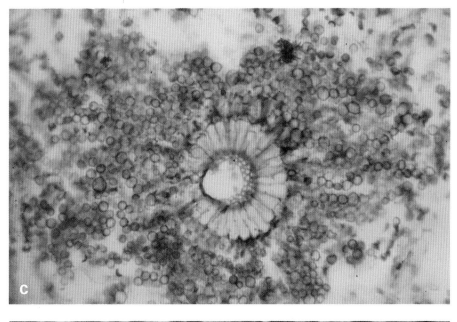

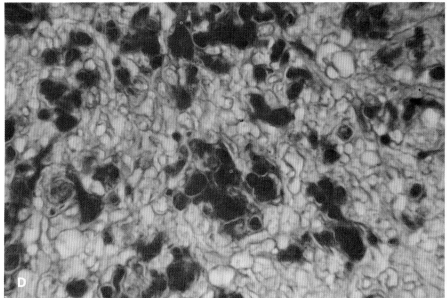

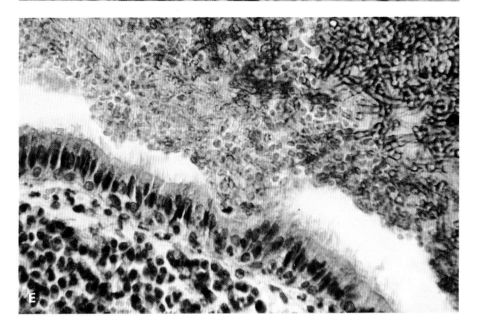

Clinical Picture

Clinically, noninvasive *Aspergillus* sinus infections present as chronic, recurring sinusitis. The symptoms, namely facial pain, headaches, a feeling of pressure between or above the eyes, obstructed nasal breathing, toothache, maxillary pain, nasopharyngeal drip, and occasionally fetor oris do not point specifically toward a mycotic infection. Rhinoscopy only reveals significant findings in the nose or choanae only after the mycotic mass has partially destroyed the lateral wall of the nose and become visible in the middle meatus (Figs. 11.32 and 11.33).

More significant than the general symptoms of sinusitis is a complaint about "feeling a foreign body" in the nose, or a report that friable masses, crusts or scabs were expelled by a sneeze. The crusts, and the secretions attached to them frequently have a foul odor. Occasionally a "moldy" odor is reported.

A mycotic infection should be suspected when patients have undergone repeated punctures and irrigations because of maxillary sinusitis and the irrigations were negative, difficult to perform because of resistance to pressure, or contained small amounts of crumbly, friable secretions.

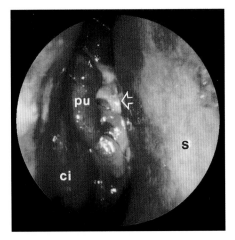 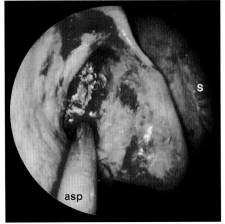

FIGURE 11.32 In this right middle meatus, masses of *A. fumigatus*, which have largely destroyed the lateral wall of the nose, can be seen advanced medially and filling the entire infundibulum. The fungal mass has eroded through the uncinate process, and is now visible between the lateral nasal wall and the septum (*arrow*). The remaining mucosa of the remnants of the uncinate process are engorged with inflammatory polyps. pu = uncinate process; ci = inferior turbinate; and s = septum nasi.

FIGURE 11.33 Note the concretion of *A. fumigatus* in this preoperative picture of a right middle meatus. The uncinate process has been injected with local anesthetic and the polypoid, hyperplastic mucosa of the head of the middle turbinate is being displaced medially by the aspirator. asp = aspirator and s = septum nasi.

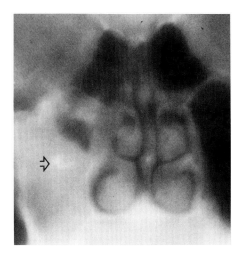

FIGURE 11.34 This is a conventional tomogram of a patient with an *A. fumigatus* fungal infection of the right maxillary sinus. Note the marked opacification of the sinus and the areas of varying radiopacity. In the central portion of the sinus there are areas of marked radiopacity, which resemble calcification (*arrow*).

Radiographic Diagnosis

In severe mycosis of the maxillary sinus, the affected sinus is usually homogeneously opaque. Occasionally, a crescent shaped air space can be identified between the fungal mass and the roof of the maxillary sinus (Figs. 11.34, 11.35, and 11.36). Approximately 50 percent of patients with *Aspergillus* mycosis show an extremely dense, circumscribed shadow, which has the appearance of a foreign body or even of a piece of metal. Occasionally, granular opaque areas are seen or there may be several pea-sized areas of increased density that are frequently misinterpreted by the radiologist as metallic, radiopaque foreign bodies, pieces of metal, aberrant dental fillings, or posttraumatic foreign bodies. At times, these changes can be recognized in the plain radiographs. At other times they can only be seen in one or two sections of a tomogram or CT scan.

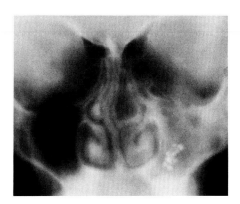

FIGURE 11.35 This is a conventional tomogram of a patient who has an *Aspergillus* mycosis of the left maxillary sinus. Note the granular appearing radiodense areas within the homogeneous opacified sinus. The ethmoid infundibulum is blocked, and there is a large concha bullosa of the left middle turbinate.

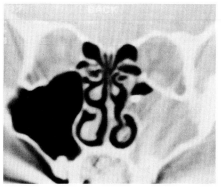

FIGURE 11.36 This is a CT of a patient who has an *Aspergillus* infection of the left maxillary sinus. The sinus is almost completely opacified with only a small apical crescent of air remaining. Note the almost metallic radiodense, lentil-sized concretion at the level of the posterior fontanelle.

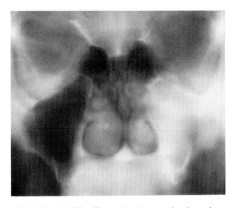

FIGURE 11.37 The clearly marked variations in radio density in this opacified left maxillary sinus are typical of *Aspergillus* mycosis.

If the presence of a foreign body can be excluded by history, then these radiopaque areas are almost pathognomonic of an *Aspergillus* infection. In the central, necrotic area of the mycotic mass calcium salts may crystalize out and establish a radiopaque area. The fungus, having a great affinity for metallic salts, may deposit heavy metals in this area. These contribute further to the radiopacity. Metals from aberrant dental fillings may also be incorporated and even pieces of dental filling materials may also be found in these radiopaque zones. Even when there are no radiopaque densities, there are typically "high and low density" areas in the affected paranasal sinus (Figs. 11.34 to 11.39).

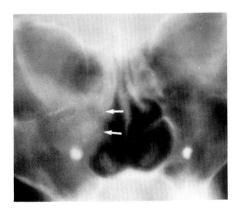

FIGURE 11.38 Bilateral *A. fumigatus* mycosis, with obvious radiopaque concretions. The lateral wall of the nose appears to have been destroyed in the area of the right uncinate process (*arrows*).

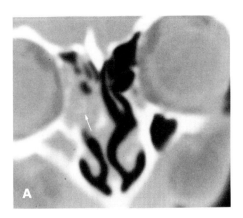

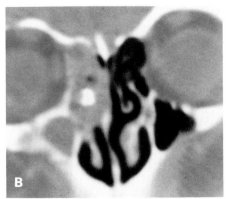

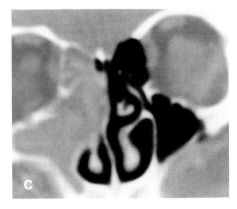

FIGURE 11.39 *A*, Severe aspergillosis of a right ethmoid and maxillary sinus. The bony details can no longer be identified in the anterior ethmoid. The *arrow* points to a mycotic concrement that is much more clearly seen in *B*. *B*, Note the now clearly visible radiodense concretion in the anterior ethmoid. *C*, There is a massive opacification of the entire ethmoid and maxillary sinus areas. Note the destruction of the bony septa and the areas of varying radiodensity. Radiographs like this can easily be misdiagnosed as a malignancy.

Definite evidence of a fungal infection may be provided by magnetic resonance imaging (MRI). In all other inflammatory diseases, the signal intensity of the paranasal sinus contents is definitely intensified in the T2-weighted studies. In mycotic disease of the paranasal sinuses, the mycotic mass appears as an optically empty space in the T2-weighted image (Figs. 11.40 and 11.41). This is primarily because of the calcium and metal deposits in the mycotic masses.

In the radiographic differential diagnosis, true foreign bodies, rhinoliths, and especially neoplasms must be excluded. Owing to its ability to destroy bony tissues by pressure and inflammatory reactions, a fungus can radiographically mimic neoplastic expansion with destruction and invasion (see Figs. 11.38 and 11.39).

FIGURE 11.40 *A*, The right maxillary sinus in this T1-weighted MRI image of a patient with *A. fumigatus* mycosis appears to be almost homogeneously opacified. *B*, In the horizontal, T2-weighted image, the periphery of the maxillary sinus demonstrates increased signal intensity, while the center appears to be almost optically empty (+). The increased signal intensity corresponds to inflamed mucosa or free secretions. The optically empty space corresponds to the mycotic concretion (for details, see text).

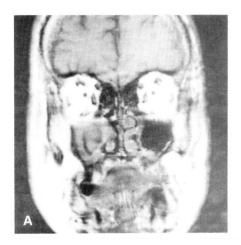
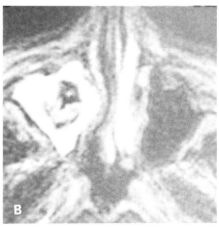

FIGURE 11.41 *A*, An MR-sequence in a patient with a cherry-sized mycotic concretion surrounded by an empyema. In the T1-weighted image, there is a homogeneous opacification of the maxillary sinus. *B*, In the T2-weighted image, there is an increased signal intensity in the area of the empyema and inflamed mucosa. The fungal ball lying in the maxilloethmoid angle appears optically empty (+).

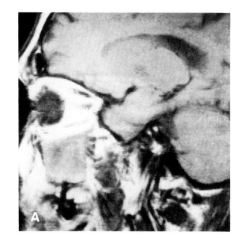
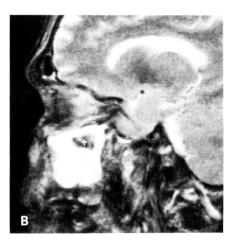

The maxillary sinus and the anterior ethmoid are by far the most frequently involved areas. Less commonly, the mycotic process may extend to involve the posterior ethmoid, the sphenoid sinus, or even the frontal sinus. Isolated involvement of any one of the paranasal sinuses is also possible (Figs. 11.42 and 11.43).

FIGURE 11.42 *A*, An air-fluid fluid level in a left frontal sinus. *B*, Note, how the radiopaque concretions of *Aspergillus* mycosis have become visible (*arrows*) in this cut 4 mm further posterior.

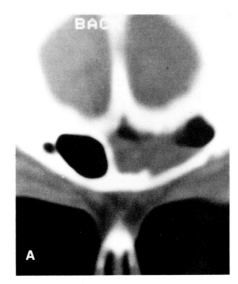
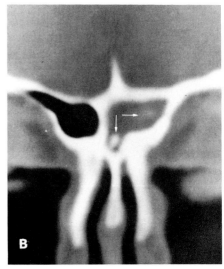

FIGURE 11.43 This is an example of an isolated fungal infection (*A. fumigatus*) in a left sphenoid sinus (*white arrows*). Endoscopic surgery was performed without any difficulty, even though the fungus had partially eroded the bony internal carotid artery canal (*black arrow*).

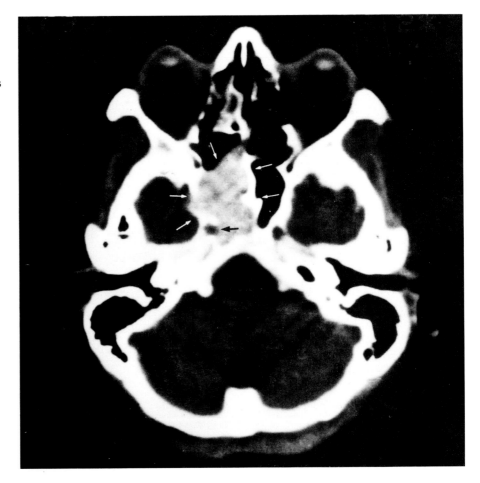

Endoscopic Diagnosis

A mycotic infection of the maxillary sinus can be diagnosed by maxillary sinuscopy through the canine fossa. The entire maxillary sinus may be filled or even tightly packed by a mass ranging in consistency from soft and buttery to friable and hard. There may be a central, smaller mycotic concretion, surrounded by purulent secretions or small, distinct mycotic concretions. The latter are usually found in the maxilloethmoid angle or in the ostium of the maxillary sinus. The mucous membrane lining the sinus may show massive polypoid changes or it may appear unremarkable if there is no inflammation. The color of the fungal mass may vary from whitish-yellow to dirty-brown or grayish-black (Figs. 11.44 to 11.47).

Occasionally mycotic concretions may be found in the hiatus semilunaris (see Figs. 11.32 and 11.33), particularly in cases where the lateral wall of the nose has already been destroyed. A biopsy of the mycotic mass and of the adjacent mucous membrane must always be obtained.

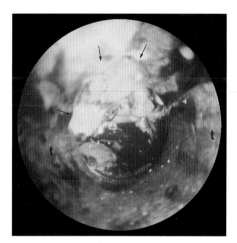

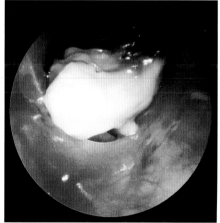

FIGURE 11.44   Right maxillary sinus endoscopy. The entire maxillary sinus is filled with buttery masses of *A. fumigatus* (*arrows*) mycosis. t = trocar sheath.

FIGURE 11.45   In this view into a right maxillary sinus, a cherry-sized fungal ball is seen in the maxilloethmoid angle. The mucosa of the sinus appears relatively normal. The fungal ball has been rotated with the trocar in order to demonstrate the layer of pus present at the site of contact of the concretion with the mucosa. In other areas, the concrement appeared to be dry.

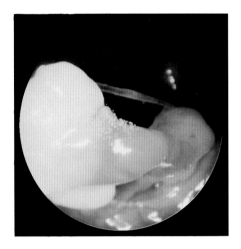

FIGURE 11.46 Fungal growth (*A. fumigatus*) on top of antibiotic ointment introduced after maxillary sinus irrigation.

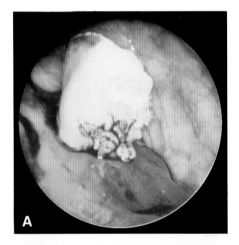

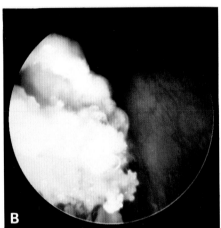

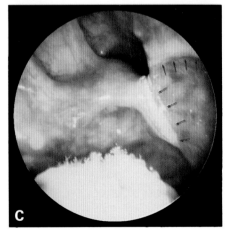

FIGURE 11.47 *A*, Note the cherry-sized fungal ball lying on top of the edematous mucosa on the floor of this right maxillary sinus. *B*, The mycelia of the fungal growth are more clearly seen in this closer view. *C*, While the ostium of the maxillary sinus was patent, it was too small for the passage of the concretion. The transportation of spores and other fungal debris can be seen clearly traveling along the secretion pathways (*arrows*).

Histologic Diagnosis

The specimen of the mycotic material can be processed in the same routine fashion as a mucous membrane biopsy. It is readily fixed, dehydrated, embedded, and stained, and special techniques are unnecessary. The fungal mycelia, the branching hyphae, the fruiting bodies, and the spores can be readily identified in the sectioned material with hematoxylin-eosin stain, although the PAS (periodic acid-Schiff) stain provides more dramatic color (Fig. 11.31).

Fungal Cultures

Unfixed fungal material should be cultured immediately, as delay increases the danger of drying and thus failure of the culture to grow. Beerwort, Sabouraud's, and Czapek's agar are recommended as culture media. Because it can take a long time for the colonies to grow in culture, incubation at 37°C must be maintained for up to 14 days. Not uncommonly, the biopsy material does not produce fungal growth, or only opportunistic fungal colonies develop. Since aspergillosis can be easily diagnosed by histology, a two-pronged diagnostic approach of both culture and histology should be followed.

Since aspergillosis is usually noninvasive, a definitive diagnosis can only be obtained from material taken from the lumen of the paranasal sinus. If only the inflammatory mucosa is examined histologically, no evidence of mycosis is likely to be found. The material recovered from the maxillary sinus should not be written off as "detritus" or as "crumbly secretions," "inspissated empyema," or "caseous material," but it must be both cultured and examined histologically.

Clinical Course and Complications

In our area, *Aspergillus* infections of the sinuses are usually noninvasive saprophytic secondary infections, although there are a few case reports of severe and even fatal complications. In addition to these noninvasive surface infections, there is also an invasive (visceral) form that may take a fulminating course, particularly in patients with decreased resistance. Orbital invasion with resultant blindness, invasion and destruction of the skull base with a fungal meningitis, and *Aspergillus* osteomyelitis with complete destruction of the maxilla have all been reported. If the central nervous system becomes involved, space occupying, intracranial aspergillomas and intracranial hemorrhages from mycotic aneurysms are the most dreaded complications. The dangers of an invasive aspergillosis in patients with decreased resistance are illustrated by some cancer patients who, following radiation therapy, died of invasive aspergillosis and not from their underlying malignancy. It has only been recently demonstrated that *Aspergillus* can produce a fungal toxin, gliotoxin, in vivo, which has a definite immunosuppressant activity.

Therapy

In those patients who have a surface growth of fungus on crusted secretions, it is usually sufficient to remove the nutritive surface, i.e., the crusts. This elimination of the initiating and sustaining conditions is usually effective. Once fungal invasion of the nasal encrustations has become established, the use of steroid containing nasal sprays and aerosols should be discontinued and the therapy should be switched to aqueous solutions and applications. The drying effect of certain steroid-containing, dosed aerosols appears to facilitate the growth of opportunistic fungi on the crusted secretions. This is a phenomenon that we have repeatedly observed.

Surgical Procedure

In most cases, the fungal masses can be removed endoscopically, even when there is a severe *Aspergillus* infection of the maxillary sinus.

If there is suspicion of maxillary sinus mycosis, the therapeutic approach should start with an endoscopic examination of the affected sinus. In positive cases, the typical, buttery-soft to crumbly-hard fungal masses are encountered. Depending upon the consistency of the mass, much of it may be evacuated through a polyethylene suction catheter. If the mass is very soft and surrounded by purulent secretions, care must be taken not to evacuate all the contents of the maxillary sinus leaving no material for histologic study and culture.

Occasionally, insertion of the trocar into the sinus is followed by bleeding from the turgid, inflamed mucous membranes with blood actually pulsating slowly from the proximal end of the trocar. In this event, careful repeated suctioning and the application of topical vasoconstrictors is indicated. It is usually possible to control the bleeding in this manner and to obtain a view of the maxillary sinus. If the fungal masses are hard, they may sometimes be broken up with the trocar or by biopsy forceps introduced through the trocar. These smaller pieces can then be removed one by one.

The trocar is always left in the maxillary sinus during any further procedures (Figs. 11.48 to 11.55). The therapeutic management of the middle meatus then proceeds in the usual way. Complete fungal casts of the middle meatus that may extend as far posteriorly as the choana are sometimes encountered. It is not unusual to find that the pressure of the fungal mass has destroyed the lateral wall of the nose, and after removal of the fungal mass from the middle meatus, a 1 × 2 cm defect in the medial wall of the maxillary sinus may be present. In this event, no additional surgical manipulation on this "window" is necessary.

FIGURE 11.48 This series of illustrations shows an endoscopic surgical procedure in a patient with a non-invasive *Aspergillus fumigatus* fungal infection of the left maxillary ethmoid sinuses. *A*, The view into the left middle meatus after resection of the uncinate process. Note the inflamed polypoid mucosa of the ethmoidal infundibulum. *B*, After removal of this polypoid mucosa, the entire anterior ethmoid can be seen to be filled with the fungal mass (*arrow*). s = nasal septum; cm = middle turbinate; and asp = aspirator. *C*, After removal of the most anterior fungal masses, copious purulent secretions drained from the frontal recess (*arrow*). cm = middle turbinate. *D*, The fungal masses were easily removed with forceps and suction. Almost all of the structures of the anterior ethmoid had already been destroyed. No bulla ethmoidalis was found. The removed fungal masses lay directly on the basal lamella of the middle turbinate. The *arrow* points to the roof of the ethmoid in the area of anterior ethmoid artery. asp = aspirator.

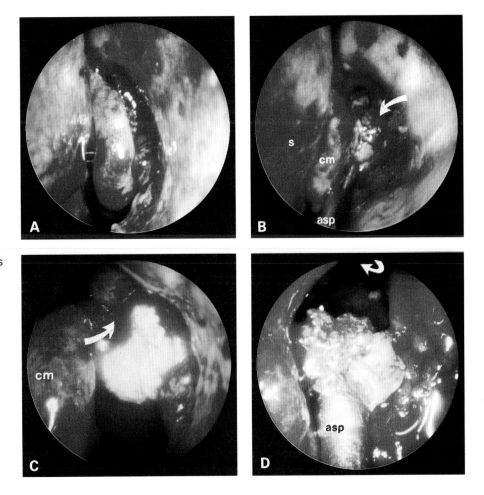

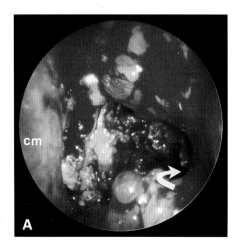 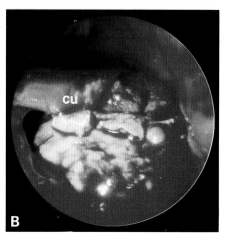 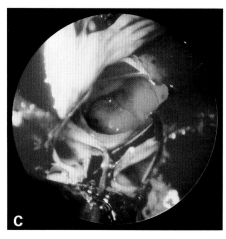

FIGURE 11.49 *A*, The view into the middle meatus after removal of the first layer of fungus. The fungal masses coming from the maxillary sinus have destroyed the lateral wall of the nose, eroded through it, and are lying adjacent to the middle turbinate. Posteriorly they extended along the basal lamella to the posterior third of the middle meatus. The *arrow* points to the natural ostium of the maxillary sinus, which had not yet been surgically enlarged. *B*, These fungal masses are now removed with a curette. cu = curette. *C*, This is followed by checking the posterior ethmoid, which is examined through the basal lamella. As the mucosa in the posterior ethmoid was normal, a more radical procedure was not required.

FIGURE 11.50 Maxillary sinus endoscopy through the canine fossa on the left side. The entire sinus cavity is packed with friable-buttery fungal masses. A portion of the fungal mass and the surrounding, purulent secretions have already been removed by suction. t = lip of the trocar sheath.

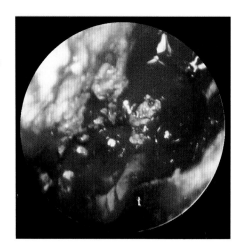

FIGURE 11.51 *A*, A view into the maxillary sinus through the canine fossa. A right angled suction tip has been introduced from the middle meatus, through the enlarged maxillary sinus ostium and additional fungal masses were removed. *B*, View into the maxillary sinus from the middle meatus, through the enlarged window. There is still a cherry-sized fungal ball in the maxilloethmoid angle. cm = middle turbinate and asp = tip of aspirator. *C*, This fungal ball is pushed toward the maxillary sinus ostium with the trocar sheath. *D*, The suction tip picks up and removes the fungal ball.

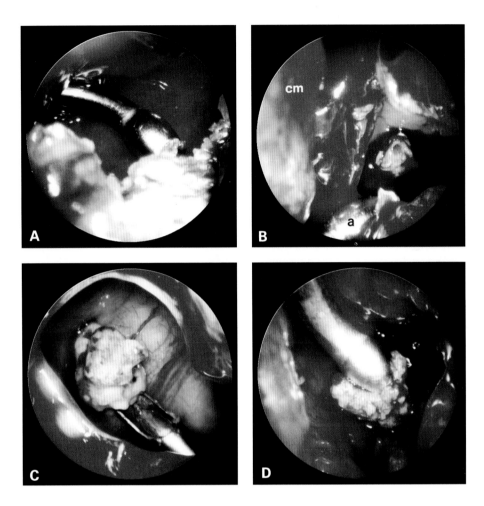

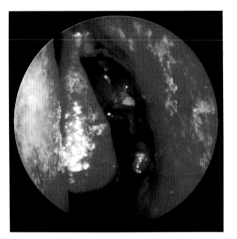

FIGURE 11.52 The view into the middle meatus after completion of the surgical procedure. No packs are placed. The distance between the middle turbinate and the lateral wall of the nose is wide enough to prevent synechia.

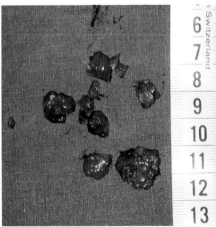

FIGURE 11.53 Part of the endoscopically removed fungal mass.

415

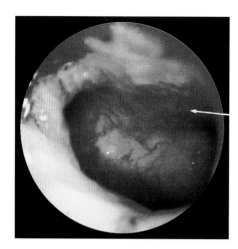

FIGURE 11.54   One week postoperatively. The mucosa appears to be almost
completely normal in this view into the
maxillary sinus from the middle meatus
with a 30 degree lens. The *arrow* demonstrates the course of the infraorbital
nerve. The blood at the upper margin of
the picture is the result of crust removal.

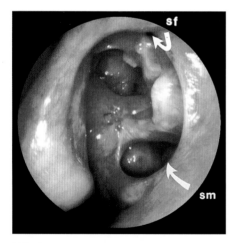

FIGURE 11.55   The appearance 3
months postoperatively. The mucosa of
the ethmoid and maxillary sinus has
returned to normal, and the paths to the
maxillary and frontal sinuses are clear.
Note the normal mucosa on the roof of
the ethmoid, which can be seen at the
top of the picture. sf = frontal sinus
ostium and sm = maxillary sinus ostium.

If the fungal masses have not yet invaded the middle meatus
through the medial wall of the maxillary sinus, the infundibulum is
opened. If required, the ethmoidal bulla is resected and the frequently
involved frontal recess attended to.

The next step is the identification and enlargement of the natural
ostium of the maxillary sinus. The harder the fungal masses and the
more they fill the maxillary sinus, the more the natural ostium should
be enlarged. Various angled suction tips can then be introduced into
the maxillary sinus through the enlarged ostium and the fungal
masses aspirated, assisted by the 30 and 70 degree nasal endoscopes.
In all manipulations, particularly with the larger suction tips, it is
advantageous to introduce the instrument without suction being
applied and to attach the suction line only after the tip of the aspirator
is within the maxillary sinus. Unless this technique is followed, and
particularly when the passages are narrow, the air being aspirated into
the tip may spray small amounts of blood or secretions onto the lens
of the endoscope, thereby obscuring vision.

The trocar introduced into the maxillary sinus through the canine
fossa has been left in place for the following reasons:

The trocar can be used to "separate" the fungal masses from the
floor and from the wall of the sinus and push them toward the
ostium, where they can then be reached with the biopsy forceps or
the suction tip and removed (see Fig. 11.51 C and D). The trocar
sheath also makes it possible to introduce a 70, 90, or even a 120
degree endoscope into the maxillary sinus, repeatedly, if necessary so
that all of the corners of the sinus can be inspected and no fungal
mass missed. The most common site for missing fungal masses is the
angle between the anterior wall and the roof and the eminentia
lacrimalis.

As soon as all of the fungal masses have been removed and the
ethmoid cleaned, the procedure is completed. The middle meatus is
not packed at the conclusion of the procedure. A final careful
inspection is necessary, so that even tiny fungal masses attached to
the surface of the mucous membranes are not overlooked. The
maxillary sinus trocar is cleaned while in situ, in order to avoid
potential contamination of the soft tissues with pus or fungal debris
during removal of the trocar. This is accomplished by leaving the
suction catheter in the trocar during its withdrawal.

If removal of the fungal masses cannot be accomplished with this
technique, or if there is reason to believe that fungal masses may be
hiding behind polypoid hyperplastic mucosa, the maxillary sinus must
be explored in the traditional fashion (Caldwell-Luc). This situation is
one of the few inflammatory conditions for which we still advocate a
traditional surgical approach to the maxillary sinus through the canine
fossa. If the *Aspergillus* mycosis is noninvasive, even with this

approach, we leave the mucous membrane alone, after the fungal masses have been removed. A window in the inferior meatus is not created since during the preceding endoscopic management of the middle meatus the natural ostium of the maxillary sinus had been enlarged (Fig. 11.56). Immediately postoperatively, no antifungal medications are introduced into the maxillary sinus or ethmoid.

FIGURE 11.56 *A* and *B* The operation in two patients in whom the mycotic involvement of the maxillary sinus was so severe that endoscopic removal was not possible. In the second patient (*B*) the maxillary sinus was completely packed with fungal masses. *C* The fungal concretions removed from the patient in *B*.

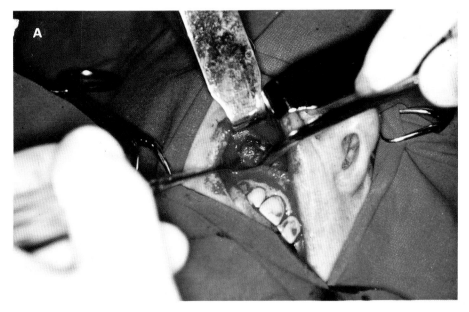

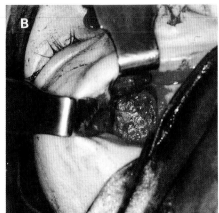

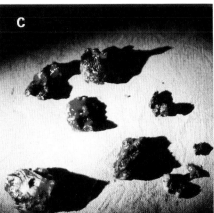

The patients are forbidden to blow their nose for 2 days (because of the trocar perforation). Postoperative antibiotics are not routinely prescribed. In cases in which an extensive empyema is found surrounding the fungal mass and there is corresponding acute inflammation of the ethmoid, we do not hesitate to use an antibiotic, since presumably all of the fungal masses have been removed. The use of an anti-inflammatory agent, e.g., diclofenac for a few days may be beneficial.

As far as the surgical approach to mycosis of the posterior ethmoid or of the sphenoid sinus is concerned, this is no different in principle from the surgical approach to any other inflammatory process in this area.

In the case of an isolated fungal infection of the sphenoid sinus, it is possible to open the anterior wall of the sinus directly along the medial edge of the turbinate and to evacuate the fungal masses (see Chapter 9).

In fungal infections of the frontal sinuses (a rare occurrence in our patient population), the endoscopic technique may have reached its limits. If only the frontal recess of the ethmoid and that part of the frontal sinus adjacent to the ostium are involved, it may be possible in individual cases to remove the fungal masses through the ostium. If, however, the entire frontal sinus, including its lateral recesses, is involved or if there is any suspicion that all the fungal masses may not be removable by this route, an anterior external approach is indicated. In the same fashion, an invasive mycosis, particularly one with a fulminating course, is not suitable for a primarily endoscopic procedure.

Postoperative Care

As with any other endoscopic sinus surgical procedure, the postoperative management following endoscopic surgery for mycotic infections is focused on the careful loosening and removal of crusts, suction removal of excessive secretions, and care of the mucous membranes to prevent synechiae and scar formation. Previously we applied local antimycotic therapy in the postoperative period, and while we rarely use this technique today, it is still occasionally of value.

While there are a number of antimycotic agents available for the local treatment of the operative field in cases of noninvasive mycosis, our personal experience is limited to clotrimazole and naftifine.

Both clotrimazole and naftifine affect the metabolism of fungi. Clotrimazole inhibits the synthesis of ergosterine, an essential component of the fungal membrane, producing a defective cell membrane that is unable to perform its normal metabolic functions, which results in the eventual dissolution of the fungal cells. This lytic effect has been demonstrated in histologic preparations of fungal concretions removed from a patient pretreated with naftifine instillations. Clotrimazole, which occasionally produces a slight superficial lysis has limited effectiveness in *Aspergillus* infections.

This mechanism of cell wall destruction is effective only when the imidazole antimycotics are able to affect the metabolism of actively growing fungal cells. Quiescent cells and spores are not affected by these compounds. In view of this, it is apparent that complete removal of the fungal masses combined with appropriate antifungal therapy (a combined surgical and medical therapy) is preferable to pharmacologic management alone. Resting fungi and the centers of large fungal masses cannot be destroyed by local antimycotic therapy.

The application of antimycotic gels in the nose or paranasal sinuses is not advisable, since many gels contain alcohol and produce an unpleasant burning sensation.

If the maxillary sinus was opened from the canine fossa and maxillary sinus endoscopy was performed by this route, no anti-mycotic should be introduced into the surgical opening until after the trocar puncture site or the window in the anterior wall of the maxillary sinus has completely closed. We have seen several long-lasting and painful infiltrations of the soft tissues of the cheek when antimycotics were instilled prior to the closure of these portals. The infiltrations occurred by the antimycotics leaking out of the sinus and into the soft tissues of the cheek through the open trocar perforation (see Chapter 13).

If the disease is invasive, the drug of choice is amphotericin B, given in doses of 0.25 mg/kg/day. In occasional cases a smaller initial dose may be advisable. The renal side effects of amphotericin B mandate caution in its use. This powerful antifungal is only indicated when there is documented invasion, a fulminating course, or a very strongly supported suspicion that this may be the case. Under no circumstances should amphotericin B be used routinely in every patient with *Aspergillus* sinusitis.

Good synergistic effects may be obtained by combining amphotericin B with flucytosine, given either orally or intravenously.

How Do *Aspergillus* Infections Arise?

Aspergillus fumigatus is universally present in the environment and its ubiquitous spores can be inhaled at any time. They are particularly prevalent in decaying organic matter, such as potting soil, humus, and hay. *Aspergillus fumigatus* is present as "mold" on numerous "spoiled" foods and on damp interior walls.

Its spores are also a normal component of ambient air and present in the dust of most houses. Even so, *A. fumigatus* is at the lower end of the frequency for fungi in the environment at our normal ambient temperatures. When incubated at 37°C however, there is a surprising amount of *A. fumigatus* growth from all of the previously mentioned potential sources, and its colonies are far more numerous than those of any other fungus.

Aspergillus does not usually grow on intact mucous membranes since it lacks enzymes that permit entry through intact skin or mucous membranes.

This fungus however, finds in diseased paranasal sinuses an ideal environment for growth. There is copious "food" in the inspissated pathologic secretions or crusts and there may even be anaerobic conditions. Chronic sinus infections provide these "ideal" conditions. The maxillary sinus, which is a hollow space where if the ostium is obstructed, pathologic secretions can accumulate or be retained. These accumulations occur either on the floor of the sinus or adjacent to the blocked ostium and may explain why these two areas of the sinus are the commonest location for *A. fumigatus* infections.

Once the fungal mass has reached a size that prevents its passage through the ostium, this mass of fungus itself may produce and sustain sinusitis.

It accomplishes this by producing a foreign body reaction or an inflammatory stimulus, possibly the result of specific toxins, pressure necrosis, and invasion. Antibiotic therapy, immunosuppression, and most commonly local antibiotic applications can promote fungal growth. The fungus can remain quiescent for years, in a vegetative state without producing any symptoms, until a recurrent sinusitis draws attention to its presence.

Many of our patients presented with the following clinical picture: ethmoid disease produced chronic maxillary sinusitis with secondary fungal superinfection. For a long time the fungus subsisted as a pure saprophyte and only became a pathogen under one of the conditions described above.

More recently, there is increasing evidence that suggests the possibility of a dental (and therefore iatrogenic) etiology. In the radiopaque areas of the fungal concretions in many cases in addition to calcium, heavy metals may also be found. These came from dental fillings or root canal packings and contained lead, titanium, bismuth, iodine, barium, and most frequently zinc. Several authors concluded that the radiopaque concretions were always the result of root canal packing materials that had found their way into the maxillary sinus and were responsible for initiating the fungal infection. Fungi have a great affinity for metallic salts that are deposited in the central necrotic areas of the concretions where they produced radiopacity in these areas.

According to these theories, zinc oxide reaches the maxillary sinus via the root canal and triggers a mycotic growth when the patient inhales fungal spores from a contaminated environment. While zinc oxide is mycostatic in higher concentrations, trace amounts are required by the fungus as a catalyst for a variety of metabolic functions and thus this salt serves as a stimulus for fungal growth.

In some cases the causal relationship between aberrant filling material and the mycosis is obvious. In one of our patients a root canal treatment was mandated by a granuloma at the tip of the root. Filling material was introduced into the previously completely normal maxillary sinus. Seven months later a significant *Aspergillus* mycosis with radiopaque concrementations was discovered in this maxillary sinus (Figs. 11.57 and 11.58).

FIGURE 11.57 *A*, In this 28-year-old patient, dental filling material was accidentally introduced during root canal treatment into a previously normal maxillary sinus. *B*, Seven months later the patient presented with a massive *Aspergillus fumigatus* mycosis. The density of the concretion (M = 2706) puts it into the range of metallic densities.

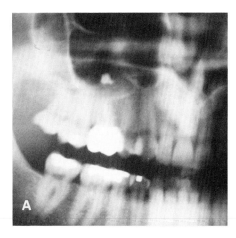 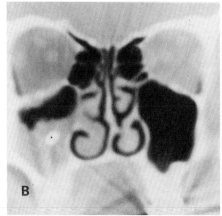

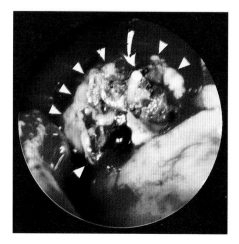

FIGURE 11.58 In another patient, a small gutta-percha cylinder (*curved arrow*) was found in the concretion (*arrow heads*). Apparently the fungal infection developed around this foreign substance.

In contrast, we have also found massive *Aspergillus* infections in patients who have been edentulous for more than thirty years.

The question of whether and how aberrant dental filling materials produce or initiate a maxillary sinus mycosis assumes particular significance, including medicolegal significance in view of the very large number of dental fillings performed these days.

Our analysis revealed high concentrations of titanium, bismuth, iodine, barium, and lead in the concretions in our patients. Zinc oxide could also be demonstrated but its concentration was the same in the periphery of the concretion as in its radiopaque center. It seems therefore, that zinc oxide is not responsible for the radiopacity of the fungal concretions. Furthermore, since zinc is found in varying concentrations in all body tissues and fluids, it is difficult to hold zinc responsible for "triggering" the mycosis.

In some of our cases, analysis of the radiopaque areas revealed that their composition was identical with that of certain dental filling materials. In other cases, with radiographically similar opacifications, an analysis of the necrotic fungal material revealed only calcium salts, mostly tertiary calcium phosphate and some sulfates. Histologic examination showed that these deposits were originally intracellular. Radiographic pictures such as Figures 11.35 to 11.39 that show variable graduations in density all the way to an almost metallic shadow support the assumption that we are dealing with a process of aggregation of radiopaque substances in the necrotic centers. The more calcium and metallic salts that are deposited, the more radiopaque the area appears.

Radiologically, cases with histochemically demonstrated filling materials in the center of the fungal mass could not be distinguished with any degree of certainty from those cases with no filling materials present.

Certain conditions must be met for the *Aspergillus* spores to remain and grow in the sinus. The transport of secretions must be significantly retarded or entirely stopped in an area of the sinus, since normal ciliary movement completely replaces the film of secretions in the maxillary sinus every 20 to 30 minutes. During this time, the spores deposited on the surface would be carried out of the sinus. A stasis of secretions, for example in the context of a viral or bacterial sinusitis, or as the result of an ostial obstruction can produce the basic conditions for the retention and germination of the fungal spores.

Aspergillosis, therefore arises as a secondary disease, superimposed upon a chronic sinusitis. The underlying inflammatory process creates ideal growing conditions, e.g., low oxygen tension, or even anaerobic conditions, low pH, optimal temperature of about 37°C, abundant nutrients, stagnating transport of secretions, and the environment of a "humidity chamber." Once the fungal masses have reached a size

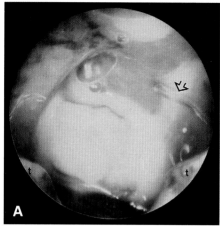
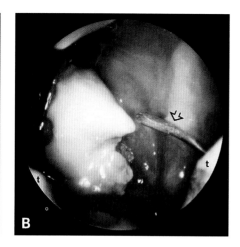

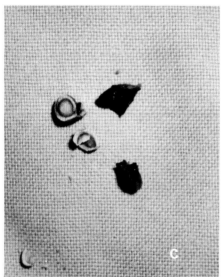

FIGURE 11.59 *A*, An empyema was found in this maxillary sinus a few months after the extraction of a left upper first molar. An oroantral fistula developed through the alveolus at the same time. arrow = indwelling sound and t = trocar sleeve. *B*, After removal of the empyema, a typical white fungal concrement is seen lying at the ostium of the maxillary sinus. arrow = sound placed through fistula and t = trocar sleeve. *C*, After removal of the concretion, a 3.5 mm "nucleus" was identified in its center. This nucleus behaved like a metal and, on section, appeared to have a rosette-like structure. Suprisingly, the analysis showed only concentric layers of fungal masses with central calcium deposits. There was *no* evidence of dental filling material.

that makes their passage through the natural ostium impossible, they become pathogens in their own right and can maintain the sinus infection. The toxins produced in vivo by the fungus are immunosuppressive and probably also myotoxic and neurotoxic. In addition to the natural dynamics of fungal development, viral or bacterial superinfections provide additional, periodic stimulation by providing increased nutrition in the form of pathologic secretions.

Mucosal damage with absent ciliary movements also favors the development of mycosis with the metallic nucleus provided by aberrant root fillings serving as a "crystallization" point for the fungal spores and hyphae. Due to the affinity of the fungus for metallic salts, these can be drawn into its metabolic pathways and deposited in the necrotic centers of the fungal masses.

We have not found any evidence that *Aspergillus* mycosis is triggered by zinc oxide. Mycotic involvement of the sphenoid and frontal sinuses and the posterior ethmoid can also not be explained on the basis of aberrant dental filling materials. *Aspergillus* infection can

423

occur elsewhere in the head and neck with no relationship to aberrant root canal filling materials. There are numerous cases, however, where such a relationship has been clearly established. Until the question of how and through what chemical components these filling materials contribute to the development of fungal sinusitis, dentists should be careful in using root canal filling materials in the vicinity of the maxillary sinus. Material that has been introduced into the maxillary sinus should be removed, whenever possible, even in the absence of symptoms or, at the least, the patient should be followed at regular intervals.

Candidiasis

The *Candida* species are yeast fungi that are pathogenic saprophytes and part of the flora of the mucous membranes of the upper gastrointestinal tract. They participate in the breakdown of organic substances with *C. albicans* being the most active member of the group. They are also found in the moist areas of skin folds particularly in the interdigital and genital areas, where they can cause intertriginous *Candida* infection.

As in the oropharynx and esophagus, *C. albicans* may become pathogenic in the nose and in the paranasal sinuses, when local or systemic factors decrease the resistance of the patient. This may be accomplished locally by injury to the mucous membranes, ulcers of any cause, or from the local application of antibiotics or cortico-steroids. Systemically, cytostatic chemotherapy, immunosuppressive therapy, and radiation for malignant diseases all contribute to the development of mucous membrane candidiasis. In such cases, the yeast cells multiply and change from a purely saprophytic yeast phase to the parasitic mycelial phase and produce the typical picture of skin or mucous membrane candidiasis.

A true, primary candidal infection of the nose and sinuses is rare. Thrush of the oral cavity and nasal mucosa of the newborn usually results from perinatal transmission from a vaginal candidal infection in the mother. As with any patient presenting with the manifestations of thrush, a patient with nasal and paranasal sinus involvement must be evaluated carefully for an underlying, predisposing, or triggering primary disease. The spectrum of underlying disease ranges from trivial infections to alcoholism, diabetes, debilitating systemic illness, malignancy, major systemic infections, and immunodeficiency diseases such as AIDS. More rarely, isolated, circumscribed patches of thrush colonization are found in small mucous membrane areas. If the fungal growth is not strictly limited to the surface of encrustations, as in Figure 11.60, the mucous membrane under the encrustation must be

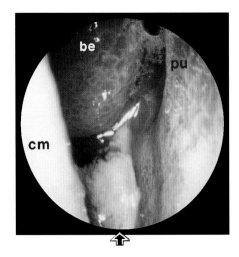

FIGURE 11.60 The large, whitish conglomeration lying between the middle turbinate, the bulla and the floor of the nose (*arrow*) in this view into a left middle meatus was proven by histological examination and culture to be *Candida*. Note the reticular pattern of the mucous membrane over the bulla. cm = middle turbinate; be = ethmoidal bulla; and pu = uncinate process.

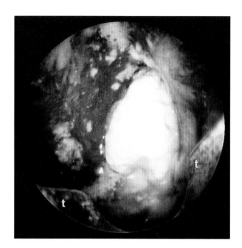

FIGURE 11.61 A view into the left maxillary sinus of the same patient. The maxillary sinus also contained whitish masses characteristic of *Candida* mycosis. A carcinoma of the lateral wall of the nose was identified as the predisposing cause. t = trocar sleeve.

carefully inspected. The patient in Figure 11.27 had used a steroid-containing nasal aerosol over a period of several months for the treatment of an allergic rhinitis.

As with candidal infections in the mouth, the mycelial patches in the nose can be wiped away, leaving an oozing and occasionally granulating mucous membrane. This area must always be biopsied in order not to miss a malignancy. We have seen several cases where *Candida* was growing on a squamous carcinoma of the maxilla or a carcinoma of the nasopharynx (Figs. 11.28 to 11.30 and 11.61).

In massive candidal infections of the paranasal sinuses, the sinuses may be packed with a soft, whitish-dirty mass (Fig. 11.61). In extreme cases of paranasal candidiasis, the sinus may be the source of a systemic *Candida* septicemia.

In diagnosing a fungal infection in nasal and paranasal sinus smears, the possibility of a mixed culture must be kept in mind. It can happen that only the secondary, opportunistic fungus shows growth and that the true pathogen does not appear in the culture (see also Table 11.1). For this reason the importance of the microscopic examination of the biopsy material can not be over emphasized. The findings are clear when the fungus can be demonstrated in the tissues, e.g., in a granuloma.

Candida is a rare cause of granuloma formation in the nasal mucosa. These lesions may be difficult to distinguish from tuberculotic lesions and therefore the diagnosis of a fungal etiology can be made only when *Candida* is identified in the granuloma. More commonly *Candida* if encountered is a secondary invader on respiratory mucous membrane granulomas or lesions produced by some other disease entity.

TABLE 11.1 Results of Culture in 48 Patients with Histologically Documented *Aspergillus fumigatus* Mycosis of the Paranasal Sinuses

n = 48	(35 females and 13 males)*
Aspergillus pure culture	*Aspergillus fumigatus* (31 cases)
Aspergillus† mixed culture	A.f + *Penicillium* (3 cases)
	A.f + *Cladosporium* (3 cases)
	A.f + *Fusarium* (1 case)
	A.f + *A. niger* (1 case)
Other pure culture	*Cladosporium* (4 cases)
	Penicillium (1 case)
	3 cases not identified
Other mixed culture	*Cladosporium* + *Fusarium* (1 case)

*Sex distribution: In cases in Graz since 1976; the ratio of female to male is 2.2:1.

†The incidence of secondary invaders emphasizes the importance of a histologic diagnosis in *Aspergillus* mycosis.

In patients who have had radiation therapy for malignancy of the upper airway or digestive tract, *Candida* is the most frequent facultative pathogen. The incidence of positive *Candida* cultures increases during radiation therapy. This finding corresponds with the common clinical observation of a high incidence of *Candida* colonization of the mucous membranes in radiation mucositis.

Therapy

In saprophytic infections of mucous membrane crusts, simple removal of the crusts, as described for *Aspergillus* infections is usually sufficient. If large areas of the mucous membrane are affected, the crusts should be carefully removed and local antimycotic therapy with naftifine or clotrimazole may be indicated. In milder, noninvasive cases ketoconazole is valuable for oral therapy. Flucytosine is also effective orally against candidiasis.

In more severe infections of the paranasal sinuses, the fungal masses must be removed surgically. Depending on the clinical picture, local irrigation with clotrimazole solution and oral medication may suffice. In cases of chronic mucous membrane candidiasis, in extensive invasion of the mucous membranes, or when specific complications are suspected, amphotericin B, with or without flucytosine, is available for intravenous therapy.

Both *A. fumigatus* and the *Candida* species can become inhaled allergens and trigger or sustain specific rhinopathies and asthma.

Mucormycoses

Representatives of the family Mucoraceae are found most commonly on moist fresh organic materials such as manure. These fungi exist primarily as saprophytes and play an important role when virgin soil is first cultivated. Occasionally they exist as parasites on plants causing mold on potatoes, apples, strawberries, and tomatoes. *Rhizopus* and *Mucor* may occasionally spoil bread and other foods. The species of *Rhizopus, Mucor,* and *Absidia* are responsible for the mucormycoses in domestic animals.

Clinical Findings

In man these fungi are occasionally found as saprophytes on cutaneous lesions or on mucous membranes. On histologic sections and in culture, they must be distinguished from the *Aspergillus* species. The hyphae of the *Mucor* fungi vary in width and usually branch off at a 90 degree angle (in contrast to the 45 degree angle of the *Aspergillus* species). The symptoms and clinical course of a noninvasive *Mucor* mycotic infection is similar to that of noninvasive *Aspergillus* infections. Sinus tomography and CT usually show areas of high and low radiopacity although the bony or metallic density described for *Aspergillus* is not found in the *Mucor* mycoses.

Under some conditions, *Mucor* infections may have a very aggressive and invasive course. Prior to the introduction of the systemically effective antimycotic agent, amphotericin B, the mortality rate of mucormycoses in diabetic patients was approximately 50 percent. Even today with amphotericin B available, the mortality rate in this group is still between 15 and 30 percent.

The most dreaded complications are the vascular ones, e.g., true or pseudoaneurysms of the cerebral vessels, arteries, and veins at the skull base. Sinus thromboses and direct invasion of the brain have also been described. Acute *Mucor* mycotic destruction of the entire maxilla has also been reported. In these cases the paranasal sinuses frequently functioned as the starting point of the infection with the fungus reaching the CNS through the orbits. The diagnosis was frequently made by an ophthalmologist, on the basis of the ocular findings.

Mucor mycoses may have a particularly dramatic and fulminating course in patients with diabetic ketoacidosis, cancer patients (following radiation or postoperatively), immunosuppressed patients (e.g., after transplantation), in infants, and in massively dehydrated, small children.

Therapy

In addition to amphotericin B, combination therapy with flucytosine may be tried since these two drugs have a synergistic effect in *Mucor* mycoses. In *Mucor* meningitis, amphotericin B may be given intrathecally, but intrathecal administration should be preceded by intrathecal administration of 10 mg of prednisolone. Because of the well-known renal toxicity of these antifungal agents, the patient's renal function must be monitored very closely. In patients with preexisting bone marrow depression, e.g., cancer patients, these drugs must be used with extreme caution. In addition to the medical therapy, every effort should be made to remove all of the affected structures. *Mucor* infections are not a primary indication for endoscopic surgery.

If the base of the skull is invaded by *Mucor* fungi or if a *Mucor* meningitis develops, then the prognosis, especially in the immunosuppressed patient is even today abysmal.

ALLERGY: ROLE OF THE MESSERKLINGER TECHNIQUE IN INHALATIONAL ALLERGIES

ENT specialists are frequently asked by patients with inhalational allergies and nasal or bronchial symptoms whether any surgical procedures are available that may supplement symptomatic or specific antiallergic therapy.

While it is obvious that IgE mediated allergies cannot be cured by any surgical procedure, the question still remains: "Are there surgical approaches that will help alleviate the allergic symptoms and that will allow the antiallergic medication to work more effectively?"

The most frequently considered surgical techniques in patients with inhalational allergies are: correction of a nasal septal deviation (Chapter 11); procedures on the ethmoid, the lateral wall of the nose, and the paranasal sinuses; procedures on the turbinates (primarily the inferior turbinate); and adenoidectomy and tonsillectomy.

All the above procedures, with the possible exception of tonsillectomy, have as their primary purpose the improvement of the nasal airways and thus affect only the *nasal* symptoms of an inhalational allergy. Clinical experience has shown that surgical intervention in the area of the ethmoid may also have beneficial effects on asthma (Chapter 13).

Since surgical intervention in these patients is not aimed at the *cause* of the problem, the indications for any surgical procedure must obviously have a direct relationship to the patient's symptoms. In cases of inhalational allergy, we do not see any indication for intervention, even in the presence of a deviated nasal septum, unless the septal deviation is definitely responsible for specific symptoms. The indications should also take into account the severity of the symptoms, since there must be a favorable surgical risk to therapeutic benefit ratio.

The nasal symptoms in allergic patients are aggravated more by abnormalities or diseases in the region of the lateral nasal wall than by a septal deviation. A number of the previously described anatomic variations can affect the ostiomeatal complex. In this respect we wish to re-emphasize the occasionally extensive pneumatization of the middle turbinate (concha bullosa). Particularly when combined with other abnormalities, e.g., a medially bent uncinate process or a large ethmoidal bulla, a concha bullosa can narrow the entire nasal airway and especially the middle meatus. With a large concha bullosa, even a minimal amount of swelling of the mucous membranes, e.g., as the result of an allergic response, may produce earlier and more severe symptoms in these patients, than in those who do not have this anatomic variation.

In those patients with documented inhalational allergy whose nasal symptoms do not respond to specific antiallergic therapy as rapidly or as completely as expected, an anatomic variation should be suspected even in the absence of clinical observations or survey radiographic findings. In individual cases, significant improvements can be obtained by relatively minor surgical procedures.

In those patients who do not have a clearly defined allergy, but who do respond positively to a multitude of allergy tests (primarily in the low RAST group), and who have nasal symptoms throughout the year, endoscopic correction of ethmoid pathology can produce a freedom from symptoms without any additional antiallergic therapy. This observation shows that a positive allergy test does not necessarily mean that the symptoms are directly or primarily allergic in nature. Positive skin or RAST tests may be present in patients who have a clinically silent predisposition to allergic responses.

In patients with massive polyposis (a very rare finding in inhalational allergies) surgical intervention may become necessary, since a purely medical regimen is unlikely to produce significant improvement and even if it does, surgical intervention significantly accelerates recovery (see Chapter 5).

Partial or total resection of the inferior turbinate, a frequent practice in many centers, is in our opinion rarely indicated. If the swelling of the turbinate is the result of an allergic response, it should respond well to specific, antiallergic therapy, without surgical intervention. If the enlargement is due to a bony hypertrophy, then the underlying condition is not allergic in origin. Mucosal swelling of the inferior turbinate is frequently a reflex response to an inflammatory process in the lateral wall of the nose. Elimination of these foci of disease frequently leads to a complete disappearance of even massive swellings of the inferior turbinate. Admittedly, these patients did not have allergies. In this group of patients, regional, geographic, or perhaps even racial differences may play a role in the reaction patterns to stimulation.

IgE mediated allergies can not be cured by surgical intervention. In individual cases and with proper indications, procedures on the lateral wall of the nose may represent a sensible form of adjuvant therapy that improves or ameliorates the nasal symptoms. In these patients, the Messerklinger technique should be regarded as an adjuvant modality to traditional antiallergic medical therapy, which may improve the symptoms, but for which very rigid criteria and indications must be observed.

The knowledge of these relationships, and particularly the ability to diagnose the frequently hidden and clinically unobservable changes are the factors that the ENT specialist should discuss with, and emphasize to, the specialists in allergy and immunology.

SEPTAL DEVIATION

A marked deviation of the nasal septum can produce significant symptoms. Such a deviation may cause obstructed nasal breathing and it may also be responsible for diseases of the paranasal sinuses (Fig. 11.62). However, clinical experience has shown that patients with massive nasal septal deviations or septal spurs may have no symptoms at all or may have their symptoms on the opposite side, i.e., the side with the allegedly better airway (Figs. 11.63 and 11.64). We are reluctant to perform routine septal surgery for diseases of the

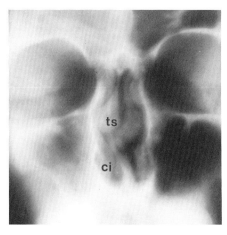

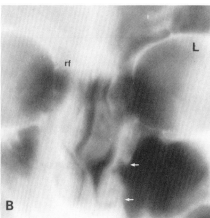

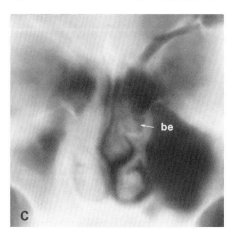

FIGURE 11.62 *A*, This patient with bilateral complaints has a severe right nasal septal deviation. The septum is in close contact with the right inferior turbinate and the septal tubercle is forced against the agger nasi. Note the marked opacification of the maxillary and frontal sinuses on the right side. ci = inferior turbinate and ts = septal tubercle. *B*, A tomographic section 5 mm further posterior in the same patient. The septum is pushed against the lateral wall of the nose along almost its entire length. While the middle turbinate is fully developed on the left side, it can not be identified on the right. The right frontal recess is opacified. On the left side there is a concha bullosa that is clearly diseased. The infundibulum is also opacified on this side, and that explains why the patient has bilateral complaints. *Arrows* indicate a patent window in the inferior meatus following a fenestration procedure several months earlier. rf = frontal recess. *C*, Another section, 1 cm further posterior. The septal deviation involves the right middle meatus, which is severely diseased. On the left, the most posterior part of the ethmoidal bulla can be identified, which is also diseased. be = bulla ethmoidalis.

lateral wall of the nose or of the related paranasal sinuses. We perform septoplasty only in extreme cases or where there is a clear indication. We have shown that most patients can be rendered symptom-free following correction of their ethmoid problems, even in the presence of a moderate or a severe septal deviation without surgical correction of the septal deviation.

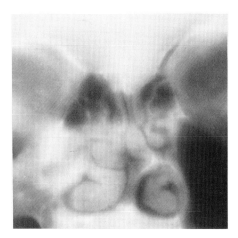

FIGURE 11.63 This patient has a marked left nasal septal deviation with septal ridge and spur formation. The symptoms however, were on the contralateral side, where there is a diseased, previously operated upon maxillary sinus and a diseased ethmoidal bulla and infundibulum. Note as an incidental finding, the difference between the two ethmoidal roofs. On the right, the roof is almost horizontal, while on the left it is very steep. This results in a significant difference in the height of the ethmoid roofs that may be of importance at the time of surgery.

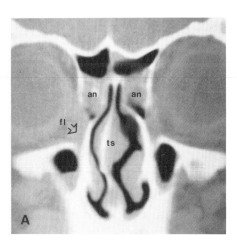 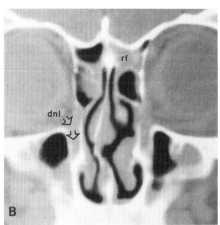

FIGURE 11.64 A, The septal tubercle is very noticeable in this patient with marked right nasal septal deviation. The septal deviation was not the cause of this patient's symptoms. There was a large diseased agger nasi cell on both sides, that caused bilateral ethmoid and frontal sinusitis. an = agger nasi; ts = septal tubercle; and fl = lacrimal fossa. B, Same patient 4 mm further posterior. Note how the frontal recess on the left side is more opaque than on the right. With such findings we see no indication for septoplasty. rf = frontal recess and dnl = nasolacrimal duct.

Our procedure in treating documented involvement of the ethmoid is as follows:

If we can pass a 4-mm endoscope and the other necessary surgical instruments past the septal deviation into the affected middle meatus, we always correct the ethmoid problem first. Naturally, the surgical procedure may be more difficult under these circumstances and it is even more important to proceed as atraumatically as possible. Injuries to the mucous membranes in the middle meatus, septum, or lateral nasal wall must be avoided. We have found it advantageous in such cases not to attempt to advance the endoscope as close to the middle meatus as possible but only close enough to get a good view of the middle meatus. As shown in Figure 11.65, it is usually possible to gain a satisfactory view of the ethmoid under these conditions.

If isolated septal ridges or spurs are in the way (Fig. 11.66), these can be resected in isolation, as part of the endoscopic procedure without performing a complete septoplasty. The mucosa surrounding the spur is injected with a local anesthetic, incised, and the spur dissected free. In most cases these isolated structures can be removed easily with a chisel or a conchotome (Fig. 11.67). The mucous membrane flaps are then approximated and gently packed for 1 to 2 days with a Merocel sponge (Fig. 11.66C).

We perform a septoplasty at the first sitting only in those cases where it is impossible to advance the endoscope or other instruments beyond the deviation. If the paranasal sinus symptoms persist and if endoscopic examination reveals the typical findings of an ethmoid problem, we then perform a therapeutic endoscopic ethmoid procedure a few weeks later at a second sitting.

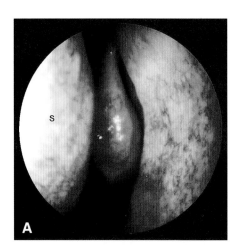 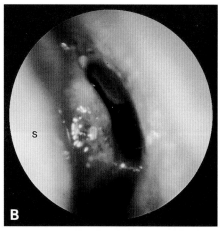 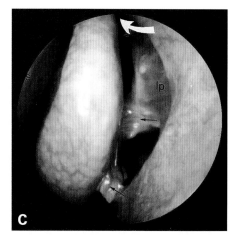

FIGURE 11.65 *A*, The view into a left middle meatus in a patient with a marked septal deviation. There is a moderately large concha bullosa of the middle turbinate and a diseased anterior ethmoid. s = septum. *B*, The same patient 3 days after endoscopic sinus surgery. There are still crusted secretions at the insertion of the middle turbinate and between the turbinate and the inferior margin of the maxillary sinus ostium. The path to the anterior ethmoid is clear. s = septum. *C*, The same patient 1 week after surgery. The mucosa has almost returned to normal. Crusted secretions are still being transported out of the maxillary sinus (*arrows*). The mucous membrane over the lamina papyracea is still somewhat edematous, but the path to frontal recess (*bent arrow*) is already open. lp = lamina papyracea.

FIGURE 11.66 *A*, The septal ridge that extends both anterior and inferior to the left middle meatus terminates in a huge septal spur that impinges on the inferior turbinate. The mucosa of the inferior turbinate is hyperplastic in this area (*arrows*). The septal spur did not obstruct access to the middle meatus, but was resected because of its impingement on the middle turbinate. s = septum. *B*, The appearance after resection of the septal spur. The mucosa has already been replaced (*arrow*). The transient contact of the septum with the middle turbinate is due to a submucosal injection on the septum. In the middle meatus the lateral lamella of the concha bullosa has already been resected and the uncinate process and the inflamed and edematous anterior surface of the bulla can be seen. *C*, At the end of the surgical procedure on the ethmoid, a small Merocel sponge was placed between the site of the resected spur and the inferior turbinate. Betnesol is being dripped onto the sponge to make it swell. The sponge was left in place for 2 days. s = septum and asp = aspirator. *D*, The appearance of the middle meatus 11 weeks postoperatively. Normal mucosa is seen and the path to the frontal recess is free.

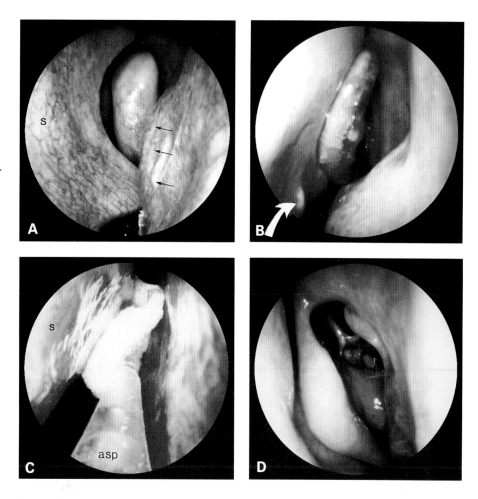

When a significant nasal septal deviation is combined with extensive bilateral nasal polyps, we may opt for a combined repair in one sitting.

The postoperative care and management of the ethmoid may be more difficult in patients with septal deviation, particularly if there are postoperative complications. Generally speaking, however, these occur so rarely that we do not consider the possibility of easier postoperative management as a sufficient indication for the routine correction of moderate septal deviation prior to an ethmoid procedure. Since we adopted this philosophy, the need for septoplasty in our patients has decreased, and it is currently well below 10 percent of all paranasal sinus procedures.

FIGURE 11.67 The jaws of a modified conchotome that is suitable for the removal of septal ridges and spurs.

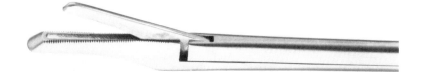

More than a third of the patients referred to us because of presumptive nasal septal problems were found to have ethmoid abnormalities as their underlying disease and could be managed without septal surgery. The dubious usefulness of routine nasal septal procedures in the treatment of sinus disease is well illustrated by the fact that many patients had already undergone unrewarding septoplasties when they were admitted for endoscopic treatment of their ethmoid disease (see Chapter 13).

REMOVAL OF FOREIGN BODIES

The endoscope is an excellent instrument for both the diagnosis and removal of foreign bodies not only from the nose but also from the hard-to-reach corners of the paranasal sinuses. The removal of dental filling material from the maxillary sinus has been discussed in Chapters 2 and 5. This can be done through a trocar sheath without "opening" the maxillary sinus. Even bulky and unwieldy foreign bodies can be simply removed with this technique. In the patient in Figure 11.68, a drill point that came loose from the dental handpiece was forcibly projected through the alveolus into the maxillary sinus. This occurred during an attempt to remove a root fragment retained following an incomplete extraction of a left upper first molar. The drill point, which was lying free in the maxillary sinus, was successfully

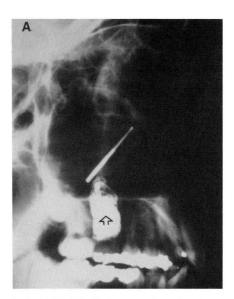
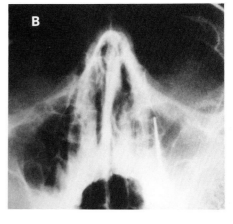
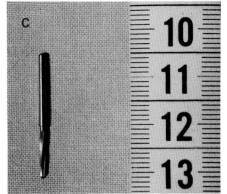

FIGURE 11.68 *A*, Survey film, lateral view. A dental drill that has entered the maxillary sinus through the alveolus of the left upper first molar can be seen in this lateral plain film. Note the radiopaque strip of packing in the dental alveolus (*open arrow*). *B*, A frontal view showing the foreign body in the left maxillary sinus. *C*, The foreign body after removal.

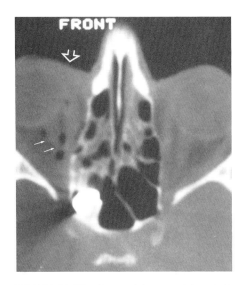

FIGURE 11.69 A metal fragment in a left Onodi cell. The splinter entered the orbit next to the eyeball (the *open arrow* points out the approximate point of entry) and passed through the orbit to enter the posterior ethmoid. Note the air within the orbit (*thin arrows*) and the potential site of injury to the optic nerve.

drawn into the trocar sheath, which had been introduced through the canine fossa. The sheath was then advanced to the posterior wall of the sinus, so that the point of the drill was entirely within the trocar sheath and could no longer slip out. The drill point was then easily grasped with forceps.

With this technique, a variety of other foreign bodies, e.g., dental root fragments, glass or metal splinters, air-gun pellets, etc., can be removed with ease provided that the diameter of the foreign body is less than the internal diameter of the trocar sheath. If the foreign body is wider than the trocar sheath, a temporary opening can be made in the front wall of the maxillary sinus and the endoscope used to remove the foreign body through this temporary opening.

In another patient (Figs. 11.69 and 11.70), a metal splinter was endoscopically removed after it had penetrated the eye and the orbit and lodged in the posterior ethmoid adjacent to the sphenoid. The foreign body had injured the optic nerve and the patient was blinded instantly. The foreign body had to be removed since infection had set in and was threatening to spread to the orbit. The metal splinter was removed transethmoidally under local anesthesia. It had lodged itself in an Onodi cell, wedged deeply into the optic nerve. It was unclear whether it was this injury that produced the damage of the optic nerve or whether the nerve was injured when the piece of metal passed through the orbit. The infection was managed satisfactorily, but unfortunately, the patient's vision did not return.

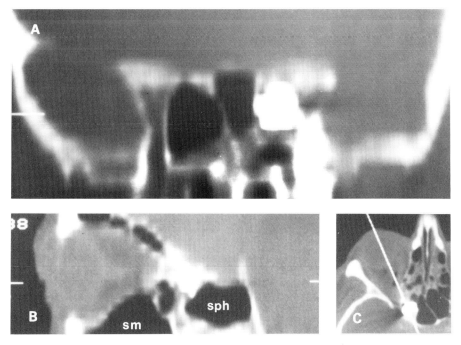

FIGURE 11.70 *A*, Frontal CT-reconstruction. The foreign body is not in the sphenoid sinus as it would appear, but instead, it is lying in an Onodi cell (*B*), that extended far laterally from the sphenoid, as shown in the reconstruction. sm = maxillary sinus and sph = sphenoid sinus. *C*, The plane in which *B* was reconstructed.

435

DETECTION AND TREATMENT OF CEREBROSPINAL FLUID LEAKS

A persistent cerebrospinal fluid (CSF) rhinorrhea is an absolute indication for the surgical repair of the leak. The most common causes for a CSF leak are direct and indirect trauma, erosion produced by an intracranial or an extracranial neoplasm, and iatrogenic causes. Fractures of the anterior fossa of the skull that penetrate the wall between the skull and the paranasal sinuses are referred to as anterior skull base injuries. These include fractures through the posterior wall of the frontal sinus, the roof of the ethmoid, the lamina cribrosa and the sphenoid sinus. Wullstein coined the term "Rhinobasal fractures" for these injuries and approximately 30 percent of all skull base fractures include injuries to the anterior skull base.

Because the fracture site is in direct contact with the outside, through the nasal passages and the paranasal sinuses, it is evident that all anterior skull base fractures must be considered as indirect, open skull-brain injuries. In dural defects and CSF leaks there is, therefore, by definition a skull-brain lesion with all the potential complications inherent in this situation. These include ascending inflammatory intracranial complications such as meningitis and brain abscess. A persistent dural fistula represents a persistent hazard for a potentially fatal purulent meningitis that may develop years after the original injury. For this reason alone, it is mandatory that such lesions be identified and documented. Occasionally it takes recurrent episodes of meningitis before the presence of a CSF leak is suspected. The episode of trauma suffered a long time ago may have been forgotten by the patient or described as only a negligible injury to which little, if any, attention was paid.

When considering the etiology of dural lesions it is important to remember that the attachment of the dura to the underlying bone is much firmer at the skull base than in any other area. This attachment is particularly tight in those areas where the vessels and nerves enter or leave the skull, i.e., in the area of the olfactory filaments or the ethmoid arteries. In these areas the dura is attached to the perineural sheath where it fixes the nerves to the bony ostia. The dura is also firmly attached to the interosseous sutures at the skull, particularly in young persons. In addition, the dura is also considerably thinner at this attachment to the skull than anywhere else along the convexity of the skull. It is particularly delicate here and therefore easily damaged over the lamina cribrosa and the crista galli. This helps to explain why anterior skull base fractures so frequently are associated with dural injuries. According to Leopold, about 10 percent of all anterior skull base fractures are accompanied by a dural injury (see Chapter 2).

For several decades, we have successfully used the following technique for the demonstration and localization of CSF leaks of otologic or rhinologic origin.

Through a suboccipital puncture, 1 ml of CSF is withdrawn and 1 ml of 5 percent Na-fluorescein solution is injected intrathecally. (The CSF sample is used for diagnostic purposes.) Subsequently, the patient is kept in the prone position with the head slightly lower than the rest of the body. This allows the dye to be distributed throughout the entire dural space, since it has a higher specific gravity than CSF. While fluorescein solution can be injected after a lumbar puncture, in this case the patient must be placed into the prone, head down position for several hours. We have had several cases, in which after lumbar injection, the fluorescein did not appear at the site of the dural lesion despite free CSF circulation and an obvious dural leak. For this reason, a suboccipital puncture technique should be used whenever possible. In our hospital the subocciptal puncture is performed by a neurologist, and is generally better tolerated by the patient than a lumbar puncture.

If there is a large CSF fistula, occasionally bright yellowish-green CSF can be seen dripping from the nose within a few minutes after the injection (Figs. 11.71 and 11.72). The patient is then placed in the supine position for endoscopic examination. The nose is sprayed with a topical anesthetic and vasoconstrictor solution (2 percent Pontocaine and phenylephrine) and the endoscopic examination can begin after 1 minute. We usually use a 4-mm 30 degree endoscope with a complementary orange filter over the eyepiece (for use with blue light).

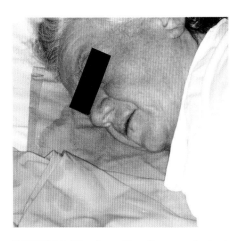

FIGURE 11.71   A positive fluorescein test in a patient with heavy CSF rhinorrhea. The exit of the dye-containing CSF from the nose is easily seen, and after only a few minutes a 20 cm area of the pad is saturated with CSF.

FIGURE 11.72   A and B, A positive fluorescein test in a relatively slight CSF rhinorrhea. Only a few drops of colored CSF appear with breath holding and straining.

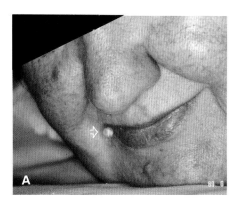

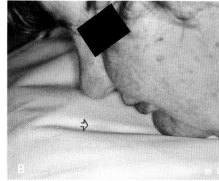

If the fluorescein test is strongly positive, even white light will show the stained CSF clearly (Fig. 11.73A and B) and allow us to follow the leak backwards to its source. At the least, the examiner can determine whether the leak originates in the lamina cribrosa, the anterior or posterior ethmoid, or the sphenoid. In a lateral skull base fracture with a CSF fistula in the area of the middle ear and an intact eardrum, the CSF may pass through the eustachian tube into the nasopharynx and simulate a CSF rhinorrhea. The endoscope makes it possible to unmask such a ''bypass.'' Thus, whenever a small pool of stained CSF accumulates in the pharynx of a supine patient, it should be removed by suction and the source of the CSF should be identified. CSF can be squeezed from the eustachian tube into the nasopharynx quite readily during swallowing.

Occasionally stained CSF can be identified behind an intact eardrum with the endoscope placed into the auditory canal. Since this CSF may have reached the middle ear by going up through the eustachian tube, the localization of the fistula and the diagnosis of the leak must be made in combination with the history and, primarily, with the tomogram.

If the CSF fistula is small and there is only a small leak of CSF at the time of the study, it may be difficult to recognize the leak and distinguish it from the watery nasal secretions of a serous rhinitis. In such cases we switch the light source to blue light to display the fluorescence of the CSF-fluorescein mixture. Even minimal traces of CSF appear under blue light as a bright whitish-green streak (Fig. 11.73C and D), while simple nasal secretions remain colorless and do not fluoresce. This blue light technique is extremely sensitive and is positive up to a dilution of 1:10 million.

FIGURE 11.73 *A*, Heavy CSF rhinorrhea from the left nostril. The cribriform plate was identified as the source. cm = middle turbinate and s = septum. *B*, There is a light but easily identified amount of CSF in the left sphenoethmoidal recess of this patient who had a basal skull fracture in the area of the posterior ethmoid. Viewed with ordinary light. s = septum and arrow = way to choana. *C*, View into a right middle meatus. The head of the middle turbinate is greatly enlarged (a concha bullosa). It was impossible to determine by ordinary white light whether the fluid between the middle turbinate and the septum (*black arrows*) was the same as the foamy secretions lateral to the middle turbinate (*white arrows*), or whether one of these secretions was CSF. s = septum. *D*, By switching to blue light, the fluid between the middle turbinate and the lateral nasal wall (*small arrows*) fluoresced and thus can be identified as CSF, whereas the secretions medial to the turbinate show no fluorescence (*open arrows*).

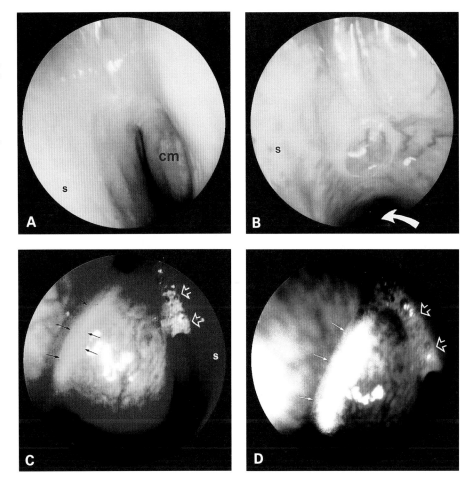

If only very small amounts of CSF are lost through the defect, it does not flow freely, but instead the CSF becomes mixed with the normal nasal secretions and is carried along the standard secretion pathways to the nasopharynx. As described in Chapter 2, the secretions from the nose and from the paranasal sinuses are "hung up" briefly at the border between the ciliated respiratory epithelium and the squamous epithelium of the oropharynx. After a brief period, gravity or the swallowing mechanism again moves the secretions onward. Consequently, this area must be carefully inspected when a CSF fistula is suspected. In the event of a negative fluorescein test, we have found it useful to place one or more small Merocel sponges into the nose for 5 to 6 hours. These sponges absorb the nasal secretions and can then be examined under blue light. Occasionally traces of fluorescein can be discovered by this method (Fig. 11.74). Electrophoretic studies of the fluid expressed from the sponges may also be informative, since fluorescein moves faster than any other substance and can be readily identified by this method.

Even when all attempts to demonstrate a CSF leak are negative, one must remember that the absence of a leak, i.e., a negative fluorescein test, and even a negative CSF specific beta-II transferrin test do not guarantee the abscence of a dural injury. A dural tear may be tamponaded for quite some time by protruding brain tissue, soft tissues, or blood clots. According to Aeberhart and Clodius, CSF leaks appear within the first 48 hours after injury in only 60 percent of cases. A CSF leak appears only within the first 3 months in about 30 percent of the patients, and even later than this, or not at all in 10 percent of all patients.

The nasal mucosa may adhere to the dural defect so tightly, that it, by itself, prevents the CSF leak. Unfortunately the mucosa is not an effective barrier to ascending infections and we have seen several such cases develop recurrent rhinogenic meningitis.

Negative CSF tests do not necessarily mean that there is no need for surgical intervention. This decision can be made only after all of the test and radiologic results and the clinical findings have been considered.

CSF fistulas following basal skull fractures are managed in the majority of cases via the proven external transethmoid route through a small incision medially in the eyebrow. This permits the exposure of the entire anterior skull base in the ethmoid and sphenoid areas, the identification of the defect, and its closure. The closure is usually achieved with lyophilized dura or fascia that is attached with fibrin-glue. In rare cases, where the management of the fistula is more difficult, e.g., in the sphenoid sinus, we use additional patches of muscle.

A dye in the CSF is helpful under these conditions, as it permits a precise localization of the leak, good control of the effectiveness of the closure, and most importantly, the identification of small areas of stained mucosa that suggest an incomplete closure and the need for further revision, even though there is no active leak at the time. We prefer the external approach to the endoscopic one, since it is impossible to determine preoperatively the full extent of the fracture with any degree of certainty. It happens with some regularity that the fracture underlying the CSF fistula in the roof of the ethmoid extends medially into the lamina cribrosa or to the crista galli or even anteriorly and superiorly to the posterior wall of the frontal sinus. It is also possible for the fracture line to extend across the midline to the opposite side so that fluorescein stained CSF appears at the left side of the nose, even though the fracture is on the right.

Postoperatively the patient is kept on strict bed rest for 1 week and forbidden from blowing his or her nose, in order not to increase the intracranial pressure. In almost 1,000 fluorescein tests during the past 18 years we have had only one serious complication. One patient had a grand mal seizure after the fluorescein was introduced suboccipitally and apparently reached the floor of the fourth ventricle.

FIGURE 11.74 *A*, A dry Merocel sponge before insertion (*above*) and after removal from the nose, damp and expanded (*below*). *B*, Two sponges showing a positive (*above*) and a negative (*below*) fluorescein test in normal white light. *C* and *D*, If the sponge fluoresces under blue light, it has absorbed some stained CSF. The picture in *C* has been taken without an orange filter, and the picture in *D* has been taken with orange filter. By using an orange filter, the effects of blue light become even more pronounced.

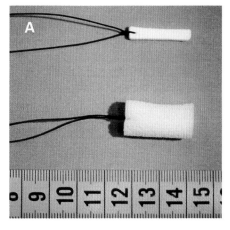
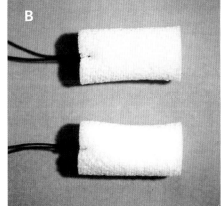
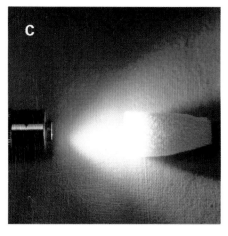
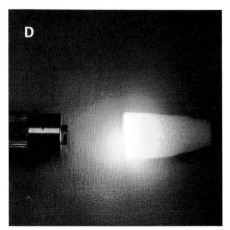

ENDOSCOPIC APPROACH TO HEADACHES AND SINUS DISEASE

Recurrent headaches can be very frustrating for both the patient who suffers from them and for the physician from whom treatment is expected. The otorhinolaryngologist is generally confronted by three different and distinct groups of headache patients:

1. Those with headaches clearly connected to sinus disease, such as inflammatory disease, neoplasm, barotrauma, or another readily identifiable sinugenic cause.
2. Those with headaches that can be traced to nonsinus causes such as migraine, neuralgias, cervical spine disorders, abnormalities of blood pressure or other vascular disorders ("ice cream headache"), temporomandibular joint disease, ophthalmic refraction problems, glaucoma, allergies, etc.
3. Those whose problems are not clear and in whom there seems to be no overt indication of sinus disease. It is this group of patients that can present a rewarding challenge for the nasal endoscopist.

TABLE 11.2 Predominant Symptoms in 100 Consecutive Patients with Sinusitis Referred to Graz ENT Department

Symptom	No. Patients
Congestion/obstruction	82
Secretion	64
Fullness/pressure— mild pain	62
Severe headaches	48

The typical triad of sinusitis symptoms includes: nasal congestion or obstruction, the presence of abnormal secretions, and headache. The distribution of the headache may be quite variable. Of 100 consecutive patients seen in our clinic with the diagnosis of acute or chronic sinusitis, 48 complained variably of headache as their predominant symptom (Table 11.2). The typical pattern of possible sinugenic headaches are pain at the top of the calvarium sometimes together with a "centrally located" or bitemporal pain, indicating possible sphenoid or posterior ethmoid disease. Pain around the glabella, around the inner canthus, "between" or "above" the eyes, or intraorbitally suggests the presence of anterior ethmoid and/or frontal sinus disease.

Sinugenic headaches may also be experienced in the area of the temples, in the temporoparietal region and also in the occipital area. The pain may radiate from the forehead or the temples to the nuchal area or may circle the head like a tight band. The pain is usually characterized as being "dull" and is combined with a feeling of pressure and fullness. In the acute cases there may be a pulsating pain, especially when the head is bent forward or when the patient is under physical stress.

Through the use of the rigid nasal endoscope the examiner may be able to identify relatively easily underlying causes such as tumors, specific diseases such as sarcoidosis, and even high and posteriorly located septal spurs. It is well established that septal spurs or deviations contacting the turbinates may cause "contact" headaches, and the mechanisms of referred pain in lesions of the septal and turbinal mucosa have also been well demonstrated.

If only one symptom of the triad prevails clinically, we still look for sinusitis if the symptom is congestion or suppurative rhinorrhea. If the symptom is headache alone and all the results of our examination seem to be normal (routine sinus radiographs, anterior and posterior rhinoscopy, nasal examination with the operating microscope, and sinus translumination), we still should consider the possibility of a sinus-related cause, especially when additional examinations by the ophthamologist, dentist, internist, neurologist, and others reveal no pathologic findings and cervical spine radiographs, electro- encephalographs, and computed tomographs of the brain are normal. Detection of disease in the narrow spaces of the lateral nasal wall hidden to casual examination, the operating microscope, and conventional radiographs is a challenging task for the endoscopist.

As we have seen, sinus disease usually starts in the middle nasal meatus. Both secretion transportation and aeration of the maxillary sinus takes place through the very narrow ethmoidal infundibulum between the uncinate process medially and the lamina papyracea laterally. Secretions then enter the middle meatus through the hiatus semilunaris. The frontal sinus drains via the frontal recess either directly into the ethmoidal infundibulum or, if the infundibulum ends in a superior blind pocket (the recessus terminalis) medially from the infundibulum, into the middle meatus. Any conditions narrowing or blocking these spaces and clefts may lead to the retention of secretions and poor ventilation and thus predispose to consequent infection of the larger, adjacent sinuses. Sometimes small localized areas of contact between the opposing mucosal surfaces in these key areas of the anterior ethmoid may lead to such a blockage, which in turn may alter nasal function. If opposing areas of mucosa come into intense contact, the beating of the cilia of these areas stops or is impeded. The mucus between these contacting areas is thus no longer transported by the cilia. This stagnant mucus provides an ideal condition for viral and bacterial growth. Depending upon the intensity and duration of such a condition, disease may spread throughout the vicinity, especially to the larger sinuses.

Most often, however, these processes remain localized to the middle meatus, causing only one of the typical symptoms of sinusitis: the feeling of pressure, congestion, and fullness; a postnasal discharge; or simply headaches. These headaches may be the result of 1) constant intense mucosal contact according to the concept of "referred pain"; 2) malventilation or nonventilation of the sinuses with resulting hypoxia, or negative pressure; 3) pressure from proliferating polyps; or 4) due to epithelial lesions and/or any combination of all of the above. This contact/pressure phenomenon, as studies carried out at our institution have shown, may be one of the factors causing the growth of nasal polyps by the local liberation of neuropeptides such as substance P as well as H-substances and seems to be a factor in mediating pain.

Time and again we find that polyps begin in the middle meatus, originating from areas of intense mucosal contact (see Chapter 5). On the other hand, when removing polyps from isolated narrow ethmoidal spaces or cells, we often find astonishingly large polyps in small niches, where they were apparently under considerable pressure, thus adding to the patient's discomfort.

Endoscopic diagnostic techniques combined with CT enable us to discover disease otherwise hidden from the eye, the operating microscope, and conventional radiographs. Some of the typical and more frequent findings in headache patients are listed in Table 11.3. Not all of these conditions should be considered as a disease per se, but they are all factors that can reduce the normally narrow spaces of the anterior ethmoid and thus give rise to areas of mucosal contact, secretion retention and malventilation and/or infection of the larger sinuses, or promote polypoid degeneration of opposing mucosal surfaces. All these conditions, even when small and circumscribed, may have one dominating clinical symptom: headache.

TABLE 11.3   Frequent Endoscopic and/or CT Findings in Patients with Sinugenic Headaches

*	Septal deviation/spurs
**	Diseased agger nasi cells
**	Diseased frontal recess

Uncinate process

**	Medially bent, contacting middle turbinate
*	Laterally bent
**	Curved anteriorly ("doubled middle turbinate")
*	Fractures (trauma, iatrogenic)

Abnormalities of the middle turbinate

**	Concha bullosa (pneumatized middle turbinate)
*	Paradoxically bent
*	Bulging into lateral nasal wall

Ethmoidal bulla

***	Large, filling middle meatus
**	Contact areas (especially polyps from turbinate sinus)
*	Anterior growth, overlapping hiatus semilunaris
**	Protruding from middle meatus

Combination of all of the above, resulting in an obstruction of the frontal recess or of other parts of the middle meatus

*	Isolated sphenoid disease

* = rare finding; ** = more frequent finding; *** = very frequent finding.

In Chapter 5 the endoscopic and CT findings are described in detail. At this point we wish to emphasize the frequency of pathologic findings in the area of the ethmoidal bulla. The ethmoidal bulla may be pneumatized (enlarged) to such a degree that it completely fills the sinus of the middle turbinate (the space in the convexity of the middle turbinate). This is one of the key findings in many headache patients. The contact between bulla and turbinate can be extensive, almost like that of gauze packing of the middle meatus. It is important to realize this condition on CT or conventional tomography, as it may be overlooked or read as normal, because there is normally no radiographic opacification of either of these structures in the case of contact headaches. A concha bullosa (pneumatized middle turbinate) can almost always be diagnosed. Frequently, there is disease in the area of contact between the bulla and the turbinate, and this area is one of the most frequent locations from which polyps originate.

The "lateral sinus" (a variable chamber above and posterior to the bulla) is another narrow ethmoidal space hidden from the eye and may only appear on CT as an area of isolated disease, the only symptom of which may be headache and a postnasal discharge.

There are cases of limited disease in the frontal recess and the infundibulum that may cause severe symptoms in the patient, and which may even be virtually unrecognized even with the endoscope. Diagnostically, these are the cases in which CT and endoscopy complement each other. Time and again we have been able to identify relatively small polyps or cysts in the depths of the infundibulum as the underlying cause for headaches of many years' standing.

As the area of the frontal recess is not always easily accessible to the endoscope, a combined diagnostic approach (CT and endoscopy) is of great importance. As mentioned earlier, agger nasi cells and concha bullosa can be pneumatized from the frontal recess. A disease of one of these structures therefore can affect the others. The frontal sinus is a common source of headaches when it is malventilated or otherwise diseased.

The typical endoscopic and radiographic findings of a diseased frontal recess are shown in Chapter 5. Sometimes only discrete signs of disease, such as a minimal amount of abnormal secretion, may be present endoscopically. Similar symptoms may occur less commonly because of scarring or synechia in the middle meatal area following surgery, nasal packing, nasotracheal intubation, or nasogastric intubation.

Unusual Lesions

There are a number of more unusual lesions that can cause sinugenic headaches. Isolated sphenoid sinus lesions such as cysts, polyps, or mycotic infection can give rise to a more "central" headache. Endoscopically, a stream of pus or viscid mucus sometimes can be seen in the sphenoethmoid recess, and sometimes it may not be possible to evaluate the sphenoid sinus ostium directly. Sphenoid sinus lesions may be recognized on a plain radiograph, but are better defined on CT.

The foramen rotundum with the second branch of the trigeminal nerve may lie in close proximity to the mucosa of the sphenoid in the event of extensive pneumatization. If the sinus is diseased, this may well affect the nerve and the patient may present with trigeminal neuralgia-like symptoms. The vidian nerve may also lie close to an extensively pneumatized sphenoid and thus be irritated in cases of sinus disease. With these possibilities in mind we can expect on occasion to unearth the underlying cause of an allegedly "idiopathic" neuralgia, which then can be treated surgically with success.

Only the endoscope and tomography helped us to detect a small cyst (see Chapter 5) sitting at the roof of the maxillary sinus on the infraorbital nerve. Conventional radiographs failed to demonstrate the cyst. The symptom of midfacial pain, which we believe originated from that cyst, had been treated medically as a trigeminal neuralgia as there was no history of any sinus infections or other sinus problems. A minor endoscopic procedure was followed by relief of the patient's problems.

When one of these possible causes of symptoms mentioned above, or combinations of these, have been identified and medical therapy has failed, then endoscopic surgery is indicated. If doubts about the indication exist, in some cases it may help to anesthetize the area of the suspected lesion (with cocaine, Pontocaine, etc.) in the office in the same way as in the operating room with cotton-tipped probes. If the patient then is free of headaches or the particular symptoms for the duration of the anesthetic, this may help the surgeon to make a decision regarding an operation in doubtful cases.

The most impressive results are usually seen in patients whose predominant symptom has been headache and in whom underlying causes such as the ones mentioned have been identified. Within a few hours of the endoscopic procedure the pain is usually gone, providing often dramatic relief despite the fact that reactive swelling, congestion, and mucorrhea may linger for several days after the procedure. For endoscopic surgeons it is therefore one of the most challenging yet rewarding tasks to identify and treat causes that underlie allegedly nonsinus-related headaches.

446

Since the patient with a sinugenic headache may not present with a typical history of sinus disease, we should investigate for underlying causes with a possible nasal and sinus causation in mind. Negative findings with anterior and posterior rhinoscopy, examination with the operating microscope and conventional radiography do not rule out a nasal or sinus causation. Diagnostic endoscopy with rigid endoscopes in many cases allows the detection of lesions hidden from the unaided eye or even from the operating microscope, although endoscopy also sometimes misses disease in particular locations even if repeatedly carried out at various intervals. Only the combination of diagnostic endoscopy with CT provides the maximum information, with one modality enhancing the accuracy of the other.

As significant symptoms can sometimes be caused by relatively small lesions, attention in examining imaging studies should not be focused exclusively on "opacifications" and/or "soft tissue masses" in the sinuses or the lateral nasal wall, but on identification of areas of possible stenoses and mucosal contact areas, like the frequent finding of a middle meatus completely "packed" by an extensively pneumatized ethmoidal bulla. This finding alone was frequently the explanation for severe headaches and a feeling of nasal obstruction.

The rhinologist should view the CTs jointly with the radiologist and explain what kind of changes and abnormalities are being searched for that may be of clinical importance.

Causes of Pain in Areas of Mucosal Irritation

No one would question the cause of pain in acute purulent sinusitis, as we all know that infections of the frontal, maxillary, and sphenoid sinuses are often accompanied by considerable pain, especially when their ostia are blocked and retention of secretions occurs, usually giving rise to a pounding pain. Divers especially know that a negative pressure due to malventilation in the larger sinuses can be very painful, with the barotrauma frequently resulting in bleeding into the affected sinuses. Studies have demonstrated that hypoxia in the sinuses is one of the factors that can give a sensation of pain.

A relatively limited mucosal lesion or area of contact can trigger severe long-standing headaches, often projecting to different dermatomes of the head. The mechanisms of referred pain in the nose and sinus area are as follows: afferent fibers from pain and other receptors in the nasal and sinus mucosa end up in the same "pool" of sensory neurons in the sensory nucleus of the trigeminal nerve as fibers serving cutaneous receptors. These two common pathways discharge along the same final neurons to a common cortical area. The cortical center cannot distinguish the original peripheral source of the impulse reaching it by this single final pathway, therefore, when the mucosa is stimulated, the afferent pain impulses may be falsely localized after reaching the sensory cortex. These are misinterpreted on the basis of previous experience as coming from the skin area from which impulses normally arrive at that point in the brain. Once having identified the corresponding bundles of nerve fibers, one can understand why lesions of the inferior turbinate may project their pain to the upper teeth or the zygoma and below the eye, and why lesions of the middle turbinate may project to the temple, the zygoma, the inner canthus and/or the forehead, etc. Knowing these pathways is a helpful diagnostic tool in localizing an intranasal lesion.

Recent advances in biochemistry and research focus on one of the more important factors involved in this phenomenon: the neuropeptides. The sensory supply of the nasal and paranasal mucosa is derived from the maxillary and ophthalmic divisions of the trigeminal nerve, which also supplies the respiratory mucosa with a dense network of adrenergic and cholinergic fibers. Most of these fibers, which control blood circulation and glandular secretion, reach the vessels and glands after passing through the pterygopalatine ganglion. Recent pharmacologic studies have revealed that there is at least a third group of mediator substances besides the neuro-transmitters noradrenalin and acetylcholine. These have been identified as the neuropeptides, with the most important one for mucosal function apparently being substance P (SP). More than 50 different types of peptides have been found so far in the central and peripheral nervous system in the human respiratory tract, the vasoactive intestinal polypeptides, the gastrin-releasing peptide, the peptide histidine isoleucine and SP have been identified, among others. Our own investigations have concentrated on SP, which was discovered as early as 1931. The analysis of the chemical structure was not achieved before the early 1970s, however. Substance P is an undecapeptide (amino acid sequence: H-Arg-Pro-Lys-Pro-Gln-Gln-Phe-Phe-Gly-Leu-Met-NH$_2$) with a strong vasodilatatory effect. It is one of the mediators of sensory and vagal afferent neurons, which are known to be unmyelinated C fibers. Tachykinin-containing nerve fibers can be found in the submucosa and in the respiratory epithelium, around blood vessels and glands, and within tracheobronchial smooth muscle. Other recent reports suggest further that tachykinins such as calcitonin gene-related peptide (CGRP) and neurokinin A coexist with SP in the C fibers of the respiratory system. They are liberated simultaneously by one action potential, enhancing the pharmocologic effects of SP: vasodilatation, plasma extravasation (''neurogenic edema''), hypersecretion, and smooth muscle contraction (of bronchial, *not* of vascular muscles). The edema is possibly enhanced by a simultaneous histamine release from mast cells, apparently triggered by the SP liberation as well.

Pain Mediation

In the neuron, substance P vesicles are transported not only toward the CNS but toward the peripheral synapses as well, thus SP can be liberated at the central and the peripheral ends of a sensory neuron. Hence, SP may mediate not only central reflexes in afferent C fibers (orthodromic impulse), but local reflexes as well (antidromic impulse), leading to a liberation of SP in the nasal mucosa. This mechanism is called the axon reflex (Fig. 11.75). Among the different receptors in the nasal mucosa served by afferent peptidergic C fibers are polymodal nociceptors, mediating pain. The peripheral stimuli may possibly be noxious, infectious, chemical, or caloric irritants or simply mechanical ones like pressure. The stimulation of these polymodal receptors leads to an orthodromic impulse via the C fibers to the CNS, mediating pain. At the same time an antidromic (running in the opposite direction) impulse may lead to a local release of SP at the synapses at vessels, glands, in the nasal mucosa, and smooth muscle contraction, contraction may occur in the bronchi. This model of SP-mediated axon reflex, with an orthodromic impulse to the CNS signaling pain and an antidromic impulse causing local reactions like neurogenic edema, could well explain why areas of mucosal contact and pressure, be they from a septal spur or a diseased stenotic ethmoidal recess, can cause pain, mucosal edema, and hypersecretion and sometimes enhance pulmonary (asthmatic) symptoms by smooth muscle contraction. This model may help us to explain why chemical irritants like cigarette smoke or changes in ambient temperature can cause mucosal swelling, hypersecretion, and headache in "hyperreactive rhinopathy" (vasomotor rhinitis), and why polyps so frequently start from areas of mucosal contact.

Capsaicin (trans-8-methyl-N-vanillyl-6-nonenamide), the pungent extract of red pepper, after repeated topical or systemic application in animal experiments leads to a selective killing of the afferent C fibers and a desensitization of the polymodal neuropeptidergic nociceptors. Substance P normally is released at the synapses of C fibers of the effector organs such as vessels and glands, where it induces a change of potential at the postsynaptic membrane and thus a stimulation of the effector cells. With the first application of capsaicin, topically or systemically, a release of SP is induced; further applications then cause a desensitization of the pain receptors and selective killing of the afferent C fibers.

Conclusions

Headaches can be of sinus origin, even if this is not suspected from the case history. Nasal endoscopy in combination with polytomography and/or CT usually reveals those causes hidden from the unaided eye, the operating microscope, and plain radiographs of the sinuses. Many anatomic variations of the middle meatus and other regions of the lateral nasal wall predispose patients to headaches by narrowing even more the already narrow ethmoidal recesses. They may give rise to areas of more or less intense contact of opposing mucosal surfaces, impeding or completely blocking ventilation and drainage of the larger sinuses. As secretion between the contacting surfaces cannot be transported away, foci or reinfections of the ethmoid system, and especially the larger sinuses, may persist.

After the identification of these underlying processes, functional endoscopic surgery with usually minimal procedures can often provide dramatic relief of symptoms that may have continued for months and years.

Recent research has identified a third system of mediators besides the neurotransmitters noradrenalin and acetylcholine; the neuropeptides. Substance P is one of the mediators controlling pain perception from polymodal receptors in the nasal mucosa via unmyelinated C fibers to the cortex. Together with this orthodromic impulse an antidromic impulse can start, releasing SP to local effector cells in the mucosa, causing a "neurogenic edema" with plasma extravasation, vasodilatation, and hypersecretion. This mechanism of simultaneous orthodromic and antidromic impulses is called the axon reflex.

The release of SP from the polymodal receptors can be triggered by various stimuli such as chemical, infectious, and thermal irritants, but also by sheer mechanical pressure. The pressure exerted on nasal mucosa in areas of contacting opposing mucosal surfaces, whether through inflammation, polyps, or mucosal swelling due to other reasons, especially in the narrow spaces of the key areas of the ethmoid where anatomic variations can cause additional stenoses predisposing to mucosal contact, can apparently be enough to trigger an SP-mediated pain sensitization via the afferent C fibers. This axon reflex can explain why an initially relatively small localized lesion may lead to a vicious cycle and on to massive symptoms. This model of "referred pain" makes it clear why the pain may not necessarily be felt at its origin, but projected to the corresponding sensory dermatomes.

The mediating function of SP can be blocked selectively by local administration of capsaicin, which desensitizes the receptors and kills the afferent C fibers without affecting other sensory structures. We

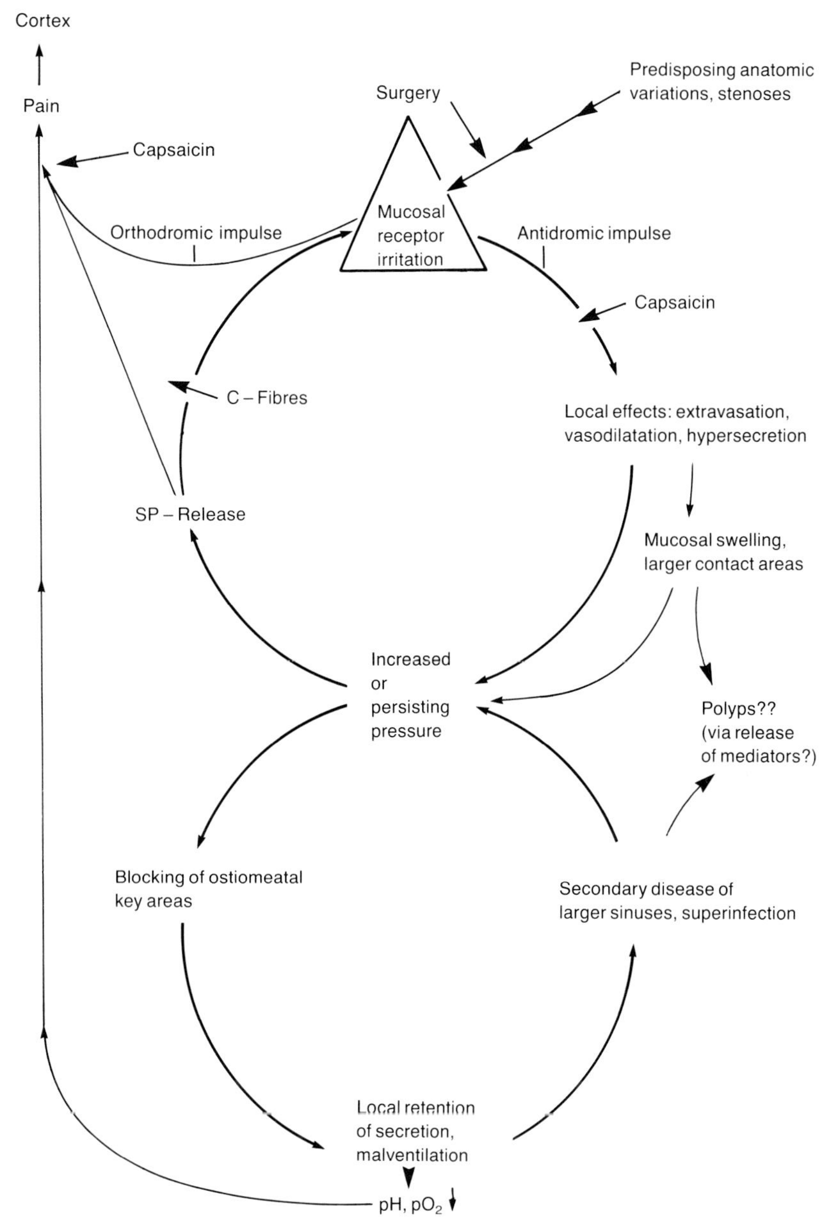

FIGURE 11.75 Schematic diagram of the Axon-reflex and its hypothetical role in ostiomeatal disease.

have tried to point out these complex interactions in a simplified schematic drawing in Figure 11.75. In patients with vasomotor rhinitis we were able to block all the symptoms, including their headaches, by topical administration of capsaicin.

Knowledge of these possible mechanisms appears to be useful in patients with cephalgia. Identification of intranasal and sinal lesions and contact areas should be carried out and surgery performed if medical treatment fails. The functional endoscopic approach with minimal trauma has given us our best results. For the future, application of capsaicin derivatives may offer an additional alternative for individual cases, although the primary aim of therapy should always be elimination of the underlying causes rather than simply amelioration of symptoms.

451

Chapter 12

ASTHMA AND SINUS DISEASE

Bronchial asthma is a very complex disease in which there are numerous factors that can either trigger or exacerbate the underlying bronchospasm. The close relationship between inflammatory paranasal sinus disease and the onset, maintenance, and exacerbation of bronchial asthma is a well documented common clinical observation. The role of sinusitis in the pathogenesis of asthma has been argued for decades and is, even today, a subject of heated controversy.

Some investigators assume that sinusitis and bronchial asthma are manifestations of the same basic disease in two different areas of the respiratory system. Even a causal relationship between sinusitis and asthma has been proposed. Others consider the appearance of sinusitis and asthma in the same patient as purely coincidental and emphasize that any surgical manipulation in the paranasal sinuses may trigger or aggravate asthmatic symptoms.

There are numerous reports concerning the sometimes spectacular improvement of the asthmatic symptoms following surgical treatment of inflammatory sinus disease. This usually entailed the removal of marked polypoid disease from the nose or large sinuses. Most reports in the literature usually assess the degree of improvement on the basis of purely subjective statements from the patient and, additionally, by a decreased requirement for asthma medication.

In order to determine whether the improved nasal airway had a "placebo effect" on the pulmonary symptoms, we studied 54 patients during 1988 and 1989. This study was performed in cooperation with specialists in pulmonary diseases. The patients ranged in age from 15 to 71 years, with a mean age of 43 years. There were 32 females and 22 males in the study. All of them suffered from perennial bronchial asthma. Most of the patients (79.6%) had intrinsic asthma. All patients had asthma for more than 1 year and all required medication for the management of their symptoms. Thirty-six patients (66.7%) were steroid-dependent and 18 patients were managed with nonsteroidal bronchodilators.

The severity of the asthma at the time of admittance to the study was determined by the frequency and intensity of the attacks, the type and amount of medication used, the frequency of status asthmaticus and the need for inpatient care, and the results of pulmonary function tests (vital capacity [VC] and forced expiratory volume [FEV_1]) performed.

On the basis of these studies, 44 of 54 patients were classified as "severe" asthmatics.

Forty-six patients (85.2%) gave a history of nasal or paranasal sinus problems, while 8 patients (14.85%) reported no previous nasal problems. Anterior rhinoscopy found no disease in the latter group. In all patients, endoscopy and routine CT performed prior to admission to the study showed clear evidence of ethmoidal disease. This was considered to be the most important criterion for inclusion into the study.

The most frequent complaint was reduced or blocked nasal breathing, with or without a reduction in the sense of smell (45 patients = 83.3%), followed by postnasal discharge (44 patients = 81.5%), persistent sniffles (36 patients = 66.7%), and headache (23 patients = 42.6%). The majority of patients with obvious nasal symptoms reported that their asthma became more severe when the sinus and/or nasal symptoms worsened. In order to prevent pulmonary complications, many patients increased their asthma medication when an upper respiratory infection or increased nasal symptoms appeared.

It was noteworthy that 72.2 percent (39 patients) reported that their nasal problems *preceded* the onset of asthma. Six patients (11.1%) reported that nasal symptoms and asthma appeared about the same time and 8 patients (14.8%) claimed that they had no nasal symptoms prior to the onset of asthma.

Thirty-four patients (63%) had one or more previous nasal or sinus procedures with 25 having undergone fenestration of the maxillary sinus and/or some radical procedure. Fourteen of these 25 patients had no improvement in their asthma following surgery. Nine reported varying degrees of improvement, lasting from 6 months to 5 years.

454

During the initial diagnostic study or during the surgical procedure, endoscopy revealed polypoid mucosal changes in the key locations of the anterior ethmoid in the significant majority of the patients. The maxillary and/or frontal sinuses were involved to a varying degree. In 70 percent of the patients, polyps were found even on anterior rhinoscopy.

On the basis of endoscopic and radiographic findings, 29 patients (53.7%) were classified as having massive nasal pathology and 25 (46.3%) as having only a slight nasal involvement. It was interesting to note that among those patients with slight nasal involvement, 21 of 25 (84%) had a history of severe asthma and that postoperatively 18 patients (72%) reported significant improvement of their asthma.

A surprisingly high percentage of the patients had a dense eosinophilic infiltrate in the surgically removed mucous membranes and a clinical picture of diffuse polypoid rhinosinusitis. In 14 cases there was definite aspirin sensitivity and in 7 more there was strong suspicion of aspirin sensitivity, although this could not be confirmed.

The endoscopic surgical procedure was adapted to the individual pathologic findings and consisted of correcting the disease in key locations and leaving the adjacent large paranasal sinuses alone. Sphenoethmoidectomy was performed in 4 cases of diffuse polypoid rhinosinusitis, but even in these cases the middle turbinate was spared unless it had been partially or totally resected during previous procedures.

There were no intraoperative complications in any of the 54 patients. Three patients required intraoperative intravenous aminophylline and/or steroids or other bronchodilator aerosols. No procedure had to be aborted because of an asthmatic attack. All procedures were performed under sedation and topical and local anesthesia.

Of the 46 patients who had massive nasal symptoms preoperatively, 37 (80.4%) showed significant improvement in their nasal symptoms within the first few days postoperatively. Thirty-three patients (61.1%) showed a marked improvement in their asthma, using the same amount of medication as before. Twenty-one patients (22.2%) had a slight to moderate improvement in their asthma and 7 patients (12.9%) had no improvement over their preoperative status. Two patients (3.8%) required a higher dose of steroids postoperatively for the control of their asthma. During the entire postoperative study period of 1 year, only one patient developed status asthmaticus. None of the other patients required hospitalization for asthma during this period.

All results were confirmed by postoperative pulmonary function tests. The comparison of preoperative and postoperative FEV_1 and VC showed a definite improvement in both parameters. The percentage of improvement was 16.3 percent for the VC and 24 percent for the FEV_1. These differences were significant statistically.

In order to get a firm end-point, the reduction in the dose of steroids was not started until 1 month after the endoscopic procedure. Thus the effects of the surgical intervention could be independently evaluated. Because of the many different bronchodilators used, these could not be individually assessed. The basic concept was that whatever medication the patient had been taking was continued unchanged for the first month before any reduction in quantity or type of medication was initiated on the basis of improved FEV_1 and VC.

Eighteen and a half percent of our patients had a recurrence of their nasal symptoms during the follow-up period and of these, the large majority had been diagnosed as suffering from diffuse, polypoid rhinosinusitis.

We believe that the results of this study permit us to draw the following conclusions.

Intrinsic asthma is related directly to diseases of the lateral nasal wall and the paranasal sinuses. More than 70 percent of the patients had nasal symptoms first and developed the symptoms of asthma later. This temporal (and causal ?) relationship cannot be denied.

Nearly all patients who had initial nasal symptoms felt that there was a relationship between the deterioration of the nasal symptoms and the appearance or exacerbation of their bronchial asthma.

In the majority of even those patients who had no subjective evidence of any nasal symptoms, diseases in the key locations of the lateral nasal wall were demonstrated by endoscopy and/or sinus CT. The findings were evidently relevant to the pulmonary disease process as shown by the improvement of the asthma following medical or surgical therapy of these allegedly ''asymptomatic'' foci of ethmoidal disease.

Patients with asthma and marked nasal symptoms should be examined and treated for the latter problem. If conservative therapy fails, surgery should be considered. More than 70 percent of patients with intrinsic asthma can confidently expect an improvement of their disease following such therapy.

Even though the nose-lung trigger effect is clear both clinically and from the history, the underlying pathomechanism—undoubtedly a multifactorial relationship—is not yet clear. The role of neuropeptides and other mediators (e.g., substance P) and substances liberated from the eosinophils are being investigated.

The presence of dense eosinophilic infiltrates in the mucosa of the diseased paranasal sinuses in asthmatic patients appears to be of significance. As we know from electron microscopic studies, the eosinophils in these patients frequently show evidence of degranulation. This is particularly characteristic of patients with diffuse polypoid rhinosinusitis and of patients with aspirin sensitivity.

Even though the clinical relationship is obvious, we unfortunately still lack any objective criteria that would permit us to predict which patients would be improved to what degree and for how long by either conservative and/or surgical therapy. In this sense, only negative predictions are possible with any certainty. A poorer therapeutic result and a less impressive clinical improvement can be expected in those patients who have diffuse polypoid rhinosinusitis, who are prone to recurrence, who have dense eosinophilic infiltrates in the mucosa of the paranasal sinuses, who have ASA sensitivity, who have been steroid dependent for several years, and who have undergone several previous surgical procedures.

The results of this study again show clearly that a reasonably certain positive result can be anticipated only when the surgical procedure is directed toward the primary disease foci in the lateral nasal wall and not toward the secondarily involved paranasal sinuses.

Chapter 13

RESULTS, PROBLEMS, AND COMPLICATIONS

RESULTS

Because of the large number of different indications for the Messerklinger technique (Table 13.1), no single unified statistic can represent the results of this technique. The results must instead be examined on the basis of the different disease entities.

An assessment of the results of surgery is further complicated by the lack of criteria that allow a truly objective measurement of "success." In numerous indications such as headache, pressure, postnasal discharge, or frequent or protracted colds with "obstructed" nasal breathing, the assessor is almost totally dependent upon the patient's subjective evaluation. Rhinomanometry has not proven useful in our hands, either as a determinant for surgery or as a measure of successful outcome. Frequently, even after extensive sinus surgery with preservation of the middle turbinate, patients show the same rhinomanometric curves postoperatively, as preoperatively even though the subjective symptoms reported by the patient are significantly improved or even eliminated, and endoscopy also frequently reveals normal mucous membranes (Figs. 13.1 to 13.4).

TABLE 13.1 Spectrum of Frequent Indications for FES

Polypoid sinusitis (60%)	Symptomatic retention cysts
Chronic and acute recurring infections of all sinuses	Orbital complications
	Sinus mycoses
Nasal obstruction	Persisting complaints after Caldwell-Luc and fenestration operations
Headaches	
Pressure feelings	Tubal dysfunctions
Postnasal discharge	Adjuvant surgery to allergy treatment
Epiphora	Antrochoanal polyps
Anosmia	Mucoviscidosis
Mucoceles of all sinuses	Sinubronchial syndrome/Asthma

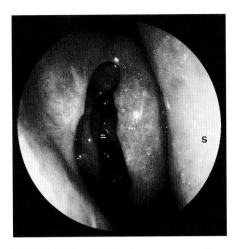

FIGURE 13.1   The ideal appearance after endoscopic surgery for ethmoid and concha bullosa disease on the right side. The entry into the middle meatus is free and the mucosa is unremarkable. s = septum.

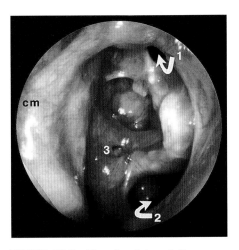

FIGURE 13.2   The view into a left ethmoid, 1 year after surgery. The path to the maxillary and frontal sinuses is free (*curved arrows 1 and 2*). The mucosa is unremarkable everywhere. At *3*, it is still possible to see the somewhat scarred opening into the ground lamella that was made to inspect the posterior ethmoid. Note that no attempt had been made to create a large and smooth operative cavity. Only the important pathologic changes were corrected. 1 = to maxillary sinus; 2 = to frontal sinus; 3 = scarred opening into the ground lamella; cm = concha media.

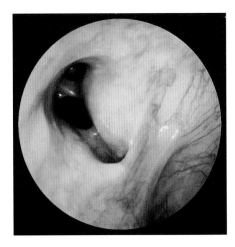

FIGURE 13.3   View into a left maxillary sinus (through a window in the inferior meatus, created during an earlier surgical procedure) approximately 2.5 years after an endoscopic ethmoid procedure. The enlarged ostium can be seen with a 90 degree lens, and through it, the unremarkable ethmoid may be seen.

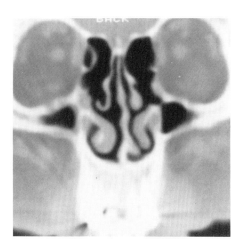

FIGURE 13.4   CT of the patient shown in Figure 13.1. This CT shows the normal appearance of the ethmoids after bilateral functional endoscopic sinus surgery in a patient who had bilateral ethmoidal sinus disease and bilateral concha bullosa. The medial lamellae of the concha bullosa serve as "normal" middle turbinates on both sides. The section plane is somewhat *anterior* to the maxillary ostium, which is just excluded on the patient's right.

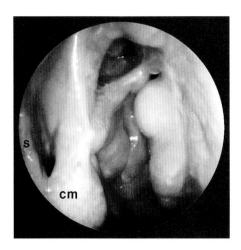

FIGURE 13.5 Abnormal mucosa, postoperatively, in a left middle meatus. Details in the text. s = septum and cm = concha media.

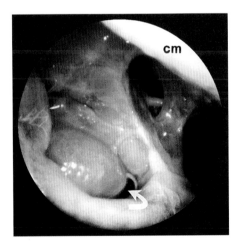

FIGURE 13.6 The postoperative persistence or recurrence of polypoid mucosal changes in a patient with diffuse polypoid rhinosinopathy is evident. The *curved arrow* shows the maxillary sinus ostium (right side). For details, see text. cm = concha media.

Since we can look into the remote corners of the paranasal sinus system and of the lateral wall of the nose in most cases postoperatively with the endoscope, it becomes apparent that the objective evaluation of the outcome is really difficult. We have seen a number of patients who were free of symptoms for years after a surgical procedure and yet whose mucous membranes were far from "normal" (Figs. 13.5 and 13.6). One can find mild inflammatory changes, polypoid thickening, crusts, and increased secretions in patients with the sinubronchial syndrome or asthma with ASA intolerance who postoperatively report a significant improvement in their nasal symptoms and even in some cases a complete disappearance of their asthma (see Chapter 12). Many of these patients were steroid-dependent preoperatively, but were able to reduce or discontinue the steroid regimen and had a significant improvement in the quality of their life.

On the other hand, there are patients whose mucous membranes appear to be perfectly normal postoperatively and whose ostia are all free and patent, yet still complain about a variety of persistent problems for which no anatomic basis can be found. In these patients, unrealistic expectations may be in conflict with reality. For this reason we now explain to the patient in great detail that the surgical procedure will not protect them from future colds and that they may even develop sinusitis again.

All this shows that it is difficult to give percentages of objective postoperative improvement and to develop meaningful statistics. How should one classify a patient whose asthma has disappeared postoperatively, whose nasal respiration is improved, but whose mucous membrane looks like that in Figures 13.5 and 13.6. Can this patient be classified on the basis of clinical symptomatology as a 100 percent success, or only as a 60 percent success on the basis of the endoscopic findings? How should the patient be classified whose mucous membranes have become completely normal, but yet who complains about a variety of inexplicable and unclassifiable residual problems? How can the results of different surgeons, perhaps using different techniques, be compared, when one of the authors does not use an endoscope postoperatively, and thus cannot see the residual changes and instead relies entirely on the patient's clinical symptoms?

There are a number of unresolved questions that indicate the difficulty in gathering statistics and in comparing the results of different authors.

In our postoperative assessment we have asked our patients to indicate a percentage improvement (see below) and we have then attempted to relate this subjective grading to our endoscopic and radiologic findings and express it as a percentage result. The statistics presented below clearly still contain a significant subjective component.

TABLE 13.2 Preceding Therapies
(500 Patients)

Frequent repeated maxillary irrigations/
   indwelling tubes
82 fenestrations and/or radical operations
   (some multiple and bilateral)
54 septoplasties
69 patients with multiple previous
   "standard" polypectomies

TABLE 13.3 Best Results from FES

Anatomic variants causing stenoses
Cephalgia
Mycoses
First procedure
Allergy: if good response to medical
   treatment
Mucoceles

During 1986 and 1987 we evaluated more than 500 patients who had endoscopic surgery from 8 months to 10 years previously and in whom the indications encompassed the widest possible spectrum (see Chapter 6). In all patients a diagnostic nasal endoscopy was performed, a careful history was taken, and a detailed questionnaire was completed by the patients and then evaluated by a third party.

Table 13.2 lists the various surgical procedures that had been performed without much success on these patients prior to their endoscopic surgery. The large number of patients whose symptoms were not improved by fenestration or Caldwell-Luc procedures is noteworthy. More than 10 percent of patients had one or more septoplasties. It was not possible to accurately determine the number of patients who had a partial resection of the middle or inferior turbinate. Most patients could not remember whether or not turbinate resection was performed as part of another procedure. Even endoscopic examination could not fully confirm these reports.

Independently from the extent and severity of the original disease process, the best operative results (Table 13.3) were achieved when the anatomic variations were identified as the basic problem. Particularly good results were obtained in those patients who were operated on because of sinugenic headaches. Eighty-eight percent of these patients reported that their symptoms had either disappeared completely or were significantly improved. (See also Chapter 11.)

Good results were also obtained in mycotic infections of the paranasal sinus, although only when the mycoses were noninvasive (see Chapter 11).

Of the 23 mucoceles of the paranasal sinuses that were treated by endoscopic surgery, the technique failed only in two cases. One patient had cystic fibrosis and an ethmoidal/frontal sinus mucocele with such thick tenaceous secretions in the lateral part of the mucocele, that they could not be removed endoscopically, and as a result, an external approach was necessary. In the second case of a large frontal sinus mucocele, an external approach had to be used. During the endoscopic procedure it was found that the orbital fat was pressed so hard into the anterior ethmoid by the pressure of the mucocele that the frontal recess could not be entered without injury to the orbit (see Chapter 9).

Allergies had no statistically significant effect on the postoperative results. As mentioned in Chapter 11, allergic rhinosinusitis is not a primary indication for an endoscopic surgical procedure. When an endoscopic procedure was performed as an adjuvant measure to manage obstruction in the middle meatus and ethmoid complex, the results were clearly better in those patients who had already shown some improvement under antiallergic medical management.

Another important factor in the success rate was whether or not the

TABLE 13.4 Postoperative Onset of Relief Following FES

Cephalgia/pain:	at once
Fullness, pressure feeling:	at once
Epiphora:	at once—days
Congestion:	days to 6 weeks
Crusts, secretion:	days to 6 weeks

endoscopic procedure was the first surgical intervention. When a number of other procedures had previously taken place, this not only made the endoscopic surgery much more difficult, but also made the postoperative assessment by both patient and surgeon more difficult. It was sometimes impossible to distinguish between residual complaints following the Messerklinger technique from those complaints which persisted from a previous procedure, e.g., a previous Caldwell-Luc procedure (see Chapter 11).

Reports from the patients showed a pattern by which certain symptoms disappeared (Table 13.4). The patients consistently reported that headaches, and feelings of fullness or pressure between the eyes disappeared immediately (within the first few hours) after the endoscopic procedure. Tearing also stopped within hours or maximally within 1 to 2 days. Postnasal drip, a symptom most patients found particularly bothersome, almost always stopped within the first postoperative day.

In a number of cases the patients reported improvement in nasal breathing, while still on the operating table. During the first few postoperative days there was again a "partial obstruction" of the nose that was due to a reactive swelling of the mucosa. In most cases the feeling of obstructed nasal breathing disappeared completely in 1 to 2 weeks. Occasionally this feeling lasted for 6 weeks. In individual cases, increased secretions and crusting also lasted up to 6 weeks.

Our worst results were obtained in those patients with diffuse polypoid rhinosinopathy (see Chapter 5). Of the 500 patients studied, 246 had more or less massive polyposis. Sixty-four of these patients showed the clinical picture of a diffuse polypoid rhinosinopathy, manifested histologically by a massive inflammatory primarily eosinophilic infiltration. In this group, slightly more than 18 percent had recurrent complaints after only a short time interval. In most cases, a few weeks of improvement were followed by increased nasal obstruction and polypoid mucous membrane changes. Local and systemic steroid therapy produced variable and unpredictable results. In some cases, repeated endoscopic procedures were followed, surprisingly, by extended periods (even years) of symptom-free intervals. This happened even though the second and third endoscopic procedures were no more radical than the first one. When we realized that this diffuse, polypoid rhinosinopathy probably represented a unique disease entity and because we were disappointed with our conservative surgical results, we started using a radical approach with resection of the middle turbinate, external approaches, total sphenoethmoidectomies, etc. We found, however, that these radical techniques did not yield statistically demonstrable better long term results than the more conservative endoscopic techniques. On the contrary, the patients had more postoperative problems after the radical surgery.

It is our impression that diffuse polypoid rhinosinopathy is a generalized disease of the entire mucous membrane of the upper (and possibly the lower) airway of unknown etiology and that there is at present no rational therapy. Management of this disease clearly requires more than surgical management (of whatever type). Ultimate therapy will probably come from the pharmacologic therapeutic realm.

We must separate from diffuse polypoid rhinosinusitis those cases of stubborn, persistent, polypoid mucosal swellings with tenaceous (purulent) secretions that can be attributed to a limited or more extensive osteitis and/or periosteitis. In these cases, a long-term specific antibiotic therapy yields excellent improvement or even complete recovery.

A second, largely unresolved problem is presented by patients whose paranasal sinus mucosa appears to be essentially normal postoperatively and yet whose complaints have not significantly improved. These patients still produce a highly viscous, rubbery secretion that cannot be completely removed by ciliary action from the paranasal sinuses and from the recesses of the ethmoid (Fig. 13.7). This picture is found primarily in patients with bronchial asthma or with the sinubronchial syndrome. Mucosal biopsies show a slight increase in the number of goblet cells, but this is insufficient to explain the dramatically increased production of secretions. The mucosal glands appear unremarkable on light microscopy. The etiology of this disorder is unknown.

Symptomatic therapy with inhaled mucolytic agents and a variety of nasal sprays occasionally produces remarkable improvements, but in most of these cases they are totally ineffective. Occasionally the secretions are so viscous that they cannot be removed with suction and a Blakesley forceps has to be used.

Radical surgical procedures have not been helpful in this situation either. To perform radical surgery in the face of essentially normal macroscopic conditions is of questionable benefit. In some severe cases we have performed a fenestration of the inferior meatus to facilitate removal of the secretions by gravity, or at least to establish an opening into the maxillary sinus for the aspirator.

The most unfavorable outlook for a surgical procedure is the combination of a diffuse polypoid rhinosinopathy and ASA sensitivity with a long history of bronchial asthma and viscous paranasal sinus secretions combined with a number of previous surgical procedures that have destroyed the anatomic landmarks and have led to extensive scar formation.

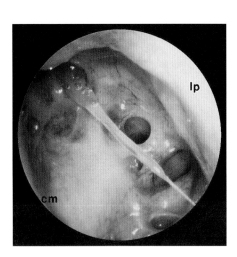

FIGURE 13.7 Tenacious secretions are shown coming from the frontal sinus in a patient with otherwise normal mucosa. For details, see text. lp = lamina papyracea and cm = concha media.

TABLE 13.5 Improvement of Symptoms: Patients' Evaluation (n = 500)

85%	Very good/good	(425 patients)
6%	Fair	(30 patients)
4.2%	Moderate	(21 patients)
4.6%	No improvement/ bad	(23 patients)

Follow-up time: 8 months to 10 years.

Table 13.5 shows the results of the examination and survey of 500 patients, who were reexamined in 1986 and 1987. Eighty-five percent (425/500) reported good or very good results. Six percent (30/500) were satisfied with the results, 4.2 percent (21/500) reported only moderate success, and 4.6 percent (23/500) reported no improvement of their symptoms postoperatively. None of the patients in the last group reported any aggravation of their symptoms postoperatively. In one patient, 1 year after endoscopic surgery, asthma appeared for the first time, but no causal relationship between this event and the surgery could be established.

The results in asthmatic patients were also encouraging (see Chapter 12). Slightly more than 60 percent of patients with intrinsic bronchial asthma reported an impressive and persistent improvement in their symptoms postoperatively and these improvements were documented by improved FEV_1 and reduced drug utilization. Twenty percent showed only transient, subjective improvement, not supported by FEV_1 changes and 10 percent reported no improvement at all in their asthma symptoms. Surprisingly the duration of the asthma symptoms preoperatively bore no relationship to the postoperative results.

Even though it is clinically obvious that endoscopic surgical management of diseases of the lateral nasal wall in patients with bronchial asthma can produce very beneficial results, there are no criteria to predict in which patient, to what extent, and for how long such improvements will occur. Despite this fact, our results and our clinical experience encourages us to operate not only in cases of massive nasal and paranasal sinus disease, but also when the changes are relatively limited (for details, see Chapter 12).

Since a number of the 500 patients in this study had their surgery up to 10 years ago, and since at that time the patients were not routinely queried about loss of smell, nor were smelling tests performed, we have no statistically meaningful information on this subject. On a purely historical basis, about 23 percent of the 500 patients indicated that they had some reduction in their sense of smell preoperatively. Many of these patients also indicated that there was a definite improvement in this parameter postoperatively. In most cases, unfortunately, no precise, retrospective measurement of either loss or improvement was possible.

PROBLEMS AND COMPLICATIONS

In 8 percent (43/500) of our patients at the time of their follow-up examination we observed synechiae of varying sizes between the head of the middle turbinate and the lateral nasal wall (Fig. 13.8). Synechiae are most likely to develop when opposing wound surfaces are created during surgery, e.g., when the head of the middle turbinate is injured during work on the anterior ethmoid. This can occur easily when the passage into the middle meatus is very narrow, e.g., when the middle turbinate has a paradoxical bend, or if the head of the middle turbinate is large and is tightly pressed against the lateral nasal wall. Opposed wound surfaces can be created during the partial resection of a concha bullosa, although the distance to the lateral nasal wall after the lateral lamella of the concha has been resected is usually great enough to prevent the formation of adhesions. An exception to this rule may occur if the remaining medial lamella of the concha bullosa is unstable because it was fractured during the procedure. In this case synechia can form at the insertion of the turbinate, which may scar the free part of the turbinate to the lateral nasal wall over a period of several weeks or months.

The presence of synechiae or adhesions does not necessarily mean that the patient will have a recurrence of symptoms. Only 20 percent (8/43) of the patients in whom we found considerable synechiae had persistent or recurrent symptoms that were attributed exclusively to the synechiae. Problems usually appeared when the synechiae constricted the entrance to the middle meatus or closed off parts of the ethmoid, causing the retention of secretions and narrowing of the ostia. If there is scar formation that directly obstructs the ostium of the maxillary sinus, the symptoms return quite quickly.

In some cases there may be only a thin anterior scarred plaque that blocks the entrance to the middle meatus (Fig. 13.9). This is enough to create the feeling of severely obstructed nasal breathing, even though the nasal cavity is completely patent and the ethmoid components, behind the synechia, are entirely unremarkable. This observation re-emphasizes the importance of unobstructed aeration of the middle meatus for the subjective feeling of free nasal airflow.

Synechiae are easily identified and managed endoscopically. They are divided and excessive scar tissue resected and a small piece of silastic or other type of stent is inserted for a few days. This small procedure usually eliminates the synechia.

The recurrence of synechiae cannot always be prevented, however. In some cases we have seen adhesions appear after many years of complete freedom from problems. Apparently, these late adhesions developed following a viral infection and concommitant epithelial lesions. Resection of the middle turbinate is not, in our opinion in-

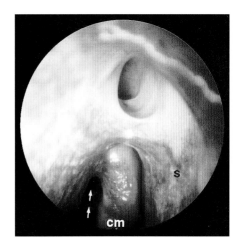

FIGURE 13.8 Postoperative adhesions between the septum, the head of the middle turbinate, and the lateral nasal wall in the area of the agger nasi are seen. The *arrows* show the entrance into the right middle meatus. s = septum and cm = middle turbinate.

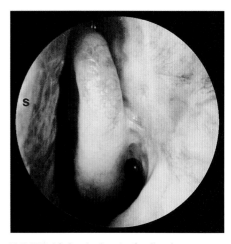

FIGURE 13.9 A sheet of adhesions are visible between the left middle turbinate and the lamina papyracea. s = septum.

dicated, since this will not solve the problem of the synechiae. If the middle turbinate is resected, synechiae may still form medially, toward the septum and can then obstruct the rima olfactoria. Furthermore, the additional trauma of the procedure (pain and bleeding) and the removal of the anatomic landmarks are unjustified.

The best prophylaxis against the development of synechiae is scrupulous attention to atraumatic surgery and the absence of injury to the mucosa of the middle turbinate.

Massively diseased ethmoidal cells or fissures, if overlooked at the time of endoscopic (or any other type of) surgery, can naturally be the reason for persistent or recurring problems (Fig. 13.10). Such cells were either incorrectly diagnosed or overlooked at the time of surgery because of increased bleeding or other reasons (e.g., uncertainty of the surgeon about the topography). This and other types of postoperative problems can be readily identified and then appropriately handled through the endoscope (Figs. 13.11 to 13.13).

The percentage of problems that could be attributed to the stenosis of an enlarged maxillary sinus ostium was surprisingly small in our study. Only 8 patients of 500 (less than 2%) had such functional stenoses. One patient had developed stenosis on three consecutive occasions, in spite of apparently correct surgical technique.

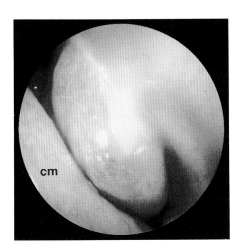

FIGURE 13.10 A diseased left ethmoidal bulla that was "overlooked" at the time of endoscopic surgery. Pus can be seen coming from a perforation in the anterior wall of the bulla. cm = concha media.

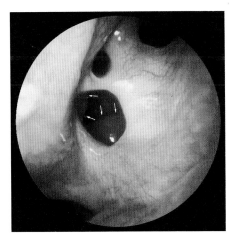

FIGURE 13.11 A view at the entrance to a left sphenoidal sinus, 3 months postoperatively (the indication for the original surgery was extensive polypoid pansinusitis). The patient continued to complain of a purulent drip into the nasopharynx. From this viewing angle it would appear that there are retention cysts inside the sphenoid sinus (arrows).

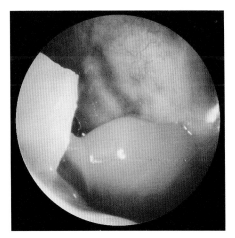

FIGURE 13.12 On closer examination, it became evident that the "retention cysts" were actually two bone fragments extending from the floor of the sphenoid sinus into its lumen that were covered by a purulent exudate. These sequestered bone spicules were probably displaced into the lumen of the sinus at the time the anterior wall of the sinus was perforated (fractured inward) and which then became necrotic. Following removal of these sequestra, the patient's recovery was uneventful.

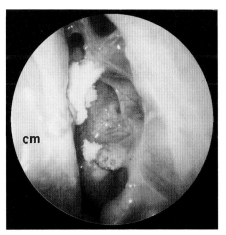

FIGURE 13.13 A left ethmoid cavity 6 months after surgery for polypoid disease. The mucosa is more or less unremarkable. There is fungal growth on crusts following excessive use of cortisone-containing nasal spray. cm = concha media.

The reepithelialization of the edges of the enlarged ostium apparently takes place rapidly. One explanation may be that the transport of secretions from the maxillary sinus once again takes place through the natural ostium and that this contributes to the more rapid healing process. Furthermore, a complete circumferential lesion of the ostium can be avoided, since the ostium is enlarged only at the expense of the anterior fontanelle. If the posterior fontanelle is also enlarged, e.g., if there is an accessory ostium in that area, the result is an ostium of 10 × 6 to 8 mm in size, which provides adequate ventilation and drainage even if it should shrink to half this size. According to our experience, a diameter of 3 mm is sufficient to provide a physiologic outlet from the maxillary sinus. In independent studies, Kennedy and his associates have also found that the natural ostium had little tendency toward stenosis. These findings suggest that enlarging the natural ostium in the middle meatus is more effective and more physiological than a fenestration in the inferior meatus. We believe therefore that Hilding's postulate: "never touch the virginity of the natural ostium" can no longer be supported. Kennedy et al have repeated Hilding's experiment in rabbits and were able to show that after surgery on the natural ostium, the transport of secretions may not be ideal in some cases, but that as in man, the secretions are transported by genetically determined pathways toward the natural ostium. Even after surgical manipulation of the ostium, the secretions leave through this aperture in practically all cases.

In the 500 patients in this study, the following additional complications were seen. In 9 patients there was definite injury to the lamina papyracea and the periorbital area with a prolapse of the orbital fat. Three of these patients had edema of the lid on the first postoperative day, while in 2 patients there was a hematoma at the inner canthus. In none of these patients was there any additional complication, such as diplopia or infection of the orbital contents. In 11 patients there was such severe intra- or immediate postoperative hemorrhage that packing became necessary. In one out of these 11 patients a posterior (Bellocq's) packing had to be inserted. This was also the only patient in whom a blood transfusion was necessary, which is at least partially because we missed preoperative diagnosis of the patient's coagulopathy.

In the 10 other cases, a repeat endoscopic procedure had to be performed because bleeding obstructed the view at the time of the initial surgery. During the last few years, the number of cases in which bleeding forced cessation of the procedure has dropped to less than 1 percent.

Intraoperative Bleeding

Normally bleeding is not a problem when local and topical anesthesia are used. If there is bleeding, it is almost never an isolated, single vessel, but is usually a generalized oozing from the edges of the mucous membranes at the site of resection. This type of bleeding can be bothersome, particularly when the operation is performed for an acute inflammatory problem with corresponding hyperemia. In most cases it is possible to stop this type of bleeding by the repeated application of Pontocaine and epinephrine soaked cotton pledgets. It is usually sufficient to introduce these pledgets into the middle meatus, under gentle pressure and to leave them there for 2 to 3 minutes. It is also usually possible to continue the procedure without undue difficulties. If it is necessary to keep the pledgets in place longer, the surgeon can operate on the other side in the interim, and not waste time waiting.

In some cases the Blakesley-Weil forceps, with built-in suction channel may be helpful (Fig. A.17). Unfortunately, the additional suction channel makes the instrument bulky and thus increases the probability of causing unintentional mucosal injury within the middle meatus. For this reason we do not use this instrument routinely.

Bipolar cautery forceps can be helpful when the bleeding comes from an individual vessel. This is most likely to occur around the ostium of the maxillary sinus or at the insertion of the middle turbinate. For capillary oozing, the placement of fingernail sized pieces of Oxycel in the area of the bleed has proven useful. Oxycel adheres well to the underlying surface and controls the oozing very effectively. Even small squirting vessels can be controlled in this fashion. For this purpose we place an appropriately shaped piece of Oxycel on a cotton applicator which is then held in place with gentle pressure with a pair of forceps. After 1 minute the cotton applicator is removed. The Oxycel usually adheres to the mucosa and stops the bleeding.

Measurements have shown that the average blood loss after bilateral surgery is less than 30 ml. The one patient who required a transfusion was not included in the calculation of this average.

Bleeding from the anterior ethmoidal artery can usually be easily identified and managed (Fig. 13.14). Pontocaine/epinephrine pledgets are also useful in this situation when applied with gentle pressure and buttressed with Oxycel. Coagulation with cautery or the placement of a silver clip are also effective measures. When required by the procedure, the anterior ethmoidal artery can usually be easily identified and avoided during the remainder of the procedure (see Chapter 3).

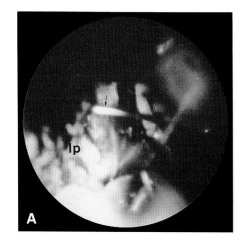

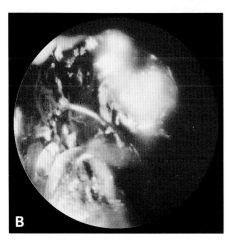

FIGURE 13.14 Intraoperative hemorrhage from the anterior ethmoid artery in a right middle meatus. Note the pulsation of the stream of blood as seen in this pair of photographs. *A*, During systole. lp = lamina papyracea. *B*, In diastole. The bleeding was easily controlled with a Pontocaine-epinephrine pledget.

In contrast, a divided anterior ethmoidal artery can produce one of the most dangerous complications in the entire field of ethmoid surgery. This happens when the vessel retracts into the orbit and continues to bleed. The resulting periorbital or intraorbital hematoma can produce all of the dreaded orbital complications, including blindness. We have seen two cases of orbital hematoma, due to injury to the anterior ethmoid artery. Within a few seconds, the eyeball protruded, became fixed and "cast in concrete." In such cases the surgeon must be prepared to perform an emergency decompression of the orbit to prevent blindness. This type of complication once again emphasizes the advantages of operating under local anesthesia. The fundus and vision can be immediately checked and the patient can give precise information concerning visual field changes. Under general anesthesia precious time may be lost in deciding whether a decompression is necessary or not, when one has to wait for the patient to wake up and be subjected to a determination of the visual fields, acuity of vision, and fundoscopic examination.

To determine whether decompression is indicated, it is helpful to have diagnostic ultrasound equipment available to locate the hematoma. The surgeon can thus determine where the hematoma is, in what direction it is expanding (periorbitally, intraorbitally, retrobulbarly), and the degree of displacement, stretching, and flexing of the optic nerve. A periorbital hemorrhage between the lamina papyracea and the periorbital area only rarely produces visual field defects or visual problems. Both of our cases were of this type and fortunately required no further surgical correction.

When the slightest evidence of visual field loss or obvious loss of vision occurs, immediate action is necessary. It is the recommendation of our ophthalmologists that the first step should be an immediate lateral canthotomy and an adjacent opening of the orbital septum (in the area of the lower lid). This allows the periorbital fat to move anteriorly, thereby decreasing the intraorbital pressure and the pressure on the optic nerve and optic vessels. After these emergency measures, the decompression of the orbit takes place with identification and control of the bleeding site. An external approach above the eyebrow may be the technique of choice.

If an intraorbital or periorbital hematoma has been demonstrated, *and* visual loss and/or impairment of the visual field have occurred, medical management with diuretics, mannitol infusion, steroid administration, etc. *alone* is not recommended.

The posterior end of the middle turbinate is another place where bleeding may originate. Because of its proximity to the sphenopalatine foramen and the mucosal vessels entering and leaving through this space, injury and hemorrhage can occur quite readily in this area. With the exception of a massively pneumatized middle turbinate, the

Messerklinger technique does not usually traumatize the area of the posterior end of the middle turbinate. On the other hand, if necessary, the sphenopalatine foramen can be identified easily with the endoscope and hemorrhage can be controlled with Oxycel and pressure.

The best way to avoid intraoperative hemorrhage is to prepare the patient carefully (control of hypertension, good sedation, topical and local anesthesia) preoperatively and to use a careful, atraumatic surgical technique. One should avoid hasty procedures in acute inflammatory situations and one should treat the patient medically until the optimal preoperative conditions have been obtained. Should there be bleeding, the repeated placement of Pontocaine/epinephrine pledgets, or other topical vasoconstrictors is usually sufficient to control the mucosal hemorrhage and to permit the procedure to continue.

The surgeon should always follow the principle that if exposure is seriously limited by hemorrhage, then the procedure must be discontinued.

It is safer to come back another day than to have an iatrogenic complication. The be-all and end-all of endoscopic surgery with the Messerklinger technique is good visibility and the ability to know at all times one's precise location in respect to the various components of the ethmoid system.

The less experienced surgeon should never try to move around the roof of the ethmoid, the lamina papyracea, or the posterior ethmoid and sphenoid area blindly or by palpation (Fig. 13.15). If one studies reports of cases where serious complications occurred (serious orbital lesions, perforation of the roof of the ethmoid, lesions to the optic nerve) most of these reports have one element in common: The procedure was performed under general anesthesia, there was bleeding, and the visibility was not good. Hence the motto: "If you cannot see: STOP!"

Since all cellular septa are not removed routinely in the Messerklinger technique to create a standardized ethmoid cavity, the danger of injury to the anterior and posterior ethmoid arteries is minimal. In the Messerklinger technique, it is not necessary to work the roof of the ethmoid with a diamond drill to an "ideal" smoothness. When this is done, the thin bony covering of the vessels may be perforated and injury to the ethmoidal vessels may occur.

In some patients with mycosis of the maxillary sinus, following the instillation of antimycotic ointments into the maxillary sinus through the enlarged natural ostium in the middle meatus, we have observed a very painful, extended inflammatory infiltration of the soft tissue of the cheek. The ointment that produced the inflammatory reactions had apparently entered the soft tissues of the cheek via the track in the canine fossa through which the trocar had been passed during pre-

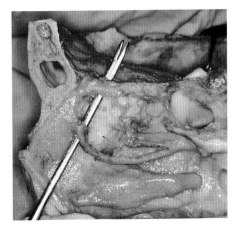

FIGURE 13.15 This dissection shows one way in which the roof of the ethmoid could be perforated. This is *not* a typical occurrence. The greater danger of perforation is not directly cranially, but medially, through the lateral lamella of the lamella cribrosa in the immediate vicinity of the anterior ethmoidal artery.

vious maxillary sinuscopy. We now wait until the fifth or sixth postoperative days, by which time the trocar perforation is always closed, before we instill antimycotic ointments. With this regimen, we no longer see this complication.

For some time now, we have stopped using any antimycotic ointments in the immediate postoperative period in cases of noninvasive mycoses. Careful removal of the mycotic masses is sufficient and specific aftercare is not required (see Chapter 11).

The spectrum of complications following maxillary sinuscopy included a transient paresthesia in the area of the infraorbital nerve that was usually limited to a small area of the upper lip and pain in the area of the upper teeth. In most cases the duration of these complaints ranged from a few days to three weeks. None of the 500 patients in this study had any persistent problems due to maxillary sinus endoscopy.

In one case a Merocel sponge, which had been placed into the middle meatus to prevent adhesions, was "forgotten." This sponge was removed 6 months later after it had caused the patient considerable problems and difficulties. Today all Merocel sponges are transfixed with a suture, which is taped to the patient's cheek. This provides an obvious warning sign to everyone that a sponge remains which must be removed. Table 13.6 summarizes the complications encountered.

Surprisingly, in none of the patients studied was there a stenosis of the nasolacrimal duct and there was no tearing. Even though we are reasonably certain that in some cases the nasolacrimal duct was injured during enlargement of the natural ostium of the maxillary sinus, this injury never led to a complete stenosis of the duct.

TABLE 13.6 Complications (500 Patients)

Orbital penetration:	9
With lid emphysema:	3
Persisting problems:	0
Bleeding (packing required):	11
(Bellocq):	1
Blood transfusion(s) required:	1
Repeated procedures due to bleeding:	10
Soft tissue infiltration after sinoscopy:	5
"Forgotten" Merocel sponge:	1

SEVERE COMPLICATIONS

All of the serious complications that occured in our centre in over 6,000 patients operated upon since 1976 are listed in Table 13.7. The problems of intraorbital hemorrhage have already been discussed in the previous section.

We know of three cases of iatrogenic CSF fistulas. Two of these cases had recurrent nasal polyposis and had undergone several previous operations. During the endoscopic procedure the ethmoid anatomy was difficult to identify because of the previous operations. The insertion of the middle turbinate was missing, there was extensive scarring and there were many adhesions. As determined retrospectively, the dura was injured in both patients at its typical weak point, namely the roof of the ethmoid at the point where the anterior ethmoidal artery exits through the lateral lamina of the cribriform plate. Some of the polyps were adherent to the dura at this point and the attempt to remove them apparently caused the dura to tear. The third patient's history revealed a basal skull fracture several years previously, although on tomography no evidence of any bony defect of the ethmoid roof was found. In this patient the perforation took place at the level of the insertion of the ground lamella at the roof of the ethmoid in the posterior aspect of the lateral sinus. It seems likely that a preexisting bony defect from the previous skull fracture was hidden by a plaque of scar tissue.

In this case, the dural defect was repaired at the same endoscopic sitting. A small piece of appropriately shaped, lyophilized dura was placed between the injured dura and the skull base. A medially based mucosal flap, from the lateral surface of the middle turbinate, was pasted over the area with fibrin adhesive. Oxycel was packed in the area under light pressure and the patient was placed on bed rest for 5 days with strict instructions against blowing his nose.

In one of the two other cases, the CSF fistula was clearly visible during the procedure. Since it was very small, it was covered with a mucous membrane flap and tamponaded with an Oxycel sponge. The hoped for spontaneous closure did not take place and a few days later an external transethmoidal closure was performed. This was successful and there were no further problems.

In the other patient, there was no evidence of a dural breach either intraoperatively or during the first 2 postoperative days. On the third postoperative day, after blowing his nose, the patient developed increasingly severe headaches. A skull X-ray film was taken that showed a marked internal and external pneumocephalus. The CSF fistula was identified with a fluorescein study and then closed from the outside through the ethmoid. In this case there were also no persistent complications.

TABLE 13.7 Severe Complications Since 1976 (Over 6,000 Patients, 3 Surgeons)

CSF leaks:	3
Pneumatocephalus:	1
Intraorbital bleeding:	2
Meningitis:	0
Partial loss of vision,	
Diplopia:	0
Blindness:	0
Fatalities:	0
Stenosis of the nasolacrimal duct:	0

To date we have not had any cases of immediate postoperative or delayed onset meningitis. None of our patients had diplopia, transient loss of vision, or blindness. There have been no deaths related to the endoscopic procedures.

We have never seen an injury to the optic nerve or to the internal carotid artery, although we are aware from the literature and from personal communications from colleagues that this may happen during an endoscopic procedure. When these cases are studied, it becomes apparent that the injuries to the optic nerve did not take place in the sphenoid sinus, where all surgeons are acutely aware of this possibility, but in the area of the posterior ethmoid (see Fig. 13.15). It is critical, therefore, to keep the anatomy and the anatomic variations of this area always in mind. One must be particularly aware of the possible existence of Onodi cells (see Chapter 3), which may extend the posterior ethmoid laterally and superiorly to the sphenoid. If the Onodi cells are massively pneumatized, not only the optic nerve, but also the internal carotid artery may bulge into the lateral or superior wall of these posterior ethmoid air cells. If the bone is extremely thin or dehiscent over these bulges, the danger of iatrogenic injury is great.

The lamina papyracea may also be thin over the medial aspect of the apex of the orbit. The surgeon should be able to distinguish between periorbital fat and diseased mucous membrane. An injury to or transsection of the optic nerve *in the orbit* directly behind the bulb is evidence of a complete disregard of the rules of the technique and ignorance of the anatomy of this area.

In the presence of large Onodi cells, it must be kept in mind that the sphenoid sinus is not located in a direct extension of the Onodi cells in a posterolateral direction. The sinus must be looked for medially and inferiorly. In the sphenoid sinus proper, any sharp or forceful removal of the mucous membranes from the lateral wall, roof, and posterior wall of the sinus must stop unless the surgeon is absolutely certain that there are no bony dehiscences or dangerous anatomic variants present.

Bony septa in the sphenoid sinus should only be removed, if at all, with extreme care and only after a careful study of the CT scans, which must be present in the operating room. These septa frequently do not run medially and may insert into a thin bony shell over the optic nerve or carotid artery. This bony shell can be easily fractured during an attempt to remove the septa and the optic nerve or the internal carotid artery may be injured (see Chapters 3 and 4).

Fortunately we have never yet been faced with a hemorrhage from the carotid artery. We believe that if the injury is punctate, the immediate application of an Oxycel sponge under pressure may have a chance to control the hemorrhage. If the injury is substantial with profuse hemorrhage, the possible emergency measures to be considered include: tight packing, manual compression of the common carotid artery in the neck against the cervical vertebrae on the affected side, and ligation of this vessel. Extensive neurosurgical exploration may or may not be adequate to prevent a life threatening situation or severe permanent CNS damage. No predictions can be made for the individual case. The success should depend on the availability of adequate collateral circulation through the circle of Willis, the immediate availability of suitable blood in sufficient quantity, and the immediate availability of a skilled neurosurgeon, etc. We know of one case where the carotid hemorrhage was transiently controlled, although unfortunately, the patient succumbed to complications within a few days.

Other intracranial complications we have heard about include penetration into the ventricular system with the instrument and an iatrogenic lesion of the communicating artery between the anterior cerebral arteries with ensuing intracerebral hemorrhage.

The most dramatic case we know of is that of a patient, in whom both optic nerves were cut and resected within the orbit immediately behind the bulb (Fig. 13.16). This case was described in the operative note as "functional endoscopic procedure." The procedure actually performed (radical surgery with resection of the middle and superior turbinate and part of the inferior turbinate) clearly was not "functional" in nature. Many of these complications, which have been attributed to the endoscopic procedure, must in reality be attributed directly to the surgeon. "Functional endoscopic paranasal sinus surgery" and "Endonasal surgery, using an endoscope" are not necessarily identical.

The Messerklinger technique is primarily a diagnostic endoscopic concept that is based upon a thorough understanding of the pathophysiology of paranasal sinus disease. With the surgical technique developed from this concept (functional endoscopic sinus surgery), almost all inflammatory diseases of the paranasal sinus system can be managed by conservative intervention. It is rarely necessary to undertake major manipulations in the large paranasal sinuses.

The Messerklinger technique can achieve a total sphenoethmoidectomy, with preservation of the middle turbinate, but the basic principles of the Messerklinger technique attempt to avoid this type of radical surgery. It is one of the basic criteria of the Messerklinger technique that unlike other techniques, *good results can be obtained with limited, functional procedures, even in severe disease states.*

The Messerklinger technique has clearly defined limitations, contraindications, and specific problems. It can produce marked improvement, but usually no cure in many cases of diffuse polypoid rhinosinopathy, asthma, mucoviscidosis, allergies, and other diseases. Since, however, the more radical procedures also provide no better long-term results

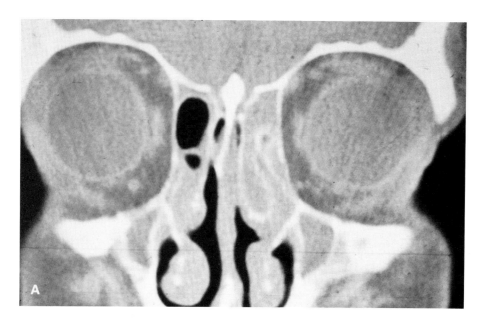

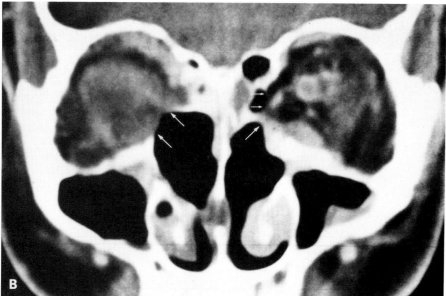

FIGURE 13.16   *A,* This shows the preoperative CT findings in the patient shown in the next two radiographs. There is moderately severe bilateral ethmoidal disease, a diseased concha bullosa on the left, and bilateral maxillary sinus shadows. *B,* In this postoperative CT it can be seen clearly that both orbits were penetrated (*arrows*). The middle turbinates were almost completely resected. *C,* In the axial CT, the consequences of the orbital perforations are visible. The optic nerve was transsected on both sides, just behind the bulb (*arrows*). (Images courtesy of DW Kennedy, MD, and SJ Zinreich, MD.)

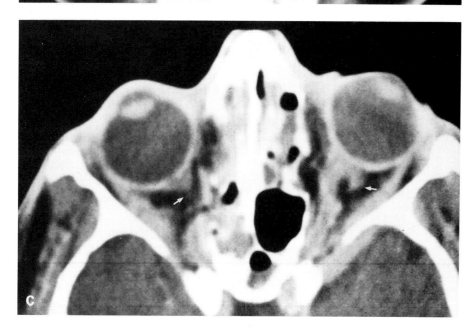

and may cause more specific complications for the patient, we believe that even in these cases the Messerklinger technique is justified as the less troublesome procedure.

The surgical aspects of the Messerklinger technique require solid training and an excellent knowledge of the anatomy of the lateral nasal wall and all of its variations. The Messerklinger technique carries all the risks and dangers of *any type of* endonasal ethmoid surgery, but when used for the appropriate indications and performed skillfully by an experienced surgeon, the Messerklinger technique has only a minimal incidence of complications.

None of the various endoscopic schools have claimed that their technique provided an easier or safer route to the ethmoid. The endoscope is not an "end" but only a means to functional therapy.

There are many excellent opportunities today to learn the endoscopic technique. Training lenses and small video cameras make it possible for the trainee to follow the diagnostic and therapeutic manipulations directly. The actual surgical procedure should be attempted only after having performed both diagnostic and therapeutic procedures many times (we recommend at least 20 to 30) on a cadaver or in anatomic preparations. Only in this way can a true familiarity with the anatomy and the anatomic variations of the area be gained. One must become thoroughly familiar with the endoscope through a number of diagnostic procedures and progress to surgical procedures only after facility in the management of the instrument and complete familiarity with the anatomic structures has been obtained. The beginner should never start out with a difficult case, e.g., a patient who has had previous surgery with severe recurrent polyposis or scar formation that distorts the anatomy. Whoever wishes to perform endoscopic surgery must be willing to practice the same careful atraumatic technique as for stapes surgery and must also be prepared to assume the sometimes extensive aftercare.

Chapter 14

DOCUMENTATION

Good documentation by photography, motion picture, or video tape is essential in all endoscopic procedures, since the surgeon works in an area that is not visible to others. Documentation serves scientific communication, research, teaching, and occasionally, medicolegal purposes.

It is sometimes extremely difficult to obtain high quality pictures in the narrow and angled clefts of the lateral nasal wall. This chapter should assist the reader in selecting the appropriate equipment and in identifying or avoiding mistakes.

STILL PHOTOGRAPHY

There are six key elements that have a decisive effect on the creation of a good endoscopic picture:

1. The camera
2. The light source
3. The light carrier
4. The lenses
5. The film
6. The photographer.

Cameras

For endoscopic photography today, 35-mm reflex cameras with "through the lens viewing" are used almost exclusively (Fig. 14.1A). These cameras are characterized by reliability and they can usually be coupled very simply with the flash unit of the light source. It is nevertheless important to consider some features of these reflex cameras very carefully.

Almost every commercially available 35-mm reflex camera can be connected to a rigid endoscope by using an appropriate zoom-adapter-lens (Fig. 14.1B). The zoom lens permits additional focusing and the selection of a smaller target area.

We have found it useful to leave the setting of the zoom lens the same for the entire series of photographs. This prevents differences in the size of the image during projection or printing of the related pictures. Using the Karl Storz variolens adapter (Fig. 14.1B), we prefer a 130-mm setting on the zoom lens since this permits maximal utilization of the center of the 35-mm slide by the endoscopic picture. Depending on the type of camera chosen and the type of light source used, there are two options: manual or automatic flash. If a light source with a manual flash is chosen, it will not be possible to have a series of pictures with different exposure times and light intensities until experience with the system makes it very clear which lens, with which light intensity is suitable for which picture. With cameras with automatic light systems, there is still regretfully the problem that the manufacturers of the different light sources make their equipment compatible only with a certain camera. This means that in selecting the camera, the selection of a light source that is compatible with the camera must also be considered.

Regardless of the camera selected, it is critically important that centerweighted lightmetering be used since with the endoscope, the illuminated area is always circular and, at best, only takes up 50 percent of the area of a 35-mm slide; precise lighting measurement can only be achieved with the centerweighted measurement technique. If the light is measured uniformly over the entire illuminated area, as is the case with some cameras, it is inevitable in automatic cameras, that the electronic sensor "waits" until the black areas outside the illuminated center get more light, even though the center is quite adequately illuminated. This results in the reflector staying up for a fraction of a second with the shutter open. This does not lead to an improper exposure, since after the flash, no appreciable light falls on the field, but it may cause the picture to be blurred, due to motion. In those cameras that give a choice between integral and spot measurement, the latter should be used every time.

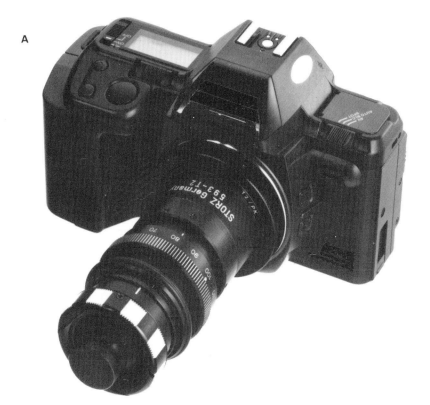

FIGURE 14.1 *A*, A 35-mm TTL camera with attached Karl Storz zoom lens adapter (70–140 mm). *B*, Top view. The focal distance recommended for the non-wide angle endoscope is 130 mm.

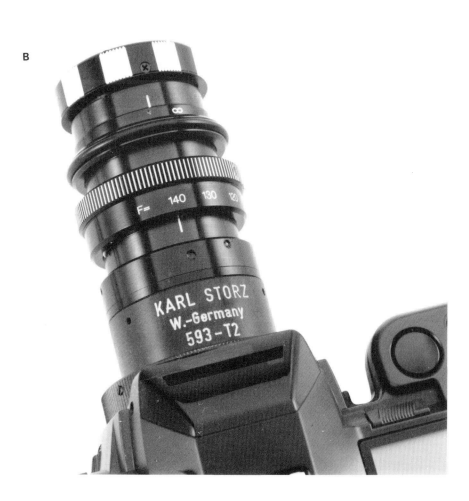

Light Sources

The light source must contain a flash generator. In the nose, even a strong halogen or xenon light is inadequate for photodocumentation. Particularly when a surgical situation is the subject of the photograph, a few drops of blood can absorb enough light to make a flash an absolute requirement. The use of more sensitive films, such as switching from the standard ASA 400 to ASA 1200, 1600, or even 3200, has not proven satisfactory in our hands. There are a number of light sources available commercially from several manufacturers. When deciding which light source to purchase, its compatibility with the electronics of the camera must be taken into consideration. Almost all illustrations in this text were taken with the Storz 600 light source (Fig. 14.2). It was used with an Olympus reflex camera with automatic flash coupling or in combination with a Nikon F3 camera with manual setting of the flash intensity.

Flash tubes must be changed from time to time as they have a limited lifespan and lose their efficiency with continued use. According to our experience the Karl Storz model 600 light source (see Fig. 14.2) and flash generator is ideal for taking pictures. This model has an acoustic signal that indicates whether the flash was sufficient for proper illumination of the field. The flash generator beeps when there was enough light and the electronics of the camera properly set the flash. This is helpful in preventing unpleasant surprises and in avoiding the discovery of inadequate lighting only after the film has been developed. The absence of the audible signal denotes the inadequacy of the light and thus one has the opportunity to take another picture of a possibly unique situation. Perhaps the angle of the lens ought to be changed, the lens brought closer to the subject, or perhaps a more light efficient lens used.

Light Cables

Since the light emerging at the end of the light cable (light carrier) is already limited by its diameter, it is more important when selecting a cable to consider the quality of the glass fibers, the color spectrum of the flash, and the intensity of the light. In principle, the light carrier can consist of glass fibers or it may be filled with a gel or a fluid. The fluid cables generally emit a harder (bluer) light that must be taken into consideration in selecting the film, in order to avoid distortion of the natural colors.

Fiber cables have a much higher attrition rate than fluid cables, since the individual fibers break easily, leading to a loss of illumination. Fiberoptic cables should therefore never be coiled, but should be stored straight, preferably hanging. Kinking must be avoided at all costs.

With fluid cables, even a simple semicircular path will lead to internal reflections and a substantial loss of light. If a loop is formed, as much as 50 percent of the illumination may be lost and this can happen easily when the cable is placed carelessly on the operating table. The human eye can compensate for this loss and the surgeon may not realize the loss of light, but it is obvious on a slide or videotape. "Insufficient light" is, therefore, not necessarily due to an inadequate output by the light source, but may be due to such a trivial cause as a loop in the cable. For photography and videotaping, the light carrier should be kept as straight as possible. In our experience, this can be best accomplished if the light source is behind the surgeon or photographer (see Fig. 8.1A).

FIGURE 14.2   All of the endoscopic illustrations in this volume were made with this Karl Storz model 600 light source and flash generator. An Olympus OM 40 camera with liquid light carrier and synchronizer cable are also shown.

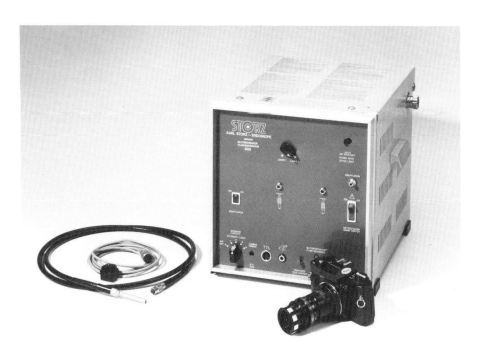

Endoscopes

Since the lenses of the endoscope are also subject to slight, but constant deterioration through repeated use, cleaning, and sterilizing, we like to keep a specific instrument devoted entirely to photographic documentation. If the same instrument must be used for diagnosis, therapy, and photography, the exit port for light at the distal end of the endoscope requires special attention.

Even minimal soiling with traces of blood and secretions results in a substantial loss of light. While this loss of light may not be noticeable to the naked eye, it may lead to underexposure on photography or videotape. The exit ports for the light fibers are the only point at the distal end of the endoscope where heat is generated (Fig. 14.3). For this reason, secretions and blood tend to dry rapidly in this area and obstruct the emergence of light. The distal lens, through which the endoscopist looks and which is not warmed, remains clear. Since the endoscopist maintains a clear view, any decrease in illumination and poor light will be blamed on the light source, the light carrier, or the photographic equipment. It is important therefore, to monitor the light exit ports at all times. This can only be done by changing the light source to its lowest setting and by withdrawing the light carrier into its sheath, so that the light output is minimal. Only in this way can the naked eye detect any dirt on the exit port (see Fig. 14.3B). This can not be done by full illumination, due to the excess light effect. While in use, the endoscope should never be placed on a dry surface, but should always be immersed in a container with warm saline to avoid the drying of blood or secretions on the distal end. The container should be lined with a thick layer of cotton to protect the lenses (Fig. 8.2B).

When an angled lens is used, it is important to realize that the exit points of light are not distributed symmetrically around the tip of the instrument (see Fig. 14.3A). If, for instance, the 30 degree lens is turned so that the view is directed laterally toward the middle meatus, the primary light path is medially, i.e., toward the septum. If the endoscope is then placed too close to the septum, it can happen that due to the strong reflection of the flash, this area will be over illuminated. When the illumination is controlled manually, this is just a nuisance, but when automatic light control is used, this may lead to the unimportant septal area being correctly illuminated and the important deeper areas of the middle meatus appearing black on the photograph from under-exposure (Fig. 14.4). It is important, therefore, that during photography the endoscopist always be fully aware of the precise location of the tip of the endoscope and the area of maximal illumination.

In general, wide angle lenses require more light to give proper illumination to the wider field of vision. In most cases, however, wide

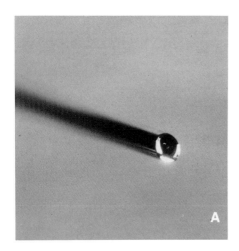

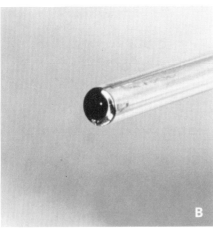

FIGURE 14.3 The distal lens of a 4-mm 30 degree endoscope. Note that when the light output from the source is reduced maximally, the asymmetric distribution of the light-carrying fibers in the shaft of the endoscope can be seen. *B*, The distal lens of the 4-mm 0 degree endoscope. Notice the traces of dried secretions and blood that can be seen in the sickle-shaped light path when the light source is maximally reduced. This debris significantly reduces the available light.

angle systems have no more light fibers than standard endoscopes. They are still suitable for the documentation of uncomplicated diagnostic problems, such as a survey photograph of the maxillary sinus. In narrow spaces and particularly if there is blood in the field, the wide angle scope has only a limited usefulness in documentation because of its limited light output.

When holding the camera attached to the endoscope, it is critical to avoid even the most minimal bending of the instrument (Fig. 14.5). Bending leads to sickle-shaped black areas and loss of the picture. The use of the endoscope handles has been particularly beneficial in this situation (see Figs. 14.12B, A.3, and A.4). They allow good photography even through a 2.7-mm endoscope, which is at best a difficult undertaking in the nose.

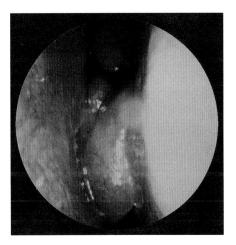

FIGURE 14.4 A typical illumination defect. The exit port of the light is too close to the inferior turbinate, which has been over exposed.

FIGURE 14.5 The 2.7-mm endoscope (30 degree lens). In the absence of a protective endoscope handle, the weight of the light carrier is sufficient to cause a slight bend in the shaft of the endoscope.

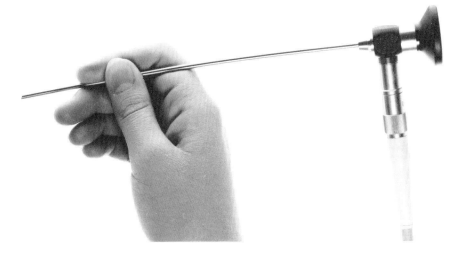

Photographic Technique

In stationary findings, e.g., the documentation of a diagnostic finding, a direct photographic technique is used. The endoscope is attached directly to the zoom lens of the camera and the selection of the target area and focusing is performed through the eye-piece of the camera (Fig. 14.6). In this technique the loss of light is minimal.

When non-stationary situations, such as surgical encounters must be recorded, where changes take place within fractions of a second, documentation can only take place by using a beam-splitting technique. This makes it possible for the surgeon to keep his hands on the endoscope and surgical instrument. There are again two possibilities. In the first one, an assistant operates the camera that is attached to the endoscope by an articulated arm (Fig. 14.7). The assistant controls the selection of the target through the eye-piece of the camera and shoots on command by the surgeon.

FIGURE 14.6 The endoscope is attached directly to the zoom lens of the camera for direct endoscopic photography.

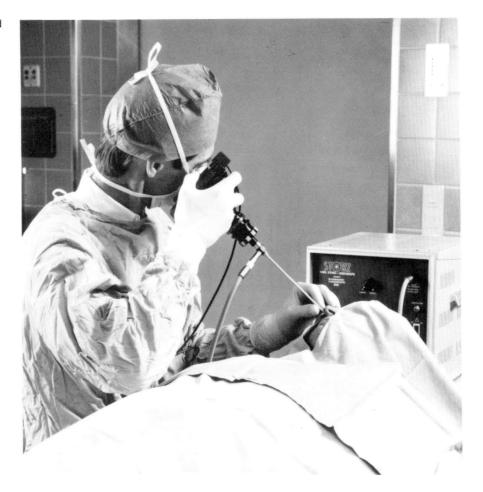

FIGURE 14.7 The articulated arm is attached to the zoom lens and the camera operated by an assistant.

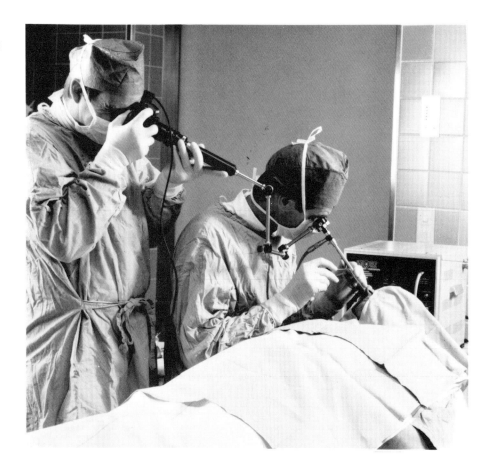

The second possibility is to place the camera, attached to the endoscope by an articulated arm, on a small table, where it can be activated by the surgeon through a foot pedal. Selection of the target and focusing must be done before the shooting begins. The disadvantage of both techniques is that in situations that require maximal illumination, the light available may be insufficient. The articulated arm causes a considerable loss of light, which is directly proportional to the number of articulations (prisms) (Fig. 14.8). To hold the loss of light to a minimum, we use a two or (for demonstration) three joint, Wittmoser articulated optical arm. The beam-splitter causes a further loss of light. In most articulated lens systems, two arrangements are possible: for observation, 50 percent of the available light goes to the surgeon and the other 50 percent to the observer or to the camera. For photographic documentation 90 percent of the light goes to the camera and 10 percent to the surgeon.

FIGURE 14.8 For indirect photography, the Wittmoser articulated optical arm with a beam-splitter is attached to the eyepiece of the endoscope. The beam can be split variously from 50:50 to 10:90 (10% to the observer and 90% for documentation).

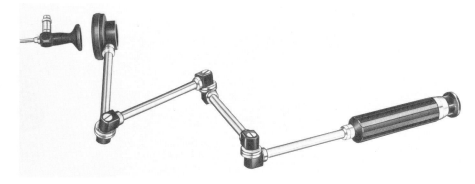

These substantial losses of light unfortunately mean that an unbroken photographic sequence is still extremely difficult and may well mean that under narrow conditions, or minimal bleeding, it becomes impossible. Even a few drops of blood absorb as much light from the endoscope as a black road surface at night and in the rain absorbs from the headlights of a car.

Film Selection

To obtain the truest color reproduction, the following factors are important. Intensity and color of the source of light used (the flash generator), the optical quality of the lenses and the condition of their surface and, most importantly, the resolution and color characteristics of the photographic film. After much experimentation, we have found the Kodak Ektachrome, ASA 400, daylight film to be the most satisfactory for making slides. All endoscopic illustrations in this volume were made with this film. More sensitive films (ASA 1600 or 3200) do not have the same accurate color rendition and they are also much more granular. We had good results in special cases when we "pushed" the Ektachrome 400, i.e., exposed it as though it were ASA 800 and then made the appropriate adjustments during the developing process. None of the illustrations in this volume were done by this technique. High quality prints can be made from Ektachrome 400 slides without much trouble and without the need for an intermediary negative.

VIDEO DOCUMENTATION

All the problems discussed in the previous section, that is, loss of light, light carrier, care of the lenses, etc. are equally valid for the production of videotapes. In contrast to the importance of the flash, here the emphasis is on the production of a uniform, constant, bright light (Fig. 14.9).

In the video camera, the decisive criteria are also the light sensitivity and the associated resolution capacity. Here also the color red is the limiting factor, since it absorbs the most light. A moderate hemorrhage may easily cause a failure of the video signal and make the tape obtained unusable.

The selection of suitable equipment is extremely difficult. There are currently a number of incompatible systems (PAL, Secam, NTSC), a number of tape formats (U-Matic, High-Band, Low-Band, VHS, Super-VHS, Beta, etc.) and an almost infinite variety of cameras and recording systems. In the area of medical use, at least at the present time, the U-matic (3/4 inch) seems to have the edge.

The most important component is the camera. The tube cameras have been replaced by the chip cameras and the first generation, 1-chip camera has already been replaced by the 3-chip camera.

The requirements for an ideal video camera for endoscopic use specify that it should be light, small, easy to use, sturdy, reliable, and affordable. Its light sensitivity should be around 5 Lux, but so far this has been achieved only by the tube cameras (e.g., Lembke 533). Currently, the best chip cameras achieve only around 10 Lux.

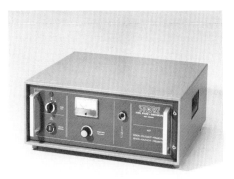

FIGURE 14.9 A variety of cold light sources for videoendoscopy. Lately we have used only the video cold light source with a 250 Watt HTI bulb.

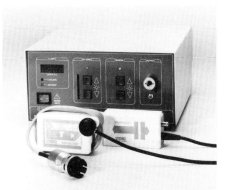

FIGURE 14.10 The Karl Storz Endopocket camera Model 536 with its chip control unit (CCU) and its power supply attached to a light source.

Without trying to make a value judgement, we have found that the Karl Storz Endopocket TV camera Model 536 met these requirements most closely (Fig. 14.10). In connection with a 45 degree angled beam splitter (Fig. 14.11) the camera can be easily attached to the endoscope and positioned so that it rests on the back of the surgeon's hand (Fig. 14.12). It takes only little additional effort to compensate for the additional weight and torque. This is most important to permit the surgeon to work without excessive fatigue. The use of endoscope handles makes the work very much easier and permits the smoother manipulation of the endoscope and the easier and less strenuous rotation of angled lenses around their long axis. It should be mentioned that the video cameras are being improved almost monthly, becoming smaller, lighter, and providing improved light sensitivity and greater resolution of detail.

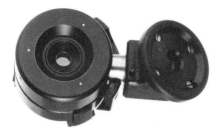

FIGURE 14.11 *A*, The Karl Storz 45 degree angled beam-splitter for use with a video camera. *B*, The camera and the eyepiece can both be independently rotated.

A

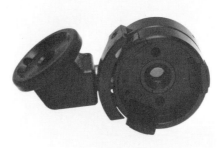

B

FIGURE 14.12 *A*, The 30 degree endoscope with a round handle and attached Endocamera. *B*, The camera should always be rotated so that it rests comfortably on the back of the surgeon's hand and thus produces practically no torque.

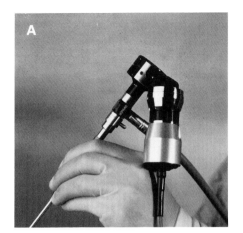
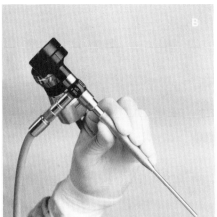

Videotaping Technique

The comments made concerning handling the instrument and utilizing the light in still photography are valid here as well. Since in endoscopic photography shadows are particularly bothersome, the endoscope must be manipulated with the greatest possible care. The distal lens must be kept free of secretions and mucus and must therefore be kept away from contact with the mucous membranes. The position of the exit port of the light beam must always be kept in mind.

When a manually adjustable light source is used, it is essential that an assistant continuously keep an eye on the television monitor and regulate the light intensity as necessary. Xenon light sources have recently become available that adjust brightness automatically, thereby avoiding over or under illumination.

Depending on the technique used in editing the tape, it may be necessary to have at least a 10 or 15 second run prior to the scene that is to be recorded, in order to have a smooth transition between scenes. It should become a routine practice to start the tape at least 10 seconds before the surgical sequence to be taped, so that the critical sequence is fully available for editing.

TEACHING MODALITIES

Endoscopic surgery provides excellent opportunities for observation and hence for teaching. By using an articulated side-arm, each diagnostic and surgical step can be directly followed and the observer has an excellent opportunity to watch every phase of the procedure. The observer must have a delicate touch, and he/she must follow every movement of the endoscope carefully while holding and guiding the side-arm so that the surgeon is not burdened with an additional weight on the endoscope (Fig. 14.13). The video camera offers the best opportunity when more than one observer wishes to follow the procedure. As shown in Figure 14.14, the procedure can be readily followed on the monitor screen, however, even the best television monitor does not provide the perception of depth that a single observer can get through the articulated side-arm. This lack of depth perception is also the reason why we have established a strict rule, never to operate from the monitor. The surgeon must have his eye at the proximal end of the endoscope and must manipulate the endoscope in the surgical field. Only in this manner can the surgeon remain truly oriented in all three dimensions.

We routinely use an endoscopic television camera in all of our procedures. We do this not only to teach trainees and demonstrate to visitors, but also to enable the scrub nurse to follow the procedure and thus be able to assist the surgeon more effectively.

FIGURE 14.13 An assistant watching through an articulated arm.

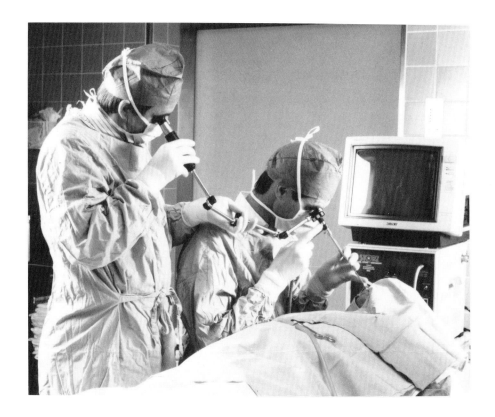

FIGURE 14.14   Observing on a monitor
screen.

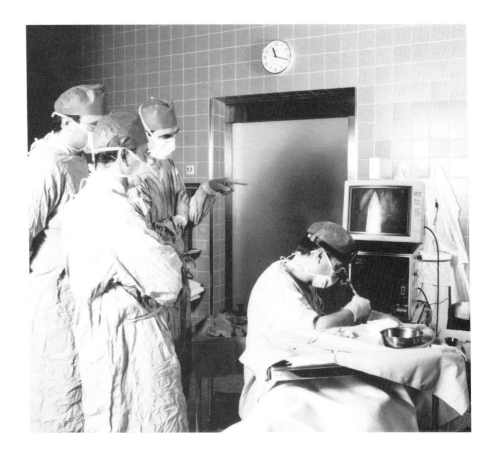

ENDOSCOPES AND INSTRUMENTS

The endoscopes and instruments illustrated in this appendix represent only a part of the equipment that we use. Only those endoscopes and instruments that we use regularly are described and their special areas of usefulness are sketched briefly.

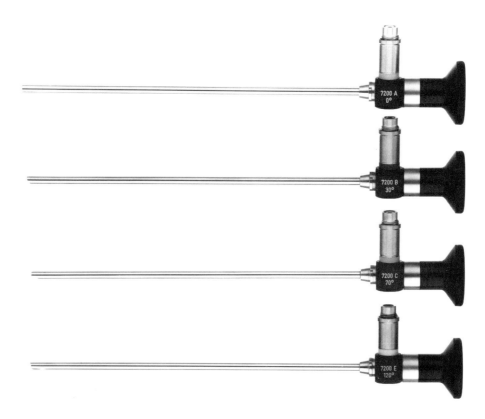

FIGURE A.1 The 4-mm endoscope that we use most frequently. The 0 degree endoscope (straight forward anterior view) is the standard scope for surgical procedures. About 80 percent of all surgical procedures are performed under the guidance of this endoscope. Because of its direct forward looking orientation, this is the only endoscope whose long axis always points in the direction in which one looks (i.e., directly along the axis of the shaft). This allows the most precise orientation. Combined with a flat handle (see Fig. A.3) it can be held securely and permits easy, motion-free photography and video documentation.

The 0 degree 4-mm nasal endoscope is also useful in maxillary sinus endoscopy for orienting the trocar sheath precisely toward the area from which a biopsy is to be taken or mucous membrane removed.

The 30 degree 4-mm diameter tele- scope also allows a forward view and can be introduced without difficulty. This endoscope is *the* diagnostic instrument of choice, and because of the orientation of its lens it allows a careful inspection of the middle meatus, the sphenoethmoidal recess, and the entire epipharynx. It is

also used in maxillary sinus endoscopy, where its wide-angle view is particularly useful. During surgery we use the 30 degree endoscope only when at the end of the procedure the anatomic landmarks have been accurately identified, and the ostium of the maxillary sinus must be enlarged for some work within the maxillary sinus. This endoscope is also very useful for working in the frontal recess. We use it in combination with a round handle (see Fig. A.4), which facilitates rotation of the endoscope around its long axis, between the fingers. The round handle makes these maneuvers much easier, particularly when the heavy liquid light carrier and a video camera are used.

The 70 degree angled 4-mm endoscope is used primarily for diagnostic purposes and in some special surgical situations, particularly in the frontal recess and in manipulations in the maxillary sinus, through an enlarged ostium. This endoscope does not allow a view along the shaft of the scope, and consequently great care and experience is necessary in avoiding contact with the mucous membranes and injury during its

introduction. As described in Chapter 7, it is frequently helpful to introduce a trocar sheath over a 0 or 30 degree endoscope to the position to be inspected with the 70 degree scope. The trocar sheath is then held fixed in this position and the 70 degree endoscope is introduced through the sheath placing it in the required position and avoiding mucosal contact during the introduction.

The 120 degree endoscope is used only during maxillary sinus endoscopy, for instance to inspect the anterior wall of the sinus through a trocar sheath introduced through the canine fossa. We do *not* use this endoscope for surgical purposes.

The illustration does not show the thinner 2.7-mm diameter endoscopes that are available with 0, 30, and 70 degree lenses. These endoscopes are used primarily in difficult diagnostic situations and in severely constricted areas (e.g., in children). We do not use them for surgical procedures. The use of handles with the slender endoscopes facilitates a more precise manipulation of the instrument and also avoids the risk of bending or kinking.

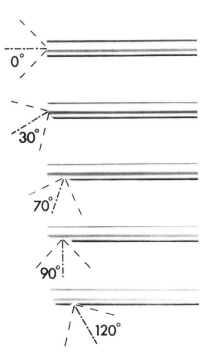

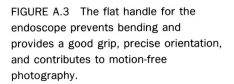

FIGURE A.2 A schematic drawing shows the direction of view with the different endoscopes. The angle of deflection is always relative to the long axis of the endoscope at its tip.

FIGURE A.3 The flat handle for the endoscope prevents bending and provides a good grip, precise orientation, and contributes to motion-free photography.

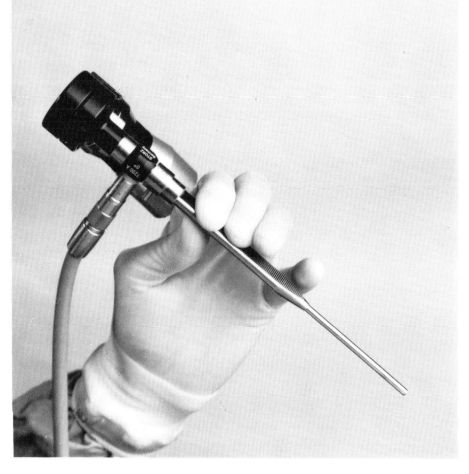

FIGURE A.4   The round endoscope handle facilitates rotation of the endoscope around its longitudinal axis. The knurled handle also promotes a good grip and precision of movement while preventing the endoscope shaft from bending.

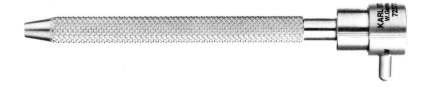

FIGURE A.5   Longitudinal section through an endoscope with traditional lens arrangement (A) and with the Hopkins rod lens system (B). In contrast to the single lens or group of lenses in the traditional system, the Hopkins system uses quartz rod lenses. These give greater clarity, more brightness and a wider angle with a scope of a smaller diameter.

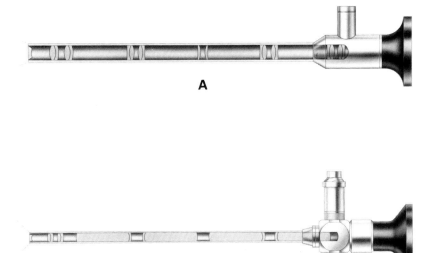

A

B

FIGURE A.6 The most commonly used suction tips. *A*, an angled surgical suction tip with a small hole in the handle so that the surgeon can control the force of suction with a fingertip. Its primary use is in diagnostic and surgical sinus procedures. The newer suction tips have a cm scale etched along the shaft, so that the approximate position of the tip can be estimated, e.g., from the anterior nasal spine. *B*, The bent nasal suction tip is used primarily to remove secretions and crusts postoperatively.

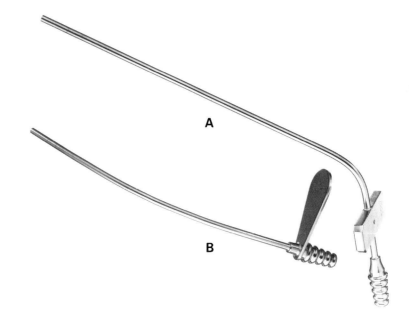

FIGURE A.7 The Freer-type suction elevator. It is most commonly used in diagnostic endoscopy for the careful displacement of the middle turbinate, when the endoscope must be introduced into the nasal passages. The suction hole in the tip of this elevator permits the simultaneous removal of secretions and thus eliminates the need to switch back and forth between a Freer elevator and a suction tip.

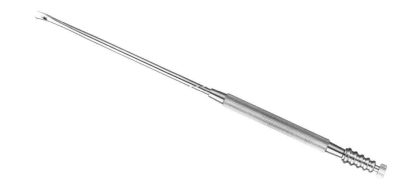

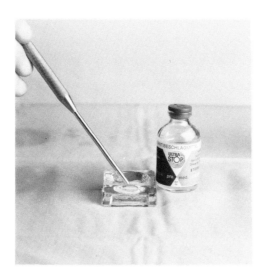

FIGURE A.8 The acrylic cup used for the application of antifog solution to the distal lens of the endoscope. The bottom of the cup is covered with a layer of cotton to protect the lens. A few drops of antifog solution are usually sufficient for the entire procedure.

FIGURE A.9 The maxillary sinus trocar used for performing maxillary sinus endoscopy through the canine fossa (and in exceptional cases, through the inferior meatus).

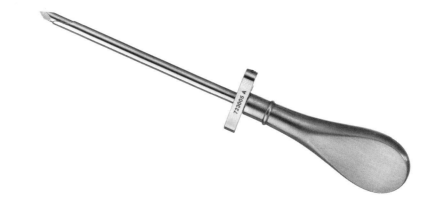

FIGURE A.10   Detail of the trocar sheath. We prefer the shovel-shaped trocar sheath. It makes both manipulations within the maxillary sinus (displacement of cysts or polyps) and introduction into the middle meatus (e.g., careful introduction into a very tight middle meatus) easier.

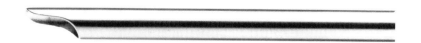

FIGURE A.11   Delicate biopsy forceps used in the removal of small cysts or polyps and for biopsy through a trocar sheath from the maxillary sinus.

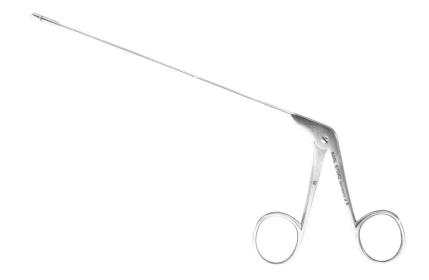

A

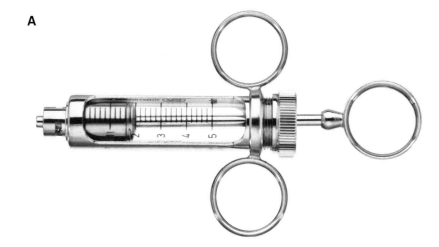

FIGURE A.12 *A*, Three-ring syringe and needle (*B*) used for the infiltration of local anesthetics. The steel wire in the needle is used for cleaning.

B

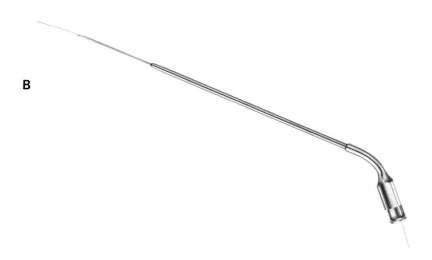

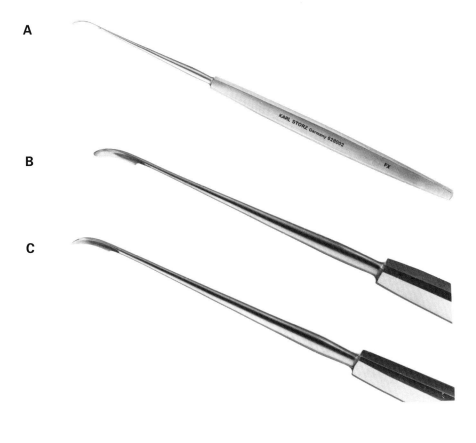

FIGURE A.13   The sickle scalpel (curved blade): available in (*B*) rounded and (*C*) pointed form. The sickle shaped scalpel is used for the initial resection of the uncinate process, opening of a concha bullosa, and for splitting the mucosa for the removal of septal spurs or ridges.

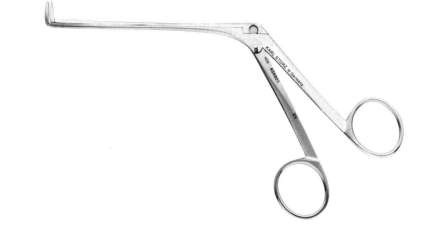

FIGURE A.14   *A*, Blakesley-Weil forceps. Jaws flex at right angle. *B*, The jaws, which are shown in detail are also available in a 4-mm longer version. The forceps are used for the preparation of the roof of the ethmoid, for work in the frontal recess and *in* the maxillary sinus, through an enlarged ostium.

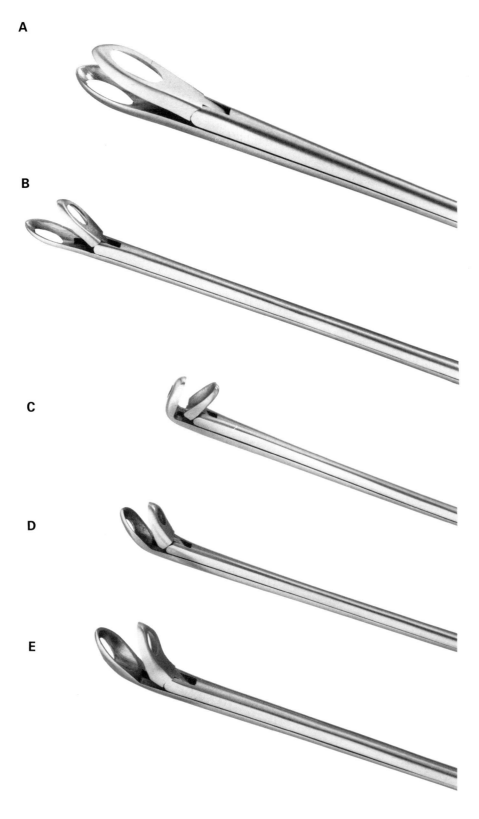

A

B

C

D

E

FIGURE A.15 The Blakesley-Weil forceps are available in a variety of sizes and shapes. *C*, The large form is used very rarely. We only use this forcep in cases of excessive polyposis, when all finer bony structures have been destroyed by chronic inflammation or by pressure from the polyps. This instrument is too large for most other purposes. Most of our procedures are performed with the delicate Blakesley-Weil forceps in its straight form (*B*) and in its flexed form (*D*).

FIGURE A.16   The flexed Blakesley-Weil forceps with built-in suction channel. The suction can be regulated with a finger. *B,* Close-up.

A

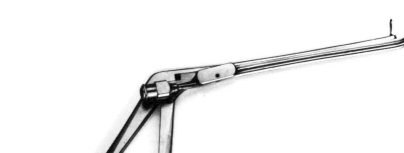

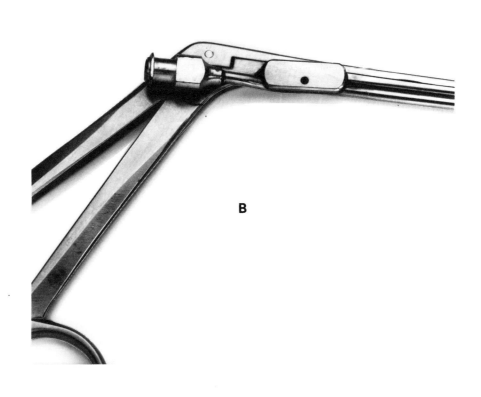

B

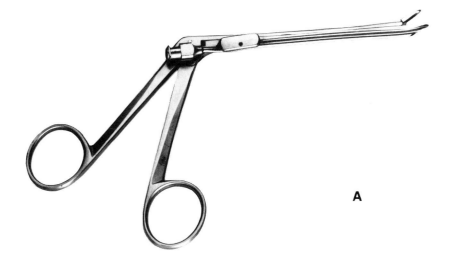

A

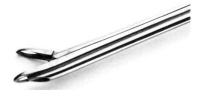

B

FIGURE A.17   *A*, The straight, delicate Blakesley-Weil forceps with built-in suction channel. *B*, Close-up. We only rarely use the suction Blakesley-Weil forceps. The primary indication for their use is extensive capillary oozing as seen in some cases of diffuse, polypoid rhinosinopathy, in complications of acute sinusitis, or in those rare cases where general anesthesia must be used.

In *B*, the oblique, recessed suction aperture can be seen at the end of the instrument. This recess is supposed to prevent the aspiration of soft tissues before they can be grasped by the jaws. Since the additional suction channel makes the instrument bulkier, it is more likely to cause undesirable injury during its introduction into the middle meatus, especially to the head of the middle turbinate.

Suction-irrigation handles are *not* used in the Messerklinger technique, since they are too bulky for more delicate manipulations. Their 5- to 6-mm diameter is also too large for safe introduction into the middle meatus. Suction irrigation is contraindicated when patients are being operated under local anesthesia as in these patients, the nasopharynx can not and should not be packed.

If the procedure is performed under general anesthesia, then increased bleeding frequently results in a demand for the suction-irrigation endoscope. In order to introduce this instrument into the middle meatus, the middle turbinate must be partially or totally resected. This leads to more bleeding and finally results in a radical procedure that should have been avoided in the first place.

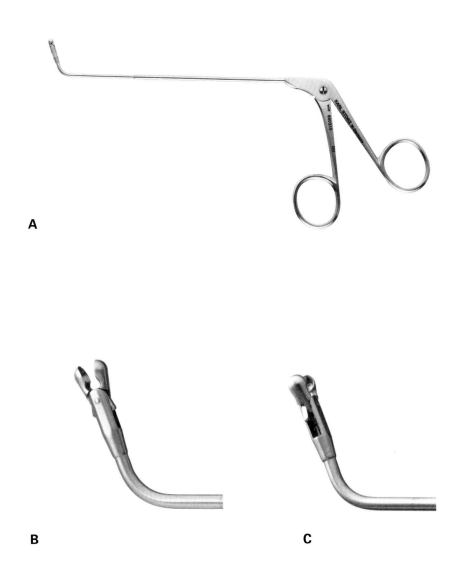

A

B   C

FIGURE A.18 *A*, Upward bent, delicate forceps. *B*, Jaws close longitudinally. *C*, Jaws close crosswise. These forceps are useful for manipulations in the frontal recess in combination with 30 or 70 degree lenses. They are also suitable for manipulations in the maxillary sinus, e.g., the removal of small polyps or the opening of cysts through the natural ostium.

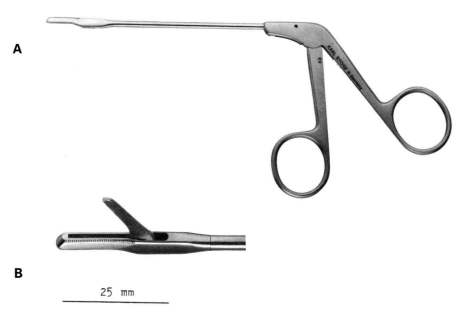

FIGURE A.19 *A*, The Struycken modified nasal cutting forceps. The jaws of these forceps are considerably more delicate than in Struycken's original model, but still strong. They are useful for opening a concha bullosa, cutting fibrous bands, septal spurs, and ridges. *B*, Close-up of jaws.

25 mm

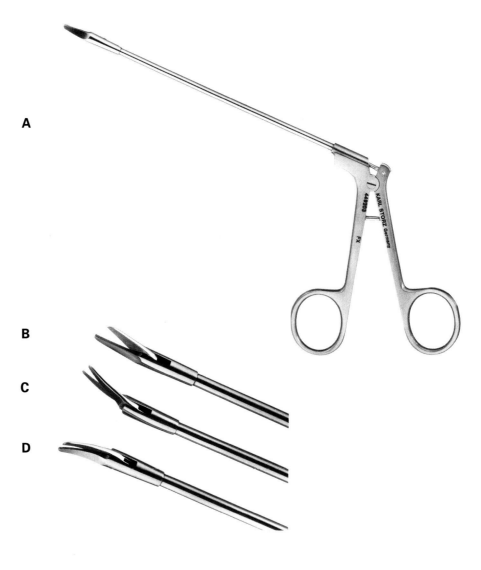

FIGURE A.20 *A*, A set of scissors for endoscopic use. *B*, Straight jaws, *C*, angled to the right, and *D*, to the left. This set of scissors is useful for opening a concha bullosa, resecting the stalks of coarse single or recurrent polyps, and for cutting fibrous strands and synechiae.

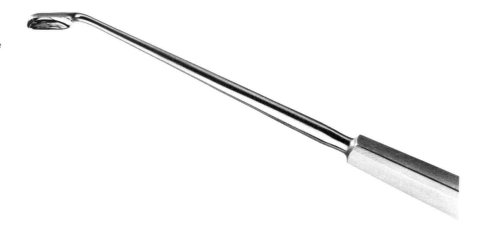

FIGURE A.21 The bent spoon is an instrument of general usefulness available in two sizes. It is used not only for locating and enlarging the ostium of the maxillary sinus, but is excellent in palpating resistances. It is also used for carefully removing fine bony lamellae in search of the ostium of the frontal sinus and for perforating the anterior wall of the sphenoid sinus.

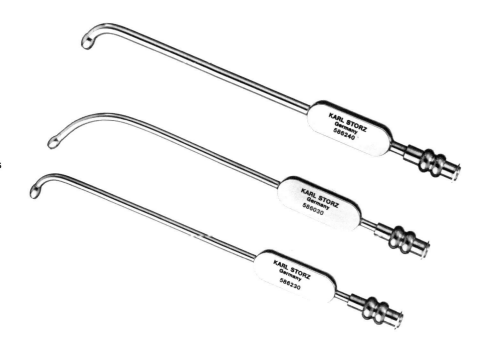

FIGURE A.22 A set of angled suction tips of different size and shape. These suction tips are used primarily for removing secretions from the maxillary sinus and from the middle meatus. Frequently, fungal masses can also be removed by suction. The thin instruments are useful primarily when the frontal recess must be entered from below a far anterior insertion of the middle turbinate.

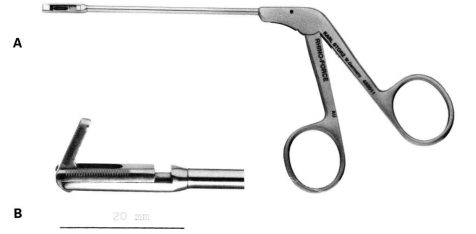

FIGURE A.23 *A,* The Stammberger-Ostrum backward cutting antrum punch. *B,* Close-up of the jaw. These back biting forceps are available in two models (sideward cutting to the right and to the left). They are used for the enlargement of the ostium of the maxillary sinus at the expense of the anterior fontanelles and for the retrograde resection of the uncinate process.

A

B

20 mm

BIBLIOGRAPHY

ARNOLD WJ, LAISSUE JA, FRIEDMANN I, NAUMANN HH, Eds. Diseases of head and neck. An atlas of histopathology. New York: Thieme, 1987.

ASHIKAWA R, KASAHARA Y, MATSUDA T, KATSUME K, YOSHIMURA S. Surgical anatomy of the nasal cavity and paranasal sinuses. Auris Nasus Larynx 1982; 9:75–79.

BAENKLER HW, DECHANT F, HOSEMANN W. In vitro histamine release from nasal mucosa upon bacterial antigens. Rhinology (Suppl) 1987; 25:17–22.

BAGATELLA F, MAZZONI A. Transnasal microsurgical ethmoidectomy in nasal polyposis. Rhinology 1980; 18:25–29.

BAGATELLA F, MAZZONI A. Microsurgery in nasal polyposis. Transnasal ethmoidectomy. Acta Otolaryngol Suppl 1986; 431:1–19.

BARNES PJ. Asthma as an axon reflex. Lancet 1986 (Feb) 1:242–245.

BAUER E, WODAK E. Neuerungen in der Diagnostik und Therapie der Nasennebenhöhlen. Arch Ohr Nas Kehlkopfheilk 1958; 171:325–329.

BOLGER WE, PARSONS DS. Treatment of recurrent sinus barotrauma in aviators: comparison of functional endoscopic and "classic" sinus surgery techniques. Am J Rhinol 1990; 3:75–81.

BRIDGER MWN, VAN NOSTRAND AWP. The nose and paranasal sinuses—applied surgical anatomy. J Otolaryngol 1978; 7 (Suppl 6).

BUITER CT. Endoscopy of the upper airways. Excerpta Med 1976.

BUITER CT. Nasal antrostomy. Rhinology (Suppl) 1988; 26:5–18.

BUSCH H. Phantom der normalen Nase des Menschen. München: JF Lehmans, 1911.

CAMPBELL TD. Twelve years experience with inferior turbinectomy. Rhinology (Suppl) 1988; 1:106.

CHRISTENSEN H. Endoscopy of the maxillary sinus. Acta Otolaryngol (Stockh) 1946; 34:404.

COLOGNOLI R. L'fundibulum ethmoidal. Anatomie, Pathologie, Chirurgie. These. Faculte Medicine de Marseille. Marseille: Pronto Offset, 1989.

COLOGNOLI R. L'fundibulum ethmoidal. Tome II. Atlas. Faculte Medicine de Marseille. Marseille: Pronto Offset, 1989.

DAVIDSON TM, BRAHME FJ, GALLAGHER ME. Radiographic evaluation for nasal dysfunction: computed tomography versus plain films. Head Neck 1989; Sept.-Oct.:405–409.

DIXON HS. Microscopic sinus surgery, transnasal ethmoidectomy and sphenoidectomy. Laryngoscope 1983; 93:440–444.

DRAF W. Endoskopie der Nasennebenhöhlen. Diagnostische und therapeutische Möglichkeiten. Berlin: Springer, 1978.

DRAF W. Die chirurgische Behandlung entzündlicher Erkrankungen der Nasennebenhöhlen. Arch Otorhinolaryngol 1982; 235:133–305.

DRAKE-LEE AB, BICKERTON R, MCLAUGHLAN P. Free histamine in nasal polyp fluid. Rhinology 1984; 22:133–138.

DRAKE-LEE AB. Nasal mast cells: a preliminary report on their ultrastructure. J Laryngol Otol (Suppl) 1987; 13:1–17.

EICHEL BS. Revision sphenoidethmoidectomy. Laryngoscope 1985; 95:300–304.

ENZMANN H, RIEBEN FW. Rhinosinusitis polyposa und Analgetikaintoleranz (Aspirinintoleranz). Laryngol Rhinol Otol 1983; 62:119–125.

FENNER T. Technik der endonasalen, endoskopisch kontrollierten Ethmoidektomie. ORL (Bern) 1984; 7:190–197.

FREEDMAN HM, KERN EB. Complications of intranasal ethmoidectomy: a review of 1000 consecutive operations (Mayo Clinic Rochester, Minn.). Laryngoscope 1979; 89:421–432.

FRIEDMAN WH, KATSANTONIS GP, ROSENBLUM BN, COOPER NH, SLAVIN R. Sphenoethmoidectomy: the case for ethmoid marsupialization. Laryngoscope 1986; 96:473–479.

FRIEDMAN WH, KATSANTONIS GP, SLAVIN RG, KANNEL P, LINFORD P. Sphenoidectomy: its role in the asthmatic patient. Otolaryngol Head Neck Surg 1982; 90:171–177.

FRIEDMANN I. Systemic pathology. Vol. 1. Nose, Throat and Ears. Edinburgh: Churchill Livingstone, 1986.

FRIEDMANN I, OSBORN DA. Pathology of granulomas and neoplasmas of the nose and paranasal sinuses. Edinburgh: Churchill Livingstone, 1982.

FRIEDRICH JP, TERRIER G. L'chirurgie sinusale maxillare endoscopic par voie endo-nasale. Aktuel Probl Otolaryngol 1984; 7:185–189.

FRIEDRICH JP. Sinus surgery by endoscopic guidance. In: Clement PAR. Recent Advances in E.N.T. Endoscopy. Brussels: Sci Soc Med Inform, 1985.

GOLDBERGER K. Die Bedeutung des Prozessus uncinatus in der Behandlung der Stirnhöhlenerkrankungen. Monatsschr Ohrenheilk Laryngorhinol 1936; 71:175–178.

GOLDING-WOOD PG. Observations on petrosal and Vidian neurectomy in chronic vasomotor rhinitis. J Laryngol 1961; 75:232.

GRÜNWALD L. Deskriptive und topographische Anatomie der Nase und ihrer Nebenhöhlen. In: Denker A, Kahler O, Hrsg. Handbuch der Hals-Nasen-Ohrenheilkunde. Bd. I. Berlin-München: Springer-Bergmann, 1925, 1–95.

GRÜNWALD L. Die Lehre von den Naseneiterungen. München: Lehmann, 1926.

HAJEK M. Indikation der verschiedenen Behandlungs- und Operationsmethoden bei den entzündlichen Erkrankungen der Nebenhöhlen der Nase. Z Hals Nas Ohrenheilk 1923; 4:511–522.

HAJEK M. Pathologie und Therapie der entzündlichen Erkrankungen der Nebenhöhlen der Nase. 5. Aufl. Leipzig: Franz Deuticke, 1926.

HAJEK M. Pathology and treatment of the inflammatory diseases of the nasal accessory sinuses. 5th Ed. Vol. II. London: Henry Kimpton, 1926.

HEERMANN H. Über endonasale Chirurgie unter Verwendung des binoculären Mikroskopes. Arch Ohr Nas Kehlkopfheilk 1958; 171:295–297.

HEERMANN J. Endonasale mikrochirurgische Siebbeinausräumung bei Blutdrucksenkung am halbsitzenden Patienten. HNO 1982; 30:180–185.

HELLMICH S, HERBERHOLD C. Technische Verbesserungen der Kieferhöhlenendoskopie. Arch Ohr Nas Kehlkopfheilk 1971; 199:678–683.

HELLMICH S. Surgery of the paranasal sinuses: the state of the art. F Med (Br) 1986; 92(4):255–265.

HELLMICH S. Bimeatal sinuscopy. Technical and diagnostic improvements. Internat Rhinology 1972; 10(1):37–42.

HILDING AC. Physiology of drainage of nasal mucous: experimental work on accessory sinuses. Am J Physiol 1932; 100:664.

HILDING AC. Experimental sinus surgery: effects of operative windows on normal sinuses. Ann Otol 1941; 50:379–392.

HILDING AC. Physiologic basis of nasal operations. California Med 1950; 72(2):103–107.

HOUSSET B. Role of free radicals in inflammatory sinus disease. Rhinology (Suppl) 1988; 5:17–22.

HSIEH V. Non-allergic rhinitis with eosinophilia (NARES): a precursor of the triad nasal polyposis—intrinsic asthma—intolerance to aspirin. Rhinology (Suppl) 1988; 1:129.

HOSEMANN W. Mukoziliärer Transport der Nasennebenhöhlenschleimhaut nach Kieferhöhlenfensterung. Arch Otorhinolaryngol (Suppl) 1985; 2:245-246.

HOSEMANN W, WIGAND ME. Örtliche Unterschiede im Gewebebild der chronisch-hyperplastischen Nasennebenhöhlenschleimhaut. HNO 1985; 33:311-315.

HOSEMANN W, WIGAND ME, FEHLE R, SEBASTIAN J, DIERGEN DL. Ergebnisse endonasaler Siebbeinoperationen bei diffuser hyperplastischer Sinusitis paranasalis chronica. HNO 1988; 36:54-59.

HOSEMANN W, WIGAND ME, NIKOL J. Klinische und funktionelle Aspekte der endonasalen Kieferhöhlenoperation. HNO 1989; 37:225-230.

ICHIMURA K, MINEDA H, SEKI A. Vascular effects of neuropeptides on nasal mucosa. Ann Otol Rhinol Laryngol 1988; 97:289-293.

JAMAL A, MARAN AGD. Atopy and nasal polyposis. J Laryngol Otol 1987; 101:355-358.

JOHANSSON P. Experimental and clinical studies of maxillary sinusitis. Thesis. Stockholm: Repro Print AB, 1988.

JORISSEN M. Ciliogenesis and ionchannels in human nasal epithelial cell cultures in vivo. Leuven University Press, Belgium, 1990.

KAINZ J, STAMMBERGER H. Das Dach des vorderen Siebbeines: Ein Locus minoris resistentiae an der Schädelbasis. Laryngol Rhinol Otol 1988; 67:142-149.

KAINZ J, STAMMBERGER H. The roof of the anterior ethmoid: a place of least resistance in the skull base. Am J Rhinol 1989; 4:191-199.

KAUFMANN E. Über eine typische Form von Schleimhautgeschwulst ("lateralen Schleimhautwulst") an der äusseren Nasenwand. Monatsschr Ohrenheilkd 1890; 1-8. Cited in: Zarniko C. Krankheiten der Nase und des Nasenrachens. Berlin: Karger, 1910.

KENNEDY DW. Functional endoscopic sinus surgery: technique. Arch Otolaryngol 1985; 111:643-649.

KENNEDY DW. Surgery of the sinuses. In: Johns ME. Complications in otolaryngology—head and neck surgery. Toronto: BC Decker, 1986, 71-82.

KENNEDY DW, ZINREICH SJ, KUHN F, SHAALAN H, NACLERIO R, LOCH E. Endoscopic middle meatal antrostomy. Theory, technique and patency. Laryngoscope 1987; 97 (Suppl 43), Part 3.

KENNEDY DW, ZINREICH SJ, KUMAR AJ, ROSENBAUM AE, JOHNS ME. Physiologic mucosal changes within the nose and ethmoid sinus: imaging of the nasal circle by MRI. Laryngoscope 1988; 98:928-933.

KENNEDY DW, ZINREICH SJ, ROSENBAUM AE, JOHNS ME. Functional endoscopic sinus surgery. Theory and diagnostic evaluation. Arch Otolaryngol 1985; 11:576-582.

KENNEDY DW, ZINREICH SJ, SHAALAN H, KUHN F, NACLERIO R, LOCH E. Endoscopic middle meatal antrostomy: theory, technique, and patency. Laryngoscope 1987; 97(Suppl 43):1-9.

KENNEDY DW, ZINREICH SJ, JOHNS ME. Functional endoscopic sinus surgery. In: Goldman J, Ed. The principles and practice of Rhinology. New York: Wiley & Sons, 1987, 879-902.

KENNEDY DW, JOSEPHSON JS, ZINREICH SJ, MATTOX DE, GOLDSMITH MM. Endoscopic sinus surgery for mucoceles: a viable alternative. Laryngoscope 1989; 99:885-895.

KENNEDY DW, SHAALAN H. A re-evaluation of maxillary sinus surgery: an experimental study in rabbits. Ann Otolaryngol 1989; 98:901-906.

KENNEDY DW, GOODSTEIN ML, MILLER NR, ZINREICH SJ. Endoscopic transnasal orbital decompression. Arch Otolaryngol Head Neck Surg 1990; 116:275-282.

KENNEDY DW, ZINREICH SJ. The functional endoscopic approach to inflammatory sinus disease: current perspectives and technique modifications. Am J Rhinol 1988; 2(3):89-93.

KESSLER L. Die Verletzungen des Gesichtsschädels und der Rhinobasis. Leipzig: Thieme, 1983.

KILLIAN G. Die Nebenhöhlen der Nase in ihren Lagebeziehungen zu den Nachbarorganen. Jena: Fischer, 1903.

KLEINSASSER O, SCHROEDER H-G. Adenocarcinomas of the inner nose after exposure to wood dust. Arch Otorhinolaryngol 1988; 245:1-15.

KOPP W, STAMMBERGER H, FOTTER R. Special radiologic imaging of the paranasal sinuses. Eur J Radiol 1988; 8:153-156.

KRAJINA Z. Advances in nose and sinus surgery. Dubrovnik: University of Zagreb, 1984.

KROEGEL C. Pathomechanismen der allergischen Entzündungsreaktion: der eosinophile Granulozyt. Allergologie 1990; 13(8):281–294.

KUMAZAWA H, ZEHM S, NAKAMURA A. CT-findings of aspergillosis in the paranasal sinuses. Arch Otorhinolaryngol 1987; 244:77–83.

KUMLIEN J. Blood flow measurements in sinus and nasal mucosa. Methodological studies with special reference to induced sinusitis in rabbits. Thesis. Stockholm: Repro Print AB, 1984.

KÜTTNER K, SIERING U, EICHHORN M. Ergebnisse und Erfahrungen bei der endoskopisch-chirurgischen Behandlung entzündlicher Nasennebenhöhlenaffektionen. HNO-Prax 1990; 15:45–52.

KÜTTNER K, SIERING U, EICHHORN M. Erfolge und Misserfolge nach endonasaler Fensterung der Kieferhöhle über den unteren Nasengang. HNO-Prax 1990; 15:45–52.

LANG J. Klinische Anatomie der Nase, Nasenhöhle und Nebenhöhlen. Aktuelle Oto-Rhino-Laryngologie. Bd. 11. Stuttgart: Thieme, 1988.

LANG J. Arteriae ethmoidales. Ursprung, Verlauf, Versorgungsgebiete und Anastomosen. Acta Anatomica 1979; 104:183–197.

LANG J. Über die Cellulae ethmoidales posteriores und ihre Beziehungen zum Canalis opticus. HNO 1988; 36:49–53.

LAYTON TB. Catalogue of the Onodi Collection in the Museum of the Royal College of Surgeons of England. Published in conjunction with the Royal College of Surgeons of England by The Journal of Laryngology and Otology. London: Headly Brothers, 1934.

LLOYD GAS. Diagnostic imaging of the nose and paranasal sinuses. London: Springer, 1988.

LOTHROP HA. Empyema of the antrum of Highmore. A new operation for the care of obstinate cases. Boston Med Surg J 1897; 136:455–462.

LUCKHAUPT H, BERTRAM G, BRUSIS T. History of paranasal sinus surgery. HNO 1990; 38:279–286.

LUND VJ. Inferior meatal antrostomy. Fundamental considerations of design and function. J Laryngol Otol (Suppl) 1988; 15:1–18.

LUNDBLAD L, LUNDBERG JM, BRODIN E, ÄNGGARD A. Origin and distribution of Capsaicin—sensitive substance P-immunoreactive nerves in the nasal mucosa. Acta Otolaryngol 1983; 96:485–493.

LUSK RP, LAZAR RH, MUNTZ HR. The diagnosis and treatment of recurrent and chronic sinusitis in children. Pediatr Clin North Am 1989; 36(6):1411–1420.

LUSK RP, MCALISTER WH, MUNTZ HR. Distribution of chronic pediatric sinus disease. 13th Congress of the European Rhinologic Society, London, England, June, 1990.

LUSK RP, MUNTZ HR, MCALISTER WH. Comparison of paranasal sinus radiographs and coronal CT scans in children. VIII ISIAN International Symposium on Infection and Allergy of the Nose, Baltimore, MD, June, 1989.

MAHALEY MS, ODOM GL. Complication following intrathecal injection of fluorescein. Neurosurg J 1966; 25:298.

MALTZ M. New instruments: the sinuscope. Laryngoscope 1925; 35:805–811.

MEES K, VOGL T. Computertomographie und Kernspintomographie des Gesichtsschädels und des Halses. Otorhinolaryngology 1989; (Suppl 1):1–40.

MERCKE U, LINDBERG S, DOLATA J. The role of neurokinin A and calcitonin gene-related peptide in the mucociliary defense of the rabbit maxillary sinus. Rhinology 1987; 25:89–93.

MESSERKLINGER W. Über die Drainage der menschlichen Nebenhöhlen unter normalen und pathologischen Bedingungen. 1. Mitteilung. Monatsschr Ohrenheilkd Laryngol Rhinol 1966; 101:56–68.

MESSERKLINGER W. Über die Drainage der menschlichen Nebenhöhlen unter normalen und pathologischen Bedingungen. 2. Mitteilung. Monatsschr Ohrenheilkd Laryngol Rhinol 1967; 101:313–326.

MESSERKLINGER W. Die Endoskopie der Nase. Monatsschr Ohrenheilkd Laryngol Rhinol 1970; 104:451–456.

MESSERKLINGER W. Technik und Möglichkeiten der Nasenendoskopie. HNO 1972; 20:133–135.

MESSERKLINGER W. Nasenendoskopie: Der mittlere Nasengang und seine unspezifischen Entzündungen. HNO 1972; 20:212-215.

MESSERKLINGER W. Hajeks atypische Hypertrophien im mittleren Nasengang und die Nasenendoskopie. Monatsschr Ohrenheilkd Laryngol Rhinol 1972; 106:481-488.

MESSERKLINGER W. Zur endoskopischen Anatomie der menschlichen Siebbeinmuscheln. Acta Otolaryngol (Stockh) 1973; 75:243-248.

MESSERKLINGER W. Zur Endoskopietechnik des mittleren Nasenganges. Arch Otorhinolaryngol 1978; 221:297-305.

MESSERKLINGER W. Endoscopy of the nose. Baltimore: Urban & Schwarzenberg, 1978.

MESSERKLINGER W. Das Infundibulum ethmoidale und seine entzündlichen Erkrankungen. Arch Otorhinolaryngol 1979; 222:11-22.

MESSERKLINGER W. Über den Recessus frontalis und seine Klinik. Laryngol Rhinol Otol 1982; 61:217-223.

MESSERKLINGER W. Die Rolle der lateralen Nasenwand in Pathogenese, Diagnose und Therapie der rezidivierenden und chronischen Rhinosinusitis. Laryngol Rhinol Otol 1987; 66:293-299.

MOLONEY JR, BADHAM NJ, MCRAE A. The acute orbit: preseptal (periorbital) cellulitis subperiosteal abscess and orbital cellulitis due to sinusitis. J Laryngol Otol (Suppl) 1987; 12:1-18.

MOSHER HP. The applied anatomy and internasal surgery of the ethmoidal labyrinths. Trans Am Laryngol Assoc 1912; 34:25-39.

MOSHER HP. The surgical anatomy of the ethmoidal labyrinth. Am Acad Ophthalmol Otolaryngol 1929; 376-410.

MOURET J. Anatomie des cellules ethmoidales. Rev Hebdo de Laryngol Otol Rhinol 1889; 3 Julliet. No. 31:913-924.

MOURET J. Rapport du sinus frontale avec le cellules ethmoidales. Rev Hebdo de Laryngol Otol Rhinol 1901; 16. No. 46:577-595.

MYGIND N, WINTHER B. Immunological barriers in the nose and paranasal sinuses. Acta Otolaryngol (Stockh) 1987; 103:363-368.

NAUMANN HH. Neue Trends in der Nebenhöhlen-Chirurgie? Laryngol Rhinol Otol 66:57-59.

OBERASCHER G, ARRER E. Immunologische Liquordiagnostik mittels Beta-2-Transferrin-Grundlagen und Methodik. Laryngol Rhinol Otol 1986; 65:158.

OBERASCHER G. A modern concept of cerebrospinal fluid diagnosis in oto- and rhinorrhea. Rhinology (Suppl) 1988; 26:89-103.

OGAWA H. Atopic aspect of eosinophilic nasal polyposis and a possible mechanism of eosinophil accumulation. Acta Otolaryngol [Suppl] (Stockh) 1986; 430:12-17.

OGAWA H. A possible role of aerodynamic factors in nasal polyp formation. Acta Otolaryngol [Suppl] (Stockh) 1986; 430:18-20.

OGINO S, HARADA T, OKAWACHI I, IRIFUNE M, MATSUNAGA T, NAGANO T. Aspirin-induced asthma and nasal polyps. Acta Otolaryngol [Suppl] (Stockh) 1986; 430:21-27.

OHNISHI T, ASHIKAWA R, TAKIGUCHI K, KAMIDE Y, TACHIBANA T. Ethmoidal nerve and artery block in endonasal sinusectomy. Rhinology (Suppl) 1987; 25:207-212.

OHNISHI T, ESAKI S, TACHIBANA T, KANETA K. Surgical treatment of recurrent mucocele of the sphenoid sinus. Rhinology (Suppl) 1990; 28:61-64.

OHYAMA M. Pathobiochemistry of chronic sinusitis. In: Myers E, Ed. New dimensions in otorhinolaryngology—head and neck surgery. Vol. 1. New York: Elsevier Science Publishers, 1985, 685-689.

ONISHI T. Bony defects and deshiscences of the roof of the ethmoid cells. Rhinology 1981; 19:195-207.

ONODI A. Die Eröffnung der Kieferhöhle im mittleren Nasengang. Arch Laryngol Rhinol 1903; 14:154-160.

ONODI A. Die topographische Anatomie der Nasenhöhle und ihrer Nebenhöhlen. Würzburg: Curt Kabitzsch, 1910.

ONODI A. The accessory sinuses of the nose in children. London: John Bale Sons & Daniellson and Würzburg: Curt Kabitzsch, 1911.

PATRIARCA J, ROMANO A, SCHIAVINO D, VENUTI A, DI RIENZO V, FAIS G, NUCERA E. ASA disease: a clinical relationship of polyposis to ASA intolerance? Arch Otorhinolaryngol 1986; 243:16-19.

PERKO D. Endoscopic surgery of the frontal sinus without external approach. Rhinology 1988; 26(Suppl 1):159.

PERNKOPF E. Topographische Anatomie. Bd 4. Topographische und stratigraphische Anatomie des Kopfes. 2. Hälfte. Berlin: Urban und Schwarzenberg, 1960.

PETER K. Vergleichende Anatomie und Entwicklungsgeschichte der Nase und ihrer Nebenhöhlen. In: Denker A, Kahler O, Hrsg. Handbuch der Hals-Nasen-Ohrenheilkunde. Bd 1. Berlin: Springer und München: Bergmann, 1925:95–136.

PETER K, WETZEL G, HEIDERICH F, Eds. Handbuch der Anatomie des Kindes. Bd 2. München: Bergmann, 1938.

PROETZ AW. Essays on the applied physiology of the nose. 2nd Ed. St. Louis: Annals Publishing, 1953.

RAHMEL U, KIETZMAN H, BRASCH J. Polyposisinvolution durch Acetylsalicylsäure-Toleranz-Induktion bei chronischer Pansinusitis polyposa. Allergologie 1989; 12(5):214–217.

RETTINGER G, CHRIST P. Visual loss following intranasal injection. Rhinology (Suppl) 1989; 9:66–72.

ROHEN JW, YOKOCHI C. Anatomie des Menschen. Photographischer Atlas der systematischen und topographischen Anatomie. Bd 1. Kopf, Hals, Rumpf. Stuttgart: Schattauer, 1982.

RUDERT H. Mikroskop- und endoskopgestützte Chirurgie der entzündlichen Nasennebenhöhlenerkrankungen. Der Stellenwert der Infundibulotomie nach Messerklinger. HNO 1988; 36:475–482.

SAKAGUCHI K, OKUDA M, USHIJIMA K, SAKAGUCHI Y, TANIGAITO Y. Study of nasal surface basophilic cells in patients with nasal polyp. Acta Otolaryngol [Suppl] (Stockh) 1986; 430:28–33.

SARIA A, ZHAO Y, WOLF G, LOIDOLT D, MARKLIN C-R, LUNDBERG JN. Control of vascular permeability and vascular smooth muscle in the respiratory tract by multiple neuropeptides. Acta Otolaryngol [Suppl] (Stockh) 1988; 457:25–28.

SARIA A, LUNDBERG JN, SKOFITSCH G, LEMBEK S. Vascular protein leakage in various tissues induced by substance P, capsaicin, bradykinin, serotonin, histamine and by antigen challenge. Naunyn-Schmiedebergs Arch Pharmacol 1983; 324:212–218.

SCHAEFER SD, CLOSE LG. Endoscopic management of frontal sinus disease. Laryngoscope 1990; 100:155–160.

SETTIPANE GA. Nasal polyps: epidemiology, pathology, immunology, and treatment. Am J Rhinol 1987; 1(3):119–126.

SIMON H. Die Fluoresceinprobe zur Diagnostik der oto- und rhinogenen Liquorfistel. Laryngol Rhinol 1970; 49:54.

STAMMBERGER H. Endoscopical diagnosis and treatment of paranasal sinus myocosis. In: Advances in nose and sinus surgery: Dubrovnik: University of Zagreb, 1984, 35–37.

STAMMBERGER H. Schleimhautveränderungen im vorderen Siebbein bei chronischer Sinusitis und NNH-Mykosen. a) Erste Mitteilung: Endoskopische und lichtmikroskopische Befunde. b) Zweite Mitteilung: Elektronenmikroskopische Befunde. Laryngol Rhinol Otol 1984; 64:107–119.

STAMMBERGER H. Endoscopic surgery for mycotic and chronic recurring sinusitis. Ann Otol Rhinol Laryngol 1985; (Suppl 119)94:1–11.

STAMMBERGER H. Unsere endoskopische Untersuchungstechnik der lateralen Nasenwand—Ein endoskopisch-chirurgisches Konzept zur Behandlung entzündlicher NNH-Erkrankungen. Laryngol Rhinol Otol 1985; 64:559–566.

STAMMBERGER H. Endoscopic endonasal surgery—new concepts in treatment of recurring sinusitis. Part I. Anatomical and pathophysiological considerations. Otolaryngol Head Neck Surg 1985; 94:143–147.

STAMMBERGER H. Endoscopic endonasal surgery—new concepts in treatment of recurring sinusitis. Part II. Surgical technique. Otolaryngol Head Neck Surg 1985; 94:147–156.

STAMMBERGER H. An endoscopic study of tubal function and the diseased ethmoid sinus. Arch Otolaryngol 1986; 243:254–259.

STAMMBERGER H. Nasal and paranasal sinus endoscopy—a diagnostic and surgical approach to recurrent sinusitis. Endoscopy 1986; 6:213–218.

STAMMBERGER H, JAKSE R. Mykotische Erkrankungen im HNO-Bereich (ausschliesslich der Hautmykosen und endemischer tropischer Sonderformen). HNO Praxis Heute 1987; 7:139–176.

STAMMBERGER H, WOLF G. Headaches and sinus disease: the endoscopic approach. Ann Otol Rhinol Laryngol 1988; 97(Suppl 134):3–23.

STAMMBERGER H, ZINREICH SJ, KOPP W, KENNEDY DW, JOHNS ME, ROSENBAUM AE. Zur operativen Behandlung der chronisch rezidivierenden Sinusitis—Caldwell-Luc versus funktionelle endoskopische Technik. HNO 1987; 35:93–105.

STAMMBERGER H, POSAWETZ W. Functional endoscopic sinus surgery: concept, indications and results of the Messerklinger technique. Eur Arch Otorhinolaryngol 1990; 247:63–76.

STANKIEWICZ JA. Complications of endoscopic nasal surgery: occurrence and treatment. Am J Rhinol 1987; 1:45–49.

STYJÄRNE P, LUNDBLAD L, LUNDBERG JN, ÄNGGARD A. Capsaicin and nicotine—sensitive afferent neurons and nasal secretion in healthy human volunteers and in patients with vasomotor rhinitis. Br J Pharmacol 1989; 96:693–701.

TAKAHASHI R. A collection of ear, nose and throat studies. Tokyo: Jikei University School of Medicine, 1971.

TAKASAKA T, KAKU Y, HOZAWA K. Mast cell degranulation in nasal polyps. Acta Otolaryngol [Suppl] (Stockh) 1986; 430:39–48.

TEATINI G, SIMONETTI G, SALVOLINI U, MASALA W, MELONI F, ROVASIO F, DEDOLA GL. Computed tomography of the ethmoid labyrinth and adjacent structures. Ann Otol Rhinol Laryngol 1987; 96:239–250.

TERRAHE K, MÜNNICH K. Gefahren und Komplikationen bei der transmaxillären Siebbein-Keilbeinhöhlenoperation. Laryngol Rhinol Otol 1974; 53:313–320.

TERRIER G. L'endoscopie rhinusinusale moderne. Lugano: Inpharzam S.A., 1978.

TERRIER G. L'endoscopie du sinus maxillare en pathologie traumatique et infectieuse. Ther Umsch 1975; 32:628.

TERRIER G, BAUMANN RP, PIDOUX JM. Endoscopic and histopathological observations of chronic maxillary sinusitis. Rhinology 1976; 14:129–132.

TERRIER G, FRIEDRICH JP. The contribution of modern endoscopy in allergic-rhino-sinusal diseases. Acta Otorhinolaryngol Belg 1979; 33(4):490–494.

TOS M. The pathogenetic theories on formation of nasal polyps. Am J Rhinol 1990; 4(2):51–56.

UDDMAN R, MALM L, SUNDLER F. Substance-P-containing nerve fibres in the nasal mucosa. Arch Otolaryngol 1983; 238:9–16.

DE VRIES N. New bone formation in nasal polyps. Rhinology 1988; 26:217–219.

WALLACE JD, ET AL. Status epilepitcus as a complication of intrathecal fluorescein. J Neurosurg 1972; 36:659.

WAITZ G, WIGAND ME. Endoscopic, intranasal surgery of inverted papillomas of the nose and paranasal sinuses. HNO 1990; 38:242–246.

WEST JM. Über die Eröffnung des Tränensackes von der Nase aus in Fällen von Dacryostenose. Verh Ver Dtsch Laryngol (Würzburg) 1913; xx:194–202.

WIET RJ, CAUSSE J-B. Complications in otolaryngology—head and neck surgery. Vol. 1. Ear and skull base. Toronto: BC Decker, 1986.

WIGAND ME, STEINER W, JAUMANN MP. Endonasal sinus surgery with endoscopical control: from radical operation to rehabilitation of the mucosa. Endoscopy 1978; 10:255–260.

WIGAND ME. Transnasale, endoskopische Chirurgie der Nasennebenhöhlen bei chronischer Sinusitis. I. Ein biomechanisches Konzept der Schleimhautchirurgie. HNO 1981; 29:215–221.

WIGAND ME. Transnasale, endoskopische Chirurgie der Nasennebenhöhlen bei chronischer Sinusitis. II. Die endonasale Kieferhöhlenoperation. HNO 1981; 29:263–269.

WIGAND ME. Transnasale, endoskopische Chirurgie der Nasennebenhöhlen bei chronischer Sinusitis. III. Die endonasale Siebbeinausräumung. HNO 1981; 29:287–293.

WIGAND ME. Transnasal ethmoidectomy under endoscopical control. Rhinology 1981; 19:7–15.

WIGAND ME, HOSEMANN W. Endoscopic ethmoidectomy for chronic sinubronchitis. Amsterdam: Elsevier, 1985, 549–552.

WOLF G, SARIA A, GAMSE R. Neue Aspekte zur autonomen Innervation der menschlichen Nasenschleimhaut. Laryngol Rhinol Otol 1987; 66:149–151.

WOLFGRUBER H. Über die Lamina cribrosa des Ethmoids. Z Laryngol Rhinol Otol 1968; 47(7):522–529.

YAMASHITA K. Pre- and postoperative evaluation of tubal dysfunction by means of endoscopy. Endoscopy of the eustachian tube. Proceedings of the International Conference on "The Postoperative Evaluation in Middle Ear Surgery" held in Antwerp on June 14–16, 1984. Ars Medici Congress Series 1984; 5:329–333.

YAMASHITA K. Pneumatic endoscopy of the eustachian tube. Endoscopy 1983; 15(4):257–259.

YAMASHITA K. Endonasal flexible fiberoptic endoscopy. Rhinology 1983; 21:233–237.

YAMASHITA K, MERTENS J, RUDERT H. Die flexible Fiberendoskopie in der HNO-Heilkunde. HNO 1984; 32:378–384.

YAMASHITA T, TSUJI H, MAEDA N, TOMODA K, KUMAZAWA T. Etiology of nasal polyps associated with aspirin-sensitive asthma. Rhinology (Suppl) 1989; 8:15–24.

ZARNIKO C. Die Krankheiten der Nase und des Nasenrachens. Berlin: Karger, 1910.

ZECHNER G. Histomorphological data on human auditory tube dysfunction. J Laryngol Otol 1981; 95:229–237.

ZINREICH SJ, KENNEDY DW, ROSENBAUM AE, GAYLER BW, KUMAR AJ, STAMMBERGER H. CT of nasal cavity and paranasal sinuses: imaging requirements for functional endoscopic sinus surgery. J Radiol 1987; 163:769–775.

ZINREICH SJ, KENNEDY DW, MALAT J, CURTIN H, EPSTEIN JI, HUFF L, KUMAR AJ, JOHNS ME, ROSENBAUM AE. Fungal sinusitis: diagnosis with CT and MR imaging. Radiology 1988; 169:439–444.

ZINREICH SJ, MATTOX D, KENNEDY DW, JOHNS ME, HOLLIDAY MJ, PRICE JC, QUINN CB, KASHIMA HK. 3-D CT for cranio-facial and laryngeal surgery. Laryngoscope 1988; 98:1212–1219.

ZINREICH SJ, MATTOX DE, KENNEDY DW, CHISHOLM HL, DIFFLEY DM, ROSENBAUM AE. Concha bullosa: CT evaluation. J Comput Assist Tomogr 1988; 12(5):778–784.

ZINREICH SJ, KENNEDY DW, GAYLER BW. CT of nasal cavity, paranasal sinuses: an evaluation of anatomy in endoscopic sinus surgery. Clear Images 1988; 2:2–10.

ZUCKERKANDL E. Normale und pathologische Anatomie der Nasenhöhle und ihrer pneumatischen Anhänge. Wien: Wilhelm Braumüller, 1882.

ZUCKERKANDL E. Normale und pathologische Anatomie der Nasenhöhle und ihrer pneumatischen Anhänge. II. Wien: Wilhelm Braumüller, 1892.

INDEX

A

Absidia spp, 426

Adhesion(s)

  as complication of endoscopic surgery, 466

  prevention of, with beclomethasone, 355

Agger nasi

  disease in, endoscopic and radiologic diagnosis

    of, 200–201

  pneumatization originating from, 162

Agger nasi cells, 62

  pneumatization of, 200

  radiologic anatomy of, 118–119

Air cells, within concha bullosa, 162

Allergy(ies)

  concha bullosa management and, 166

  endoscopic surgery for, results of, 462

  inhalation, role of Messerklinger technique in,

    428–429

Amphotericin B

  for invasive mycotic infections, 419

  for *Mucor* infections, 427

Analgesics, use of, 322–323

Anesthesia

  general, 333, 362

  infiltrative, 330–332

  local, 311

    advantages of, 332–333

    premedication for, 322–324

  for maxillary sinuscopy, 235

  topical, 328–330

    for diagnostic endoscopy, 147, 156, 187

Aneurysm(s), mycotic, 411

Antibiotic ointment, polyp or cyst filled with, 250

Antibiotics

  postoperative use of, 371

  for sinusitis, 278

Antifog solution, 148, 289

Antihistamines, postoperative use of, 371

Anti-inflammatory therapy, for sinusitis, 278

Antimycotic agents

  for infections, 418–419

  instillation of, following maxillary sinuscopy, 243

Antrochoanal polyp, 227

  components of, 346

  endoscopic surgery for, 346–349

Aspergillosis, of paranasal sinuses, 400–424

  clinical course and complications of, 411–412

  clinical picture of, 404

  conditions giving rise to, 419–424

  ecology and physiology of, 400–403

  endoscopic diagnosis of, 409–410

  fungal cultures in, 411

  histologic diagnosis of, 411

  incidence of, 400

  radiographic diagnosis of, 405–408

  treatment of, 412

    postoperative care following, 418–419

    surgical procedure in, 412–418

Aspergillus fumigatus, 398

  ecology and physiology of, 400–403

  growth of, 401

    environment for, 402

Aspergillus fumigatus fungus ball, 250

Aspergillus versicolor, 399

Aspirators, nasal, 150

Asthma

  intrinsic, 453, 456

  severity of, determination of, 454

  and sinus disease, 453–457

  treatment of, 457

Asthma granulomata, 260

B

Beck procedure, 356

Beclomethasone, adhesion prevention with, 355

Beclomethasone nose drops, postoperative use of,

  371–372

Biopsy forceps, for maxillary sinuscopy, 234

Bipolar cautery forceps, for intraoperative bleeding, 469

Blakesley suction forceps, 315

Blakesley-Weil forceps, 294, 314, 338

Bleeding

from carotid artery, as complication of endoscopic surgery, 474

during endoscopic surgery, 288

following maxillary sinuscopy, 244

intramucosal petechial, in maxillary sinus, 248

intraoperative

as complication of endoscopic surgery, 469–472

prevention of, 471

mucosal, during maxillary sinuscopy, 239

postoperative, as complication of endoscopic surgery, 468

Blood clots

in maxillary sinus, 248

postoperative removal of, 369, 372

Bony crests, in frontal sinus, mucus transport over, 20

Bozzini system, for nasopharyngeal inspection, 2

Bronchial asthma. See also *Asthma.*

sinusitis and, 453

Bulla ethmoidalis. See *Ethmoidal bulla (bulla ethmoidalis).*

Bulla frontalis (frontal ethmoidal cell), 55, 85

radiologic anatomy of, 116

Bulla lamella

bony bulge produced by, 62

pneumatization of, 57

C

C fibers, 19

and pain mediation, 449

selective killing of, 449

Calcitonin gene-related peptide, 448

Caldwell-Luc procedure

complaints following, 395

failure of, 381–398

conclusions drawn from, 394–395

endoscopic findings in, 382–389

radiologic findings in, 390–391

secretion transport in, 392–393

surgical therapy for, 396–398

symptoms of, 381–382

mucoceles as complication of, 365

radical, 394

Camera(s)

attached to endoscope, 485

used in still photography, 479–481

video, requirements of, 489–490

"Canalis semilunaris," 76

Candida albicans, 424

Candidiasis, 424–426

treatment of, 426

Candle, as light source, for early endoscopes, 4

Capillary oozing

as complication of endoscopic surgery, 469

postoperative, 369

Capsaicin, 449

Carcinogen(s), mycotoxins as, 399

Carotid artery

injury to, as complication of endoscopic surgery, 474

relationship of sphenoidal sinus to, 67–68, 210

Catheters, polyethylene, for maxillary sinuscopy, 234

Cephalosporin, postoperative use of, 371

Cerebrospinal fluid (CSF), leaks of, 436–441

demonstration and localization of, 437–440

treatment of, 440–441

Cerebrospinal fluid fistula, 437–441

as complication of endoscopic surgery, 473

Children

acute sinusitis in, complications of, endoscopic surgery for, 362–364

choanal polyps in, 227

concha bullosa in, 160

diagnostic endoscopy in, 156

maxillary sinuscopy in, 232

Choanal polyp

endoscopic and radiologic identification of, 227–229

endoscopic surgery for, 346–349

vs. polyposis, 227

Cholesterol cyst, 246

Ciliary sweep, divergence in, 260

Cilium (cilia)

abnormal, 259–260

beating of, 18, 25

optimum pH and temperature for, 26–27

postmortem, 27–28

in viscous mucus, 26

compound, 260

function of, factors affecting, 26–27, 27

Cleft(s)

ethmoid, definitions of, 50–51

of lateral nasal wall, 76–87

Clotrimazole, for mycotic infections, 418–419

"Cobbler's sphere," in early endoscopy, 4

Cocaine, use of, as anesthetic, 147, 330

Cold, chronic, vs. malignancy, 262–264

Computed tomography (CT)

advantages of, 108, 112

of combined paranasal sinus disease, 212–215

vs. conventional tomography, 108–114

diagnostic, of sinus diseases, 444–445

high resolution, 112

indications for, 145–146

of paranasal sinuses, 96–101

preoperative, 145

scheduling of, 146

technique of, 98–100

three-dimensional reconstructions from, 114

Concha bullosa

air cells within, 162

endoscopic and radiologic diagnosis of, 160–169

endoscopic examination of, 166

endoscopic surgery for, 350–355

vs. normally convex middle turbinate, 172
occurrence of, 160
pathologic findings among, 162, 164
and predisposition to sinus disease, 164
site of origin of, 162
superior turbinate, 168
Conchoscope, Wertheim's, 6
Conchotome, Struyken, 352
Contact headache, 443
Conventional tomography
vs. computed tomography, 108–114
of paranasal sinuses, 92–95
technique of, 94
Corticoids, postoperative use of, 371
Corticosteroid ointments, postoperative use of, 370–371
Cotton pledgets, 322
left in operating field, complications of, 378
vasoconstrictor-soaked, 188
Cribriform plate (lamina cribrosa), 52, 70
polyps attached to, 226
radiologic anatomy of, 122
Crista galli, radiologic anatomy of, 118
CT. See Computed tomography (CT).
Cultures, fungal, 411
Cyst(s)
at base of skull, 359
cholesterol, 246
expansion of, into maxillary sinus, 248
false, filled with antibiotic ointment, 250
frontal sinus, endoscopic surgery for, 358
as indication for maxillary sinuscopy, 245–246
maxillary sinus, opening of, 240
mucous membrane, secreting, 359
retention, 217, 246, 247
Cystoscope, development of, 6, 8

D
de Lima procedure, 394
Decompression
emergency, for intraoperative bleeding, 470
problems of, ethmoidal disease and, 248
Decongestant, for frontal sinusitis, 195
Density, measure of, Hounsfield unit as, 96
Dental materials, fungal infections and, 420–422
Dental root filling material, in maxillary sinus, 250
Diffuse polypoid rhinosinopathy, 224, 226
endoscopic surgery for, results of, 463–464
etiology of, 231
histologic findings in, 260–261
Diffuse polypoid rhinosinusitis, postoperative changes in, 377
Discharge instructions, to patient, 379
Documentation, of endoscopic procedures, 479–493
by still photography, 479–488
as teaching modality, 492–493
by video photography, 488–491
Drainage, of paranasal sinuses, 17–24
Droperidol, 323

Drug therapy, postoperative, 370–372
"Ductus naso-frontalis," 51
Dura, injury to, as complication of endoscopic surgery, 473
Dysesthesia, following maxillary sinuscopy, 243

E
Edema
mucosal, 230
neurogenic, substance P and, 230–231, 448
Electricity, as light source, for early endoscopes, 4
Emphysema, of soft tissues of cheek, following maxillary sinuscopy, 243
Empyema
conservative management of, 278
frontal sinus, 195
Encrustations
mycotic, 398
postoperative removal of, 372
Endoscope
4.0-mm 30 degree, for maxillary sinuscopy, 234
30 and 70 degree, introduction of, 286
antifog solution for, 148, 289
camera attached to, 485
flexible fiberoptic, 12
insertion and manipulation of, 284, 286–287
lenses of, 484
rigid, nasal examination with, 442
suction-irrigation, 289
switching of, during surgery, 289
types of, 2
used in photodocumentation, 484–485
zero degree
advantages of, 290
introduction of, 292
Endoscope table, 324–325
Endoscopic procedures, documentation of, 479–493
by still photography, 479–488
as teaching modality, 492–493
by video photography, 488–491
Endoscopic surgery, 283–319
for antrochoanal polyps, 346–349
complication(s) of, 466–477
diseased ethmoidal cells as, 467
hemorrhage as, 468
injury as, 468
intraoperative bleeding as, 469–472
severe, 473–477
stenosis of maxillary sinus ostium as, 467–468
synechiae as, 466–467
for complications of acute sinusitis, 362–364
for concha bullosa, 350–355
contraindications to, 275–277
difficulties, tips, and tricks in, 311–319
for ethmoid disease in sinubronchial syndrome, 344–345
for frontal sinus cyst, 358
for fungal masses, 412–418
general anesthesia for, 333

for hyperplastic inferior turbinate, 360–361
identification of frontal recess in, 314–315
identification of maxillary sinus ostium in, 315
identification of point for perforation of ground lamella in, 312–313
identification of site of insertion of uncinate process in, 312
identification of sphenoidal sinus in, 313–314
indications for, 273–275
infiltrative anesthesia for, 330–332
instrument manipulation in, 284–289
for isolated disease of frontal sinus, 356–357
local anesthesia for, 311
  advantages of, 332–333
for meningoencephalocele, 359
for mucoceles, 365–367
for nasal and paranasal sinus problems, in asthmatic patients, 455–456
as one-handed procedure, 284
orbital injuries in, 316–317
pain in, 318–319
patient information prior to, 321–322
patient positioning for, 324–326
for polypoid rhinosinusitis, 336–343
preparations for, 321–333
principles of, 283–284
for removal of foreign bodies, 434–435
results of, 459–465
technique and options in, 290–311
topical anesthesia for, 328–330
  premedication for, 322–324
Endoscopy
  diagnositic, of mycotic infections, 409–410
  diagnostic
    avoidance of injury during, 148
    in children, 156
    of concha bullosa, 160–169
    of deviated nasal septum, 156–159
    of ethmoidal bulla, 180–183
    instruments for, 148
    nasal, 145
    patient signals during, 150
    preparation for, 147
    steps in, 150–156
    technique of, 148–156
    of uncinate process, 173–179
    of variations of middle turbinate, 170–173
  historical aspects of
    of nose, 1–13
    of paranasal sinuses, 9–11
Environment, for fungal growth, 402
Epinephrine, as anesthetic, for endoscopic surgery, 328, 330
Epinephrine pledgets
  for ethmoidal artery bleeding, 469
  for frontal sinusitis, 278
Epiphora, 200
Ethmoid bone
  anatomy of, 52–53
  disease of, surgical therapy for, 396–398

roof of
  ethmoidal artery and, 70–76
  preoperative considerations for, 143
Ethmoid clefts, definitions of, 50–51
Ethmoidal artery
  anterior
    clinical and surgical significance of, 74–76
    dura mater surrounding, 74
    identification of, 73
    topographical relationships of, 70, 72
  bleeding from, as complication of endoscopic surgery, 469–470
  roof of ethmoid bone and, 70–76
Ethmoidal bulla (bulla ethmoidalis), 57, 60
  endoscopic and radiologic diagnosis of, 180–183
  enlargement of, symptoms of, 180
  and lateral sinus, 62
  pneumatization of, 180
  polyps originating in, 217
  preoperative considerations for, 142
  radiologic anatomy of, 121
  removal of, in treatment of sinubronchial syndrome, 344–345
  resection of, 297–298
  sinusitis and, 182
Ethmoidal canal (orbitocranial canal), 72
Ethmoidal cells
  behavior of, 65–66
  diseased, as complication of endoscopic surgery, 467
  frontal, 55, 85, 116
  supraorbital, 184
Ethmoidal disease
  decompression problems and, 248
  in sinubronchial syndrome, endoscopic surgery for, 344–345
Ethmoidal infundibulum, 35, 50, 60, 76
  configuration of, 80–81
  disease of
    endoscopic and radiologic diagnosis of, 185–193
    endoscopic clues in, 185
    endoscopic examination of, 186–187
    opening of, steps in, 292, 294–295
    posterior border of, 80
    preoperative considerations for, 142
    three-dimensional space of, 78–82
    variations of, 81
"Ethmoidal labyrinth," 52
Ethmoidal prechambers
  infection in, 37
  role of, 35–44
Ethmoidal sinus
  leiomyosarcoma of, 264
  mucoceles of, 366
  mucociliary transportation from, 31–32
  mycotic infection of, surgical approach to, 418
  posterior, 65–66
    disease of, endoscopic and radiologic diagnosis of, 204–207
    location of, 204

pneumatization of, 204–205

surgical approach to, 300, 302

Ethmoidal sulcus, 73

Ethmoidal turbinates, embryologic development of, 54–56

Ethmoturbinal bones, 55

Eustachian tube, function of, secretary disturbances and, 33–34

Eye

injury to, during surgery, 316–317

lens of, radiation dose to, 102–103

F

False passages, creation of, following maxillary sinuscopy, 244

Fenestration procedure

complaints following, 395

failure of, 381–398

conclusions drawn from, 394–395

endoscopic findings in, 382–389

radiologic findings in, 390–391

secretion transport in, 392–393

surgical therapy for, 396–398

symptoms of, 381–382

Fentanyl, 323

Fiber cables, 483

Fiberoptic cables, 483

Fibrosarcoma, of middle meatus, 264

Film selection, for photography, 488

Fistula

cerebrospinal fluid, 437–441

as complication of endoscopic surgery, 473

oro-antral, with maxillary sinusitis, 250

Flash tubes, 482

Fluid cables, 483

Flunitrazepam, 323

Fluorescein test, for cerebrospinal fluid leak, 437–438

Fontanelles, nasal, 60

Forced expiratory volume (FEV$_1$), preoperative vs. postoperative, in asthmatic patients, 455

Foreign body(ies), removal of, 434–435

from maxillary sinus, 240

Foveolae ethmoidales, 70

Frontal ethmoidal cell (bulla frontalis), 55, 85

radiologic anatomy of, 116

Frontal headache, 359

Frontal infundibulum, 35, 82. See also Frontal recess.

Frontal recess, 35, 82–87

anatomic configuration of, 84–85

diseased

endoscopic and radiologic diagnosis of, 194–199

repair of, 358

enlargement of, 308

identification of, in endoscopic surgery, 314–315

medial border of, 84

opening of, 305–307

polyps originating in, 217

posterior wall of, 84

preoperative considerations for, 142

radiologic anatomy of, 116

Frontal sinus

bony crests in, mucus transport over, 20

cyst of, endoscopic surgery for, 358

diseased, isolated, endoscopic surgery for, 356–357

dual, development of, 55

infection of

mechanism for, 42–44

secondary, 194

mucoceles of, 366

mycotic infection of, surgical approach to, 418

secretion transportation in, 30–31

trephination of, 356

Frontal sinusitis

endoscopic diagnosis of, 195

management of, 195–196

conservative, 278

Fungal concretions, 401

Fungal cultures, 411

Fungal hyphae (mycelia), 401

Fungal infections. See Mycotic infections.

Fungus ball, in maxillary sinus, 250

Furrows, nasal turbinates preceeded by, 54, 56

G

Ganglion pterygopalatinum, 18

Gas, as light source, for early endoscopes, 4

Gasogene, as light source, for early endoscopes, 4

Gel phase, of mucus, 17

Gliotoxin, 399, 412

Goblet cell metaplasia, 256

Granulomatous infiltrations, following maxillary sinuscopy, 243

Gray (Gy), as unit of measure, 102

H

Haller's cells, 202–203

Handles, special, for endoscope insertion and manipulation, 284, 286

Hasner's valve (plica lacrimalis), 119

observation of, 152

Hay fever, concha bullosa and, 16

Head, positioning of, for endoscopic surgery, 324

Headache(s)

contact, 443

frontal, 359

nonsinus-related, 446

sinugenic

causes of, 443–444

endoscopic and CT diagnosis of, 444–445

endoscopic approach to, 442–451

results of, 462

mucosal lesion causing, 447–449

and pain mediation, 449

unusual lesions causing, 446–447

in sphenoidal sinus disease, 208

Hematoma, as complication of endoscopic surgery, 468

Hemorrhage. See *Bleeding*.

Hiatus semilunaris, 50, 60

   mucosal changes of, 186

   two-dimensional formation of, 76–77

Hiatus semilunaris superior, 62, 77

Histologic diagnosis, of mycotic infections, 411

Hounsfield unit (HU), 96

Hyperplastic inferior turbinate, endoscopic surgery
   for, 360–361

Hypersecretion, mucus flow during, 25

Hyphae, fungal, 401

I

Immunoglobulin E (IgE) mediated allergies,
   428–429

Indwelling tube, for chronic maxillary sinusitis,
   complications caused by, 249

Infection(s)

   of ethmoidal prechambers, 37

   of maxillary and frontal sinuses, mechanisms for,
     42–44

   mycotic. See *Mycotic infections*.

Infiltrative anesthesia, for endoscopic surgery,
   330–332

Infundibular cells, 58

Infundibulum, ethmoidal. See *Ethmoidal
   infundibulum*.

Inhalation allergy(ies), role of Messerklinger
   technique in, 428–429

Injection, of anesthetic, 330–331

Instrument(s)

   manipulation of, in endoscopic surgery, 284–289

   for maxillary sinuscopy, 233–234

Interlamella cells, 64

Interlaminary cells, 162

Interturbinal meatus, 57–58

Irradiation, tissue and organ sensitivity to, 102–103

K

Kerosene lamp, as light source, for early
   endoscopes, 4

Kodak Ektachrome ASA 400 daylight film, 488

L

Lamella, ground

   identification of, 300

   perforation of, identification of correct point for,
     312–313

Lamina cribrosa (cribriform plate), 52, 70

   radiologic anatomy of, 122

Lamina papyracea, 52, 66

   injury to, as complication of endoscopic surgery,
     468

   polyps attached to, 226

Leiomyosarcoma, of ethmoidal sinus, 264

Lens

   of eye, radiation dose to, 102–103

   zoom, 480

Lidocaine, as anesthetic, 330

Light cables, 482–483

Light source

   for early endoscopes, 4

   for still photography, 482

   for video photography, 491

Limelight, as light source, for early endoscopes, 4

Linear tomography, of paranasal sinuses, 92

M

Magnetic resonance imaging (MRI), of paranasal
   sinuses, 104–107

Malignancy, chronic cold vs., 262–264

Markusowsky speculum, 6

Maxilla, destruction of, *Aspergillus* osteomyelitis
   and, 411

Maxillary sinus

   cysts of, opening of, 240

   dental root filling material in, 250

   endoscopic view of, 156

   endoscopy of, 232–252. See also *Maxillary
     sinuscopy*.

     historical aspects of, 9–11

   examination of, antrochoanal polyp removal and,
     346

   fontanelles of, accessory ostia in, 22–24

   foreign body removal from, 240

   fungus ball in, 250

   infection of, mechanism for, 42–44

   inflammation of. See *Maxillary sinusitis*.

   manipulation in, 240–242

   mucoceles of, 365–366

   mucous membrane changes in, 384, 386, 390–391

   mycotic infection of, surgical approach to,
     413–418

   renewal of mucus layer in, 19

   reversible mucosal changes in, 146

   secretion transportation in, 28–30

   septations of, 252

   squamous cell carcinoma of, 250, 264

Maxillary sinus ostium

   accessory, 178

     mucus transport over, 22–24

   enlargement of, 308

   identification of, in endoscopic surgery, 315

   secretion transport via, 30

   stenosis of, as complication of endoscopic
     surgery, 467–468

   visibility of, after resection of uncinate process,
     296

Maxillary sinuscopy, 232–252

   ciliary reflex phenomenon during, 27

   complications of, 242–244, 472

   endoscopic findings in, 245–252

   indications for, 232

   instillation of antimycotic substances following,
     243

   instrumentation for, 233–234

   patient tolerance of, 239

   technique of, 235–239

Maxillary sinusitis

   conservative endoscopic management of, 281

indwelling tube for, complications caused by, 249

oro-antral fistula with, 250

role of Haller's cells in, 202

Maxilloturbinal bone, 55

Mayo stand, 325

Mechanical obstruction, altered drainage routes
due to, 33–34

Meningitis, fungal, 411, 427

Meningoencephalocele, endoscopic surgery for, 359

Meperidine (pethidine hydrochloride), 322–323

Merocel sponges

left in operating field, complications of, 378, 472

postoperative removal of, 372

Messerklinger technique

as diagnostic endoscopy concept, 475

indications for, 459

limitations of, 475, 477

results of, 459–465

role of, in inhalation allergies, 428–429

of sphenoethmoidectomy, 283–284

surgical aspects of, 477

MRI (magnetic resonance imaging), of paranasal
sinuses, 104–107

Mucocele(s)

endoscopic surgery for, 365–367

of paranasal sinuses, 365–366

endoscopic surgery for, results of, 462

Mucociliary clearance system, 20

optimal function of, 26

Mucociliary transportation

from ethmoidal and sphenoidal sinuses, 31–32

from lateral nasal wall, 32

Mucosa

edema of, 230

engorgement of, postoperative, 377

movement of, 17–18

mucus blanket of, 17

swelling of

in combined paranasal sinus disease, 212, 214

mucus transport and, 24

on uncinate process, 178

Mucosal glands, regulation of, by parasympathetic
nerve fibers, 18

Mucosal lesion(s)

causing sinugenic headache, 447–449

mucus transport over, 20

Mucoserous nasal glands, 17

Mucous ball, 247

Mucous membranes

changes in, of maxillary sinus, 384, 386, 390–391

cysts in, secreting, 359

histologic findings of, 253–261

polypoid

changes of, 216

removal of, in treatment of rhinosinusitis, 339

polypoid changes of. See also Polyps.

postoperative evaluation of, 461

Mucus. See also Secretion(s).

gel and sol phase of, 17

quantity and composition of, 18

renewal of, in maxillary sinus, 19

transport of

in frontal sinus, 30–31

in maxillary sinus, 28–30

over accessory ostia, 22–24

over bony crests in frontal sinus, 20

over mucosal lesions, 20

viscous, ciliary action in, 26

Mucus plug, vs. polyp, 222

Multidirectional tomography, of paranasal sinuses,
93

Mucor spp, 426

Mucormycoses, 426–427

clinical findings in, 426–427

treatment of, 427

Mycelia (fungal hyphae), vegetative vs.
nonvegetative, 401

Mycotic infections, 398–427

complications and dangers of, 399

endoscopic surgery for, results of, 462

identification of, MRI scan in, 106

of nose and paranasal sinuses, 398

Mycotoxins, 399

N

NARES (nonallergic rhinitis with eosinophilia), 231

Nasal aspirators, 150

Nasal fontanelles, 60

Nasal glands, mucoserous, 17

Nasal meatus, middle

endoscopic entry into, 152

endoscopic examination of, 154–155

through trocar sheath, 155

fibrosarcoma of, 264

pathology of, endoscopic repair of, 388

sinus disease in, 443–444

Nasal pathology

in asthmatic patients, 454

endoscopic and radiographic findings of, 455

endoscopic surgery for, 455–456

improved, placebo effect of, on pulmonary
symptoms, 453–455

Nasal septum, deviation of. See Septal deviation.

Nasal speculum, historical aspects of, 6

Nasal turbinate(s). See Turbinate(s).

Nasal vestibule, endoscope in, 286

placement of instrument parallel to, 287

Nasal wall, lateral

bony structures of, 54–69

clefts and spaces of, 76–87

embryology of, 54–59

ethmoidal bulla of, 60

mucociliary transportation from, 32

uncinate process of, 60

Nasofrontal duct, 35, 82. See also Frontal recess.

Nasolacrimal duct, endoscopic examination of, 152

Nasopharynx

blood-tinged secretions of, postoperative, 370

endoscopic examination of, 150–151

inspection of

devices used in, 1–2
postoperative, 369
Nasoturbinal bone, 55
Neoplasms, benign vs. malignant, differential
diagnosis of, 262–267
Nervus canalis pterygoidei, 18
Nervus petrosus major, 18
Nervus petrosus profundus, 18
Neuralgia
improvement in, following recovery from
ethmoid disease, 397
midface, 206
trigeminal, atypical, 210
Neuroblastoma, 264
Neurogenic edema, substance P and, 230–231, 448
Neurokinin A, 448
Neuropeptides, 448–449
Nikon F3 camera, 482
Nonallergic rhinitis with eosinophilia (NARES), 231
Nonsinus-related headache, 446
Nonvegetative mycelia, of fungus, 401
Nose. See also *Nasal* entries.
neoplastic changes in, 263
Nucleus salivatorius superior, 18
Numbness, temporary, following maxillary
sinuscopy, 242

O
Obstruction, mechanical, altered drainage routes
due to, 33–34
Oil lamp, as light source, for early endoscopes, 4
Ointments, corticosteroid, postoperative use of,
370–371
Olympus reflex camera, 482
Onodi cells, 65–66, 68, 204, 474
radiologic anatomy of, 130, 138
"Operculum conchae mediae," 50
Optic nerve
injury to, as complication of endoscopic surgery,
474
relationship of sphenoidal sinus to, 67–68, 138,
210
Orbit
fungal invasion of, 411
injury to, in endoscopic surgery, 316–317
Orbitocranial canal (ethmoidal canal), 72
Organ sensitivity, to radiation, 102–103
Oro-antral fistula, with maxillary sinusitis, 250
Osteomyelitis (Pott's puffy tumor), 356
Ostium (ostia)
of maxillary sinus. See *Maxillary sinus ostium.*
of sphenoid sinus, 67
spiral transportation of secretion toward, 31
Oxycel, for capillary oozing, 469
Oxycel mesh, for capillary oozing, 369

P
Pain
causes of, mucosal irritation and, 447–449
intraoperative, 318–319, 322, 332

Papilloma(s), inverted, 264
Paranasal sinus(es). See also *Ethmoidal sinus;
Frontal sinus; Maxillary sinus; Sphenoidal sinus.*
aspergillosis of, 400–424. See also *Aspergillosis, of
paranasal sinuses.*
candidiasis of, 424–426
diseases of
differential diagnosis of, 262–267
endoscopic and radiologic diagnosis of, 212–215
fenestration and Caldwell-Luc procedures for,
failure of, 381–398. See also under specific
procedure.
histologic findings in, 253–261
inflammatory, ethmoidal infundibulum in, 185
drainage and ventilation of, 17–24
endoscopy of, historical aspects of, 9–11
evaluation of
by computed tomography, 96–101
by conventional tomography, 92–95
by conventional X-rays, 89–91
imaging techniques used in, 89–143
by magnetic resonance imaging, 104–107
inflammatory diseases of, ethmoidal
infundibulum in. See also *Ethmoidal
infundibulum, disease of.*
mucoceles of, endoscopic surgery for, results of,
462
mucormycosis of, 426–427
mucosal lining of, 76
mycotic infections of, 398–427
pathologic changes in, eustachian tube
dysfunction and, 33–34
problems of, in asthmatic patients, endoscopic
surgery for, 455–456
radiologic anatomy of, 116–132
important variants in, 133
preoperative considerations in, 142–143
viscous rubbery secretions of, 464
Parasympathetic nerve fibers, regulation of mucosal
glands by, 18
Patient
discharge instructions to, 379
positioning of
for CT scan, 99
for endoscopic surgery, 324–326
preoperative information for, 321–322
Penicillic acid, 399
Penicillin, postoperative use of, 371
Penicillium spp, 399
Pethidine hydrochloride (meperidine), 322–323
Petroleum lamp, as light source, for early
endoscopes, 4
pH
of normal nasal mucous, 17
optimum, for ciliary beating, 27
Photography
still
cameras for, 497–481
documentation of endoscopic procedures by,
479–488

film selection for, 488

light sources for, 482

technique of, 486–488

video

documentation of endoscopic procedures by, 488–491

equipment for, 488–489

light source for, 491

technique of, 490–491

Plane of investigation, in CT scans, 98

Pledgets

cotton, 322

left in operating field, complications of, 378

vasoconstrictor-soaked, 188

epinephrine, 278, 469

of topical anesthesia, 328

Plica lacrimalis (Hasner's valve), 119

observation of, 152

Pneumatization

of agger nasi cells, 200

of ethmoidal bulla, 180

of inferior turbinate, 168

of middle turbinate, 160. See also Concha bullosa.

of posterior ethmoidal sinus, 204–205

of superior turbinate, 168

of uncinate process, 178

Pneumosinus dilatans, 160

Polyethylene catheters, for maxillary sinuscopy, 233

Polyp(s)

antrochoanal, 227

components of, 346

endoscopic surgery for, 346–349

appearance of, 218

attached to cribriform plate or lamina papyracea, 226

choanal

endoscopic and radiologic diagnosis of, 227–229

vs. polyposis, 227

concha bullosa and, 166

with copious pus, removal of, 363

cystic, expansion of, into maxillary sinus, 248

endoscopic and radiologic diagnosis of, 216 232

in ethmoidal infundibulum disease, 187

false, filled with antibiotic ointment, 250

formation of

etiology of, 216, 230–232

on uncinate process, 176

in frontal recess disease, 194

vs. inverted papilloma, 264

massive, 220

medial to middle turbinate, site of origin of, 218

mucous membrane, 256

vs. mucus plug, 222

pendulated, 242

prolapse of, into sphenoethmoidal recess, 220

recurrent, 226

site of origin of, 217

small, 216

in sphenoidal sinus disease, atypical

surgical intervention for, indications of, 220

Polypoid rhinosinopathy, diffuse, 224, 226

endoscopic surgery for, results of, 463–464

etiology of, 231

histologic findings in, 260–261

Polypoid rhinosinusitis

diffuse, postoperative changes in, 377

endoscopic surgery for, 336–343

Polypoid sinusitis, posterior ethmoid involved in, 204

Polyposis

vs. choanal polyps, 227

recurrent, 224

uncomplicated, 216

Pontocaine

as anesthetic, for endoscopic surgery, 328

for frontal sinusitis, 278

for purulent sinusitis, 281

Postoperative care, 369–379

discharge instructions as, 379

drug therapy in, 370–372

local, 372–376

problems and complications in, 377–378

serious complications during, 378

Pott's puffy tumor (osteomyelitis), 356

Premedication, for local anesthesia, 322–324

Promethazine, 322–323

Pterygoid canal (vidian nerve), 206

Pterygoid process, 206

R

Rad, 102

Radiographic diagnosis, of mycotic infections, 405–408

Radiology, conventional, of paranasal sinuses, 89–91

Ramus ascendens, 54

Ramus descendens, 54

Rathke's pouch, remnant of, 150

"Recessus frontalis," 50

"Recessus suprabullaris," 87

"Recessus terminalis," 40

Reepithelialization, following surgery, 376

Reflex camera(s), 35-mm, 479–480

Retention cysts, 217, 245, 247

Rhinomanometry, 459

Rhinorrhea, cerebrospinal fluid, 436–441

demonstration and localization of, 437–440

treatment of, 440–441

Rhinoscopy, 6

Rhinosinopathy, diffuse polypoid, 224, 226

endoscopic surgery for, results of, 463–464

etiology of, 231

histologic findings in, 260–261

Rhinosinusitis

concha bullosa and, 166

polypoid

diffuse, postoperative changes in, 377

endoscopic surgery for, 336–343

Rhizopus spp, 426

Ridges, septal, 157, 158

S

Salpingoscope, 8

Salpingoscopy, 8

Sarcoidosis, mucous membrane changes in, 262

Secretion(s). See also *Mucus*.

  abnormal, in ethmoidal infundibulum disease,
    187–188

  blood-stained, 262, 264

  disturbances of, eustachian tube function and,
    33–34

  foamy, during endoscopy, 150

  postoperative removal of, 372

  in sphenoidal sinus disease, 208

  staining of, 28

  viscous rubbery, 464

"Secretion expressways," phenomenon of, 27

Secretion transportation, 17–47

  from concha bullosa, 162

  in frontal sinus, 30–31

  in maxillary sinus, 28–30

  pathology of, 25–27

  pathways of, 27–34

  phenomenon of, following fenestration failure,
    392–393

  principles of, 17–27

Sedatives, use of, 322–323

Septal deviation, 156–159, 430–434

  concha bullosa and, 160

  correction of, 157–158, 432–433

  endoscopic and radiologic diagnosis of, 156–159

  septoplasty for, 157–158, 432–433

    postoperative care following, 433

Septal ridges, 157, 158

Septal spurs, 157, 158

Septoplasty, 432–433

  postoperative care following, 433

Sickle knife, 292

Sinubronchial syndrome, 222

  ethmoid disease in, endoscopic surgery for,
    344–345

Sinugenic headache. See *Headache(s), sinugenic*.

Sinus(es). See also named sinus.

  inflammation of. See *Sinusitis*.

  polyposis of, 216. See also *Polyps*.

"Sinus concha," 172

Sinus disease

  asthma and, 453–457

    treatment of, 457

  concha bullosa and predisposition to, 164

  headaches associated with, endoscopic approach
    to, 442–451

  treatment of, improved asthmatic symptoms
    with, 435–455

Sinus lateralis, 87

  disease of, endoscopic and radiologic diagnosis
    of, 184

  ethmoidal bulla and, 62

  polyps originating in, 217

Sinus ostium. See *Ostium (ostia)*.

Sinus problems, endoscopic solutions to, 335–367

Sinusitis

  acute

    complications of, endoscopic surgery for,
      362–364

    histologic findings in, 253

  bronchial asthma and, 453

  conservative endoscopic management of, 278–281

  and ethmoidal bulla, 182

  frontal

    endoscopic diagnosis of, 195

    management of, 195–196

    conservative, 278

  maxillary. See *Maxillary sinusitis*.

  polypoid, posterior ethmoid involved in, 204

  as symptom of fungal infection, 404

  triad of symptoms of, 442

  vasoconstrictor-soaked cotton pledget for, 188

Skull, cysts at base of, 359

Slice overlapping, in CT scans, 98

Sol phase, of mucus, 17

Speculum, Markusowsky, 6

Sphenoethmoidal recess, 32, 33

  endoscopic view of, 208

  polyp prolapse into, 220

Sphenoethmoidectomy, by Messerklinger
    technique, 283–284

Sphenoidal sinus, 67–68

  disease of, endoscopic and radiologic diagnosis
    of, 208–211

  identification of, in endoscopic surgery, 313–314

  lateral wall of, bulges in, 67–68

  mucociliary transportation from, 31–32

  mycotic infection of, surgical approach to, 418

  optic nerve passing through, 138

  ostia of, 67

  pneumatization of, 67, 132

  polypoid changes in, 217

  radiologic anatomy of, 132

  surgical approach to, 302, 304–305

Sponge, Merocel

  left in operating field, complications of, 378, 472

  postoperative removal of, 372

Spurs, septal, 157, 158

Squamous cell carcinoma, of maxillary sinus, 250,
    264

Stenosis

  of inferior meatal fenestrations, 382

  of maxillary sinus ostium, as complication of
    endoscopic surgery, 467–468

Sterigmatocystine, 399

Still photography, documentation of endoscopic
    procedures by, 479–488. See also *Photography*.

Storz, Karl, Endopocket TV camera, 490

Storz, Karl, model 600 light source, 482

Storz, Karl, variolens adapter, 480

Struyken conchotome, 352

Substance P, 19

  amino acid sequence of, 448

  liberation of, in nasal mucosa, 449

  and neurogenic edema, 230–231, 448

pharmocologic effects of, 448–449

Suctioning, postoperative, of clots, crusts, and secretions, 372–373

Sunlight, as light source, for early endoscopes, 4

Supraorbital ethmoid cells, 184

Supreme concha, 168

Synechiae, as complication of endoscopic surgery, 466–467

T

Tachykinins, 448

Takahashi forceps, 314

Teaching modality(ies), still and video photography used as, 492

Temperature, optimum, for ciliary beating, 26–27

Three-dimensional reconstruction techniques, from CT data, 114

Tissue sensitivity, to radiation, 102–103

Tomography

computed. See also *Computed tomography (CT).*

of paranasal sinuses, 96–101

conventional

vs. computed tomography, 108–114

of paranasal sinuses, 92–95

technique of, 94

Topical anesthesia

for diagnostic endoscopy, 147, 156, 187

for endoscopic surgery, 328–330

Torus lateralis, 62, 298

Trigeminal neuralgia, atypical, 210

Trocar with sleeve

70 degree endoscope and, insertion of, 286

for maxillary sinuscopy, 233

insertion of, 236, 238

removal of, 239

Tuberculosis, mucous membrane, 262

Turbinate(s)

endoscopic examination of, 152, 154

ethmoidal, embryonic development of, 54–56

inferior

hyperplastic, endoscopic surgery for, 360–361

pneumatization of, 168

middle

bleeding from, as complication of endoscopic surgery, 470–471

"doubled," 173

ground lamella of, 62–64

normally convex, vs. concha bullosa, 172

paradoxically bent, 170

pneumatization of, 160. See also *Concha bullosa.*

radiologic anatomy of, 126, 129

sagittal groove formation of, 172

"triangular," 172

variations of, endoscopic and radiologic diagnosis of, 170–173

superior, pneumatization of, 168

Turbinate sinus, 77, 172, 180

diseased, 297

polyps originating in, 217

U

Uncinate process, 60

anatomic variations of, 173–174

changes in, 176

endoscopic and radiologic identification of, 173–179

identification of site of insertion of, 312

incision and removal of, in treatment of polypid rhinosinusitis, 337–338

mucosa on, 178

perforations in, 178

pneumatization of, 178

polyp formation on, 176

polyp originating in, 217

radiologic anatomy of, 120

radiologic assessment of, 175

resection of, 292, 294–295

septal ridges or spurs in, 174

strength of, 176

V

Valsalva maneuver, 43

Vasoconstrictors, use of, in diagnostic endoscopy, 147

Vasoconstrictor-soaked cotton pledget, for sinusitis, 188

Vegetative mycelia, of fungus, 401

Ventilation, of paranasal sinuses, 17–24

Video camera, requirements of, 489–490

Video photography, documentation of endoscopic procedures by, 488–491. See also *Photography.*

Vidian nerve (pterygoid canal), 206

Vital capacity (VC), preoperative vs. postoperative, in asthmatic patients, 455

W

"Water lens," in early endoscopy, 4

Wertheim's conchoscope, 6

X

Xenon light source, for video photography, 491

X-rays

conventional, of paranasal sinuses, 89–91

postoperative, 376

Z

Zinc oxide, mycotic growth and, 421, 423

Zoom lens, 480